The Global HIV Epidemics among Sex Workers

The Global HIV Epidemics among Sex Workers

Deanna Kerrigan, Andrea Wirtz, Stefan Baral, Michele Decker, Laura Murray, Tonia Poteat, Carel Pretorius, Susan Sherman, Mike Sweat, Iris Semini, N'Della N'Jie, Anderson Stanciole, Jenny Butler, Sutayut Osornprasop, Robert Oelrichs, and Chris Beyrer

THE WORLD BANK
Washington, D.C.

ISBN (paper): 978-0-8213-9774-9
eISBN (electronic): 978-0-8213-9775-6
DOI: 10.1596/978-0-8213-9774-9

Cover painting: "Untitled" by Raimundo Rubio, 1998. Oil on canvas, 52 by 52 in., World Bank Art Collection.

Cover design: Naylor Design

Library of Congress Cataloging-in-Publication Data
The global HIV epidemics among sex workers/ by Deanna Kerrigan ... [et al.].
p. ; cm.–(Directions in development)
Includes bibliographical references.
I. Kerrigan, Deanna. II. World Bank. III. Series: Directions in development (Washington, D.C.)
[DNLM: 1. HIV Infections--epidemiology. 2. HIV Infections--prevention & control--Statistics. 3. Human Rights--Statistics. 4. Sex Workers--Statistics. 5. World Health--Statistics. WC 503.41]
614.5'99392--dc23

2012042473

Contents

Boxes

Figures

Maps

Tables

Acknowledgments

This Economic and Sector Work was undertaken by the World Bank under the Project P124113, "The Global Epidemics of HIV in Sex Workers." Support from UNAIDS under the UBW Trust Fund is gratefully acknowledged.

The project was conducted by a World Bank core team from the Health, Nutrition and Population Unit (HNP), Human Development Network: Iris Semini, N'Della N'Jie, Anderson Stanciole and Robert Oelrichs (Task Team Leader) with the Johns Hopkins Bloomberg School of Public Health, Center for Public Health and Human Rights: Deanna Kerrigan, Andrea L. Wirtz, Stefan D. Baral, Michele R. Decker, Laura Murray, Tonia Poteat, Carel Pretorius, Susan Sherman, Mike Sweat, and Chris Beyrer.

Sutayut Osornprasop contributed substantially to the section on Thailand. Additional World Bank staff members who provided technical input throughout the project include F. Ayodeji Akala, Katie Bigmore, Marelize Görgens, Jody Kusek and David Wilson. The team also thanks the following World Bank Staff for their expert and constructive criticism during the course of the work: Enias Baganizi, Daniel Cotlear, Eva Jarawan, Ajay Tandon, Damien de Walque and Ethan Yeh. Thanks are also due to Nicole Klingen (Manager) and Cristian Baeza (Director) of HNP for their careful support and guidance.

The work was undertaken in cooperation with the United Nations Population Fund. The close consultation and collegiate partnership of Jenny Butler is particularly acknowledged, as well as the financial support of UNFPA to the global stakeholder consultation, which centrally informed this analysis.

We thank Ying Ru Lo (World Health Organization), Mariangela Simão (UNAIDS) and Clancy Broxton and Billy Pick (USAID) for their helpful technical inputs. Futures Institute and the leadership of John Stover and Lori Bollinger are also thanked for their contribution of the updated Goals model and technical support during mathematical modeling and cost analyses.

The team wishes to very gratefully acknowledge that consultation took place with sex worker organizations in the process of developing this report, although they do not endorse it: the Global Network of Sex Work Projects, the Asia-Pacific Network of Sex Workers, Empower (Thailand), Africa Sex Work Alliance (Uganda), The Red Umbrella (Namibia), International Committee on the Rights of Sex Workers in Europe, SZEXE, Movimiento de Mujeres Unidas (Dominican Republic), and Aproase (Mexico). Gregory Mitchell, Jose Miguel de Olivar, Lilia Rossi, Sonia Correa, Angela Donini, the Brazilian Prostitutes' Network, Carmen Lucia Paz (Brazilian Prostitute's Network), Gabriela Leite (Davida), Cristina Camara and Richard Parker. Sheri Lippman and Carlos Laudari, in addition to Juny Kraiczyk, Ivo Brito, Ronaldo Hallal, and Mauro Siqueira from the Brazilian Ministry of Health, generously assisted in gathering cost data in Brazil. We would also like to acknowledge inputs and consultation from Larry Gelmon and colleagues at the University of Manitoba in Kenya as well as Dallas Swendeman and colleagues from the University of California at Los Angeles.

Other contributors from the Johns Hopkins School of Public Health are thanked for their support: Pamela S. Lilleston who contributed to the policy review and analysis; Kate Muessig and Madeleine Schlefer who contributed to the global epidemiology review; Dina Fine Meron who contributed to the country description for Thailand; Shirin Kakayeva who provided translational support for the Ukraine cost data synthesis; and Sara Coleman who conducted the literature review for the HIV prevention intervention cost-effectiveness data among sex workers.

This work was supported by a team from the International Bank for Reconstruction and Development / The World Bank. The findings, interpretations, and conclusions expressed in this paper do not necessarily reflect the views of the Executive Directors of The World Bank or the governments they represent. The World Bank does not guarantee the accuracy of the data included in this work. The boundaries, colors, denominations, and other information shown on any map in this work do not imply any judgment on the part of The World Bank concerning the legal status of any territory or the endorsement or acceptance of such boundaries.

Abbreviations

AIDS	Acquired Immune Deficiency Syndrome
ANC	antenatal care
ART	antiretroviral therapy
CDC	Centers for Disease Control
CI	Confidence Interval
CIDA	Canadian International Development Agency
FSW	female sex worker
GFATM	The Global Fund to Fight AIDS Tuberculosis and Malaria
HBV	Hepatitis-B virus
HCT	HIV counseling and testing
HCV	Hepatitis-C virus
HIV	Human immunodeficiency virus
IBBSS	Integrated Bio-behavioral Surveillance Survey
JHU	Johns Hopkins University
LMIC	low and middle income countries
MOT	modes of transmission
MSM	men who have sex with men
MSW	male sex worker
NGO	nongovernmental organization

NSWP	Global Network of Sex Work Projects
OR	Odds Ratio
PEPFAR	The United States President's Emergency Plan for AIDS Relief
PLHIV	people living with HIV
PMTCT	prevention of mother-to-child transmission
RDS	Respondent Driven Sampling
STI	sexually transmitted infection
UNAIDS	United Nations Joint Programme for HIV/AIDS
UNFPA	United Nations Population Fund
UNGASS	United Nations General Assembly Special Session (on HIV/AIDS)
UNICEF	United Nations Children's Fund
USAID	United States Agency for International Development
WHO	World Health Organization

Executive Summary

Rationale

Since the beginning of the epidemic sex workers have experienced a heightened burden of HIV. Unfortunately, sex workers' HIV and health-related risks and rights have often gone unattended and global resource allocation related to HIV prevention, treatment and care has not been based on rigorous analysis in terms of the evidence related to sex work and HIV.

Objectives

To inform an equitable, effective, and sustainable response to HIV which promotes and protects the human rights of sex workers, the following questions were addressed in this analysis, focusing largely on female sex workers from lower and middle income countries:

- What is the *global burden of HIV* among sex workers? How do sex worker HIV burdens compare to the general population? How does this vary by region?

- How does the *policy and social context* shape sex workers' HIV risk across geographic settings? How does this context influence the provision and coverage of HIV services?

- To what extent can *comprehensive HIV prevention at-scale* among sex workers modify HIV transmission dynamics among sex workers and the general population?

- What are the most *cost-effective HIV prevention,* treatment, and care interventions in the context of sex work? What combinations of services are most cost-effective?

- Given this evidence, what are the implications for *allocative efficiency in HIV prevention programs*?

- How does *violence against sex workers* affect their health and human rights and HIV transmission dynamics among sex workers and the general population across settings?

- What has been the role of *sex worker leadership* in promoting the human rights of and reducing the burden of and risks for HIV infection among sex workers across contexts?

Methods

To answer these questions a strategic combination of epidemiologic, social science, mathematical modeling and cost-effectiveness research methods were utilized and findings from these respective analyses were integrated to inform future policy and program recommendations.

To document the global burden of HIV we conducted a systematic review of the epidemiologic literature on HIV prevalence among sex workers across geographic settings, assessing variation per region as well as conducting comparisons in the burden of HIV with the general population.

To provide further depth not only on the epidemiology but also the social and policy context of HIV-related risks and the response to HIV among sex workers in a given setting, we conducted eight country case studies across geographic regions. These case studies highlight the experiences of diverse populations of and settings for sex work. We also conducted comparative analysis related to the role of sex worker leadership and participation in the response to HIV in three of the country case study settings, including the experiences of Brazil, India, and Thailand.

We conducted mathematical modeling, using the Goals model, and cost-effectiveness analysis to examine the impact of community empowerment-based, comprehensive HIV prevention and the expansion of earlier initiation of ART (CD4<350 cells/mm^3) on trends in new HIV infections among female sex workers and the general population and their relative cost-effectiveness for Brazil, Kenya, Thailand, and Ukraine. We also modeled the impact of reducing violence against sex workers on new HIV infections among both sex workers and the adult general population.

Given the limited epidemiologic and evaluation data available among male and transgender sex workers, mathematical modeling and cost-effective analyses focused on female sex workers.

Results

The Epidemiology of HIV Among Sex Workers

Data from 111 studies in 50 countries among approximately 100,000 sex workers met the inclusion criteria for this systematic review. For each country, HIV prevalence data among female sex workers was pooled and weighted by sample size. Background HIV prevalence among adult women (15–49 years) in the general population was calculated by using UNAIDS and United States Census Bureau Data. Meta-analysis documenting the increased odds of being HIV positive among sex workers versus women in the general adult population was conducted and is depicted in the figure below.

- Overall HIV prevalence among female sex workers was 11.8% (95% CI 11.6–12.0).

- HIV prevalence among female sex workers varied significantly by region, with the highest prevalence found in sub-Saharan Africa with a pooled prevalence of 36.9%.

- Across regions, HIV prevalence among female sex workers was 13.5 times the overall HIV prevalence among the general population of women 15–49 years old.

Table ES.1   HIV Prevalence among Female Sex Workers vs. Adult Women across Geographic Regions: Meta-Analysis of the Increased Burden of HIV Experienced by Female Sex Workers

Region	Number of countries	Sample size of HIV positive female sex workers	Sample size of female sex workers	Pooled HIV prevalence (95% CI)	Background prevalence	Pooled odds ratios (95% CI)
Asia	14	3323	64224	5.2% (5.0–5.3)	0.18%	29.2 (22.2–38.4)
Eastern Europe	4	331	3037	10.9% (9.8–12.0)	0.20%	n.a.

(continued next page)

Table ES.1 *(continued)*

Region	Number of countries	Sample size of HIV positive female sex workers	Sample size of female sex workers	Pooled HIV prevalence (95% CI)	Background prevalence	Pooled odds ratios (95% CI)
Latin America and the Caribbean	11	627	10237	6.1% (5.7–6.6)	0.38%	12.0 (7.3–19.7)
Middle East and North Africa	5	17	959	1.7% (0.94–2.60)	0.43%	n.a.
Sub-Saharan Africa	16	7899	21421	36.9% (36.2–37.5)	7.42%	12.4 (8.9–17.2)
By Country Prevalence (Prev.)						
Very low/ Low prev.	21	3561	69729	5.1% (4.9–5.3)	0.17%	24.5 (19.1–31.3)
Medium/ High prev.	26	8627	28075	30.7% (30.2–31.3)	5.47%	11.6 (9.1–14.8)
Total	50	12197	99878	11.8% (11.6–12.0)	13·5 (95% CI 10.0–18.1)	

Source: Authors.
Note: CI = confidence interval; Prev. = prevalence; n.a. = not applicable; Meta-Analysis of Prevalence does not include Afghanistan, Laos, and Albania.

Country Case Studies

External Validity

The purpose of the country case studies was to provide a strategic selection of the geographical and epidemiological diversity of the global HIV epidemic. They were systematically selected by the following process: 1) the development of a list of countries providing as much regional representation as possible, covering concentrated and generalized epidemics and a range of country incomes; 2) a comprehensive review of the available evidence— regarding both epidemiology and

Box ES.1   What is Empowerment-based, Comprehensive Prevention?

Community empowerment-based approaches to comprehensive HIV prevention among sex workers rely on sex worker leadership to address social and structural barriers to HIV prevention, health and human rights. Key components of community empowerment-based approaches include the promotion of social cohesion and collective action among sex workers and efforts to facilitate their social inclusion and political participation. Traditional elements of HIV prevention such as community-led, peer education efforts, condom distribution, and HIV/STI screening and management are also common components of a community empowerment-based approach which works to attend to structural, behavioral and biomedical aspects of sex workers' vulnerability to HIV.

Source: Authors.

interventions; and 3) a selection of eight countries to arrive at a list that was practical in size and covered countries where there were sufficient quality data to conduct the analyses. While limited in number, the case studies provide in-depth analyses, and important insights into regional and global trends regarding HIV prevention in the context of sex work.

In each of the eight country case studies the importance of the legal framework, policy and social context surrounding sex work was documented, whereas in places where sex work is criminalized the response to HIV has often been stymied and limited by structural forces including stigma, discrimination and violence against sex workers.

- In settings where sex work is recognized as an occupation an enabling environment is created whereby stigma and discrimination against sex workers can be directly addressed and access to HIV prevention and treatment services facilitated.

- The coverage of HIV prevention services among sex workers is low, with generally less than 50 percent of sex workers reporting access to basic prevention services.

- Few systematic HIV prevention interventions were documented for male and transgender sex workers or for the clients and partners of sex workers.

Additionally, consistent condom use between sex workers and their regular intimate partners and clients was significantly lower than that between sex workers and new clients across the countries investigated, indicating the need for further research and programming in this area.

Modeling the Impact of Comprehensive HIV Prevention for Sex Workers

Mathematical modeling demonstrated that scaling up HIV prevention and treatment services including a community empowerment-based approach to comprehensive HIV prevention for sex workers combined with the scale-up and earlier initiation ART among all adults has a significant impact on HIV among sex workers and the general population across settings and epidemic scenarios. Benefits were observed across four epidemiologically diverse countries: Brazil, Kenya, Thailand, and Ukraine.

- Expanding a community empowerment-based approach to comprehensive HIV prevention intervention among sex workers has demonstrable impact on the HIV epidemics among female sex workers, cumulatively averting up to 10,800 infections among sex workers across epidemic scenarios within a five-year time span.

- Across epidemics, the expansion of community empowerment-based comprehensive HIV prevention among sex workers demonstrates additional impact on the adult population, up to 20,700 infections may be averted among adults within five years.

- Impact of a community empowerment-based approach to comprehensive HIV prevention among sex workers is greatest in countries, such as Kenya, where HIV prevalence is high among adults in the general population and female sex workers.

- Early initiation of ART among the adult population demonstrates an impact on HIV infection among sex workers if they have equal access to HIV testing and treatment. An empowerment-based approach could also help enable ART expansion among sex workers through community-based outreach and social mobilization strategies.

In Figures ES.1 and ES.2, one sees the impact of increasing access to community empowerment-based, comprehensive HIV prevention services among female sex workers in Kenya on both sex workers and the general population in terms of HIV prevalence over the next five years (The impacts observed in the other modeled countries are presented in Chapter 4.).

Figure ES.1   Modeling Scale-up of a Community Empowerment-based Comprehensive HIV Prevention in Kenya: New HIV Infections among Sex Workers

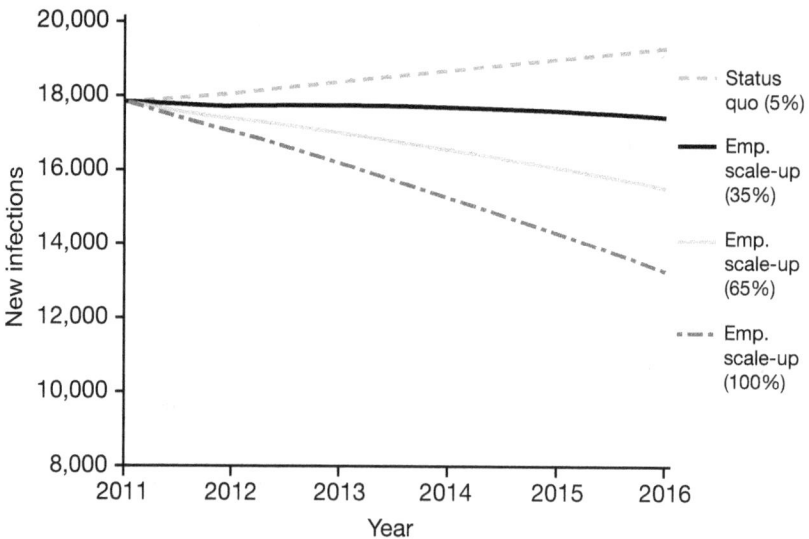

Source: Authors.
Note: Emp. = empowerment-based; ART coverage is maintainted at 2011 levels.

Figure ES.2   Modeling Scale-up a Community Empowerment-based Approach to Comprehensive HIV Prevention in Kenya: New Infections among the Adult Population

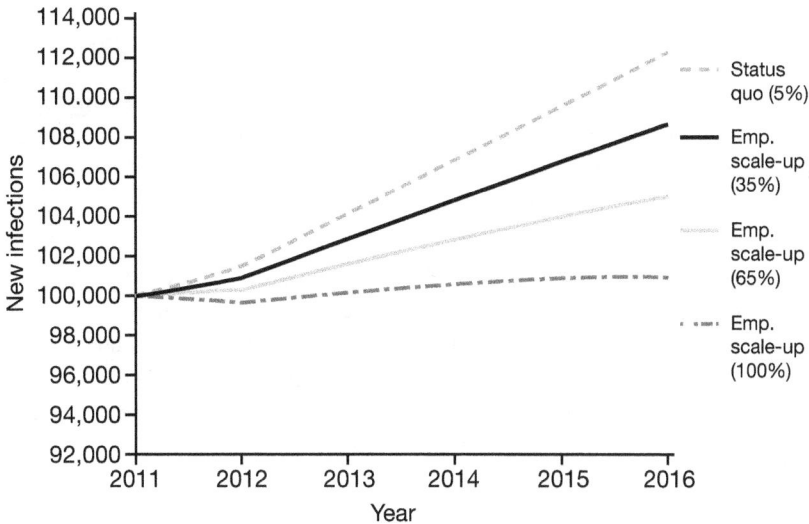

Source: Authors.
Note: Emp. = empowerment-based; ART coverage is maintainted at 2011 levels.

Cost-effective Comprehensive HIV Prevention for Sex Workers

Cost analyses demonstrate the cost-effectiveness of scaling up HIV prevention and treatment among sex workers.

- The cost per client for the community empowerment-based, comprehensive HIV prevention intervention among sex workers ranges from $102 to $184.

- When averted HIV-related medical care costs are removed the net 5-year national cost of the community empowerment intervention is significantly reduced and in Ukraine and Kenya net costs show cost savings of $39M and $8.6M respectively.

- The cost per HIV infection averted for community empowerment-based comprehensive HIV prevention is a function of prevalence: lowest in Ukraine ($1,990) and Kenya ($3,813) and highest in Thailand ($66,128) and Brazil ($32,773).

When the community empowerment-based comprehensive HIV prevention intervention is conducted in the context of earlier initiation of ART provision the cost-effectiveness is reduced modestly. This effect is explained by reductions in population-level HIV incidence driven by the ART program; cost per infection increases when there are fewer infections to avert. Below one sees the cost per HIV infection averted across the four countries in the context of earlier initiation of ART among adults over the next five years— demonstrating how overall and sex worker HIV prevalence and country labor costs influence the cost per HIV infection averted.

Implications for Allocative Efficiency in HIV Prevention Programs

It has been noted that the allocation of national prevention funding is frequently grossly mismatched to the distribution of new infections that could be averted, and the cost effectiveness of the interventions - and this is especially true for sex workers. Prior analyses by the Global Fund to Fight AIDS, Tuberculosis and Malaria for example suggestion that only 3% of funding in that round went to prevention programs targeting sex workers through that mechanism in Round 8. There is a good justification based on the analyses presented herein to more equitably allocate HIV prevention funding to interventions focused on sex workers such as the comprehensive community empowerment intervention.

Figure ES.3   Cost per HIV Infection Averted: Cumulative Due to the Expansion of the Community Empowerment-based Prevention Interventions for Sex Workers, in the Context of Earlier ART Initiation among Adults, 2012–16

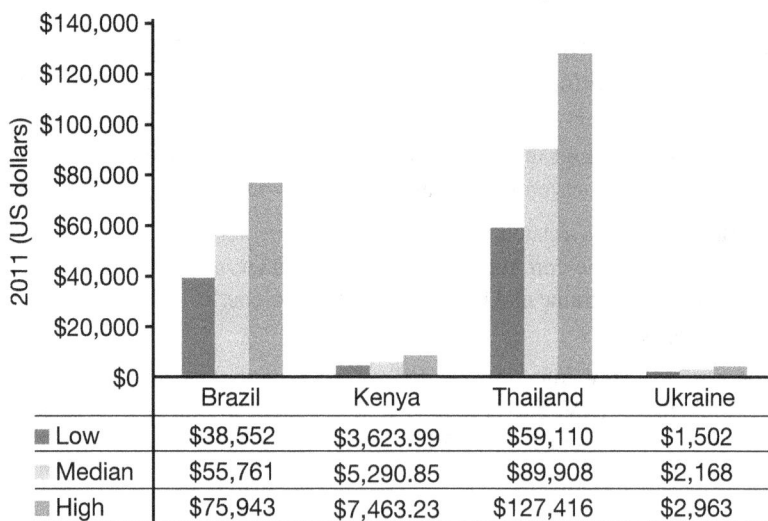

	Brazil	Kenya	Thailand	Ukraine
▪ Low	$38,552	$3,623.99	$59,110	$1,502
▪ Median	$55,761	$5,290.85	$89,908	$2,168
▪ High	$75,943	$7,463.23	$127,416	$2,963

Source: Authors.

Modeling the Impact of Violence against Sex Workers

Findings demonstrate the urgent need to address violence against sex workers to protect their human rights and reduce HIV among both sex workers and the adult general population even in the context of expanded ART coverage.

• In Kenya, reductions in the prevalence of violence against female sex workers could avert over 5,300 new infections among sex workers and 10,000 new infections among adults.

• In Ukraine, reductions in the prevalence of violence against sex workers could avert over 1,400 new HIV infections among sex workers, and over 4,000 in the adult population within a five-year time span.

In Figure ES.4 and ES.5, HIV prevalence and new infections trends for Ukraine for both sex workers and the general population are presented in the context of declines in violence against sex workers.

Figure ES.4   HIV Prevalence among Female Sex Workers in the Context of Declining Prevalence of Violence in Ukraine

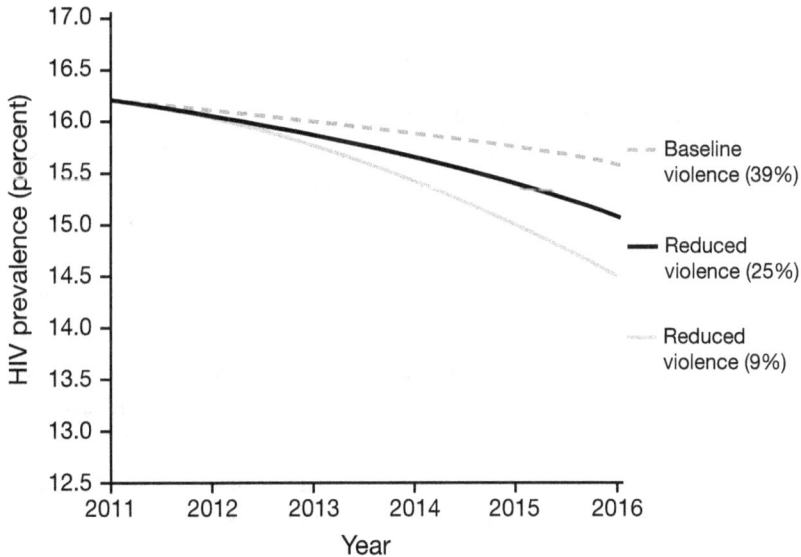

Source: Authors.

Figure ES.5   Trends in New Infections among Adults in the Context of Declining Prevalence Against Sex Workers in Ukraine

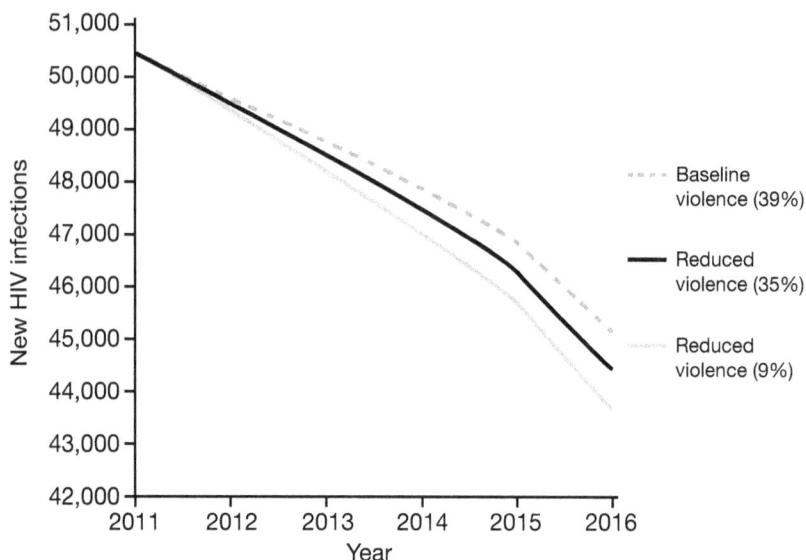

Source: Authors.

Sex Worker Leadership and Responding to HIV

Comparative analysis from country case studies showed that sex worker leadership has played an integral role in community empowerment-based responses to HIV and the promotion of sex workers' human rights.

- The nature and role of sex worker leadership in the response to HIV within a given country varies significantly across socio-political and geographic settings.

- Where sex worker organizations have partnered with government actors, the response to HIV among sex workers has been particularly effective and sustainable.

- Support for sex worker rights organizations in critical to a sustained and effective response to HIV and the promotion of sex worker's human rights and health.

Conclusions and Recommendations

The findings of this study provide important practical tools for policy makers inside and outside the World Bank. The evidence generated builds a case for increased resource allocations for HIV prevention and care among sex workers. However it should be noted that the recommendations of the report are program technical recommendations rather than final public policy recommendations for investment—due to the absence of appropriate economic and fiscal analyses at this time. A comprehensive review of the current global knowledge shows the effectiveness of best practice, evidence-based interventions that can be implemented in World Bank operations. Economic analysis indicates that the returns on these investments will be substantial in a broad range of country scenarios—evidence which can guide discussions with budget decision makers in client countries, and with development partners.

Specifically, Key Policy Relevant Findings Include:

- HIV prevalence is significantly higher (13.5 times greater in pooled analyses) across geographic settings among female sex workers than among women in the general adult population. However service coverage levels for HIV prevention services among sex workers are low (generally <50%). HIV prevention services for male and transgender sex workers are almost non-existent, as are programs for male clients.

- HIV incidence can be significantly reduced among sex workers and the general population across settings by scaling up community empowerment-based, comprehensive HIV prevention services and earlier initiation of ART.

- Where sex worker rights organizations have partnered effectively with government the response to HIV among sex workers has been particularly effective and sustainable. This has meant prevention services which involve significant sex worker leadership in their design and implementation and which attend to structural barriers to safe sex.

- Empowerment-based, comprehensive HIV prevention among sex workers is cost-effective, particularly in higher prevalence settings where it becomes cost-saving. The cost per client for the intervention ranges from $102 to $184, with Ukraine having the lowest and Brazil the highest cost per client. Labor costs are the major expense, and account for the majority of variation across countries.

- Violence, stigma and discrimination against sex workers are extremely prevalent. By reducing violence against sex workers, additional significant HIV prevention gains in terms of new infections averted will also be observed across settings. Addressing violence, stigma and discrimination against sex workers is also a human rights imperative.

- There is a good justification based on the analyses presented herein to more equitably allocate HIV prevention funding to interventions focused on sex workers, such as the comprehensive community empowerment intervention.

Authors' Note on Limitations of the Report

The analysis that follows has both strengths and limitations. While the executive summary and conclusions of the report emphasize its strengths and unique contributions it is also important to acknowledge the limitations of the analysis.

The total project implementation period was less than one year. This necessarily impacted on the nature and scope of the consultative process and the extent of data collection for the analysis. A Technical Advisory Group comprised of representatives from the World Bank, UNFPA and other donor agencies, and the Network of Sex Work Projects was formed to provide advice and feedback to the project's primary technical implementation team at JHU. UNFPA and the World Bank held a two day community consultation in Thailand with NSWP members representing all regions, JHU faculty, WHO, the UNAIDS Secretariat and USAID to discuss the shape, scope and status of the analysis. Further consultation was held with sex worker organizations on the draft case studies in respective countries, where possible.

While specific consultative efforts were undertaken, the process of project implementation in terms of time and resources available did not allow for in-depth input and discussion between the researchers and members of community-led sex worker organizations. Nor were there sufficient resources, technical or material, available to help local sex worker organizations to fully review and provide feedback on documents shared with them. In turn, these limitations influenced both the nature and depth of subsequent analyses.

There are also several important conceptual and methodological limitations to be considered. For example, with regard to the mathematical modeling we chose to model the impact of universal access to treatment for HIV at the CD4 counts <350 cells/mm^3 eligibility criteria and its impact on HIV transmission dynamics among sex workers and the general population. However, it is widely understood that sex workers disproportionately suffer from experiences of stigma and discrimination that limits their access to HIV treatment services. Hence, a limitation of the models presented are the lack of comprehensive attention to the role of such structural constraints which may significantly impede the ability to achieve the reductions in HIV incidence modeled here in real-world settings - particularly in the context of criminalization.

Additionally, the GOALS model, which is a deterministic model, is one of several mathematical models available and is based on the available demographic, sexual behavior, and HIV/STI data available which may be limited in some countries for sex workers or not fully account for the diversity in these data points across different types of sex workers within a given setting. Additionally, the model developed did not take into account "upstream" HIV transmission patterns and dynamics, such as HIV infections averted among the clients or other sexual partners of sex workers as a result of their improved access to HIV prevention and treatment services.

With regard to the cost-effectiveness analysis several limitations must also be acknowledged. The community-empowerment based prevention intervention implemented in Brazil that was utilized for the costing analysis was a unique intervention in that it was part of an international research study and partnership. The model of community empowerment that was appropriate in this context is not necessarily the same model that would be appropriate in another setting.

Additionally, in the Brazilian context the government provided ongoing clinical services for HIV and STI and access to condoms. Hence, these costs were not included in the cost per participant calculated. Another limitation of this analysis was the extrapolation of costs from the Brazil base-cost model to other settings. Country specific costing exercises of interventions tailored to given settings would improve this aspect of the analysis.

Given these limitations in terms of process and methodology it is essential that future research into this area allow for sex worker organizations to more meaningfully participate in the decision-making process regarding model inputs and parameters, as well as support them to partner with researchers in collecting cost and others types of data, and reviewing and providing feedback to the technical team.

CHAPTER 1

Introduction

Since the beginning of the epidemic sex workers have experienced a heightened burden of HIV across settings, despite their higher levels of HIV protective behaviors (UNAIDS, 2009). Unfairly, sex workers have often been framed as "vectors of disease" and "core transmitters" rather than workers and human beings with rights in terms of HIV prevention and beyond.

By gaining a deeper understanding of the epidemiologic and broader policy and social context within which sex work is set one begins to quickly gain a sense of the complex backdrop for increased risk to HIV among sex workers. This backdrop includes the critical role of stigma, discrimination and violence faced by sex workers, as well as, the importance of community empowerment and mobilization among sex workers to address these regressive forces.

Unfortunately to date, sex workers' HIV-related risks and human rights have often gone unattended and global resource allocation (Global Fund, 2011) and funding and investment recommendations related to HIV prevention, treatment and care have not been based on rigorous analysis in terms of the evidence specifically related to sex work (Schwartländer et al 2011).

This analysis, in turn, seeks to inform a holistic and evidence-based response to HIV among sex workers in lower and middle income countries by responding to the following key questions:

- What is the *global burden of HIV* Among sex workers? How do sex worker HIV burdens compare to the general population? How does this vary by region?

- How does the *policy and social context* shape sex workers' HIV risk across geographic settings? How does this context influence the provision and coverage of HIV services?

- To what extent can *comprehensive HIV prevention at-scale* among sex workers modify HIV transmission dynamics among sex workers and the general population?

- What are the most *cost-effective HIV prevention*, treatment, and care interventions in the context of sex work? What combinations of services are most cost-effective?

- How does *violence against sex workers* affect their health and human rights and HIV transmission dynamics among sex workers and the general population across settings?

- What has been the role of *sex worker leadership* in promoting the human rights of and reducing the burden of and risks for HIV infection among sex workers across contexts?

To answer these questions a combination of epidemiologic, social science, mathematical modeling and cost-effectiveness research methods were utilized and findings from these respective questions were integrated to inform future policy and program recommendations.

To document the global burden of HIV we conducted a systematic review of the epidemiologic literature on HIV prevalence among sex workers across geographic settings, assessing variation per region as well as conducting comparisons in the burden of HIV with the general population.

To provide further depth not only on the epidemiology but also the social and policy context of HIV-related risks and the response to HIV among sex workers in a given setting, we conducted eight country case studies across geographic regions including Asia, Africa and Latin America.

To assess the current state of the evidence regarding HIV interventions among sex workers we relied on WHO sponsored systematic reviews on distinct types of HIV prevention interventions among sex workers including a community empowerment-based approach to comprehensive HIV prevention, as well as, the current peer reviewed literature for topics such as the impact of earlier initiation of antiretroviral therapy (ART) (CD4<350 cells/mm^3) on HIV transmission.

Among a sub-set of four of our eight case study countries, we conducted mathematical modeling, using the Goals model developed by and coordinated with the Futures Institute, and cost-effectiveness analysis to examine the impact of a combination of community empowerment-based HIV prevention and earlier initiation of ART on trends in new HIV infections among sex workers and the general population and their relative cost-effectiveness. These countries included: Brazil, Kenya, Thailand, and Ukraine, selected to represent geographic and epidemic diversity. We also model the impact of reducing violence against sex workers and its impact on new HIV infections among sex workers and the general adult population in these countries.

Lastly, we conducted a comparative analysis of three of the case study countries (Brazil, India, and Thailand) to examine the critical role of sex worker leadership, participation and partnership, in promoting the health and human rights of sex workers and in responding to the heightened burden of HIV infection experienced among sex workers across these diverse settings.

It is important to note that sex work is understood here as work and specifically as consensual commercial sex between adults (UNAIDS, 2011). In turn, this analysis does not address issues associated with minors involved in commercial sex or issues associated with human trafficking which go beyond the scope of this report and the aforementioned definition of sex work.

It is also imperative to acknowledge and highlight that sex workers include women, men, and transgendered persons. Additionally, sex work takes on many forms, including establishment and non-establishment based sex work, and sex work which occurs directly between a sex worker and her client and that which involves a third party which may profit from her work.

The eight country case studies work to highlight the experiences of diverse populations of and contexts for sex work across settings. Given the limited epidemiologic and intervention evaluation data available among male and transgender sex workers, however, our collaborative team (JHU, World Bank, UNFPA, and NSWP) determined that the systematic review, mathematical modeling and cost-effective analyses would focus on female sex workers.

Throughout the process of this analysis as a whole, the participation of sex worker perspectives and sex worker organizations such as NSWP and their regional partners has been critical by providing documents and resources, input and consultation throughout the analytical process.

References

The Global Fund to Fight AIDS, Tuberculosis and Malaria. 2011. "Global Fund HIV Investments Specifically Targeting Most-at-Risk Populations: An Analysis of Round 8" (2008). *Phase 1.* Geneva, Switzerland.

Schwartländer, B., Stover, J., Hallett T., Atun, R., Avila, C., Gouws, E., Bartos, M., Ghys P. D., Opuni, M., Barr, D., Alsallaq, R., Bollinger, L., de Freitas, M., Garnett, G., Holmes, C., Legins, K., Pillay, Y., Stanciole, A. E., McClure, C., Hirnschall, G., Laga, M., Padian, N.; Investment Framework Study Group. 2011 "Towards an improved investment approach for an effective response to HIV/AIDS." *The Lancet.* 377 (9782): 2031–41.

UNAIDS. 2009. UNAIDS Guidance Note on HIV and Sex Work. Geneva.

UNAIDS. 2011. UNAIDS Advisory Group on HIV and Sex Work. Geneva.

CHAPTER 2

Review of the Epidemiology of HIV among Sex Workers

Introduction

Key Themes

- A systematic review was conducted based and identified 111 studies across 50 countries with data from approximately 100,000 sex workers.
- The overall HIV prevalence among female sex workers across all regions was 11.8% (95% CI 11.6–12.0).
- HIV prevalence among female sex workers varied significantly by region
- The highest HIV prevalence among sex workers was found in sub-Saharan Africa with a pooled HIV prevalence of 36.9%.
- Across all regions, HIV prevalence among sex workers was 13.5 times the prevalence among the general population of women 15–49 years old.

While the relative burden of HIV varies per geographic and epidemic context, sex workers are often found to be at significantly increased vulnerability to HIV through biological, behavioral, and structural risks (UNAIDS 2009).

Sex workers generally have higher numbers of sexual partners and concurrent sexual partnerships as compared to their counterparts in the general population. However, their HIV-related protective behaviors, including high rates of consistent condom use, are generally several times greater than condom use rates among the general population (UNAIDS, 2009).

Despite these higher levels of HIV protective behaviors among sex workers, legal and policy environments and unsafe and non-enabling working conditions often place them at significantly higher risk for HIV infection (UNAIDS 2011).

In order to assess the relative burden of HIV infection among sex workers as compared to the general population of adults across settings, a systematic review was conducted based primarily on the peer-reviewed literature related to HIV infection among sex workers from the last five years.

Findings from the review which follows provide a clear picture of the current global and regional burden of HIV infection among sex workers focusing here on female sex workers given the significantly larger evidence base available for this subset of sex workers across contexts.

Methods

Search Strategy

Electronic searches PubMed, EMBASE, Global Health, SCOPUS, PsycINFO, Sociological Abstracts, CINAHL (Cumulative Index to Nursing and Allied Health Literature), Web of Science, and POPLine were carried out in June 2011. The focus was on studies published in the last 5 years with inclusion criteria being studies published between January 1st, 2007, and June 25, 2011. Articles and citations were downloaded, organized, and reviewed using the QUOSA information management software package (Version 8.05. Waltham, MA) and EndNote (version X4, Carlsbad, CA). The search included medical subject headings (MeSH) terms for HIV or AIDS, and terms associated with sex work (prostitute [MeSH] or "sex work" or "sex work*" or "female sex worker" or "commercial sex worker").

Other data sources included national surveillance system data reports, including AIDS indicator surveys (AIS), demographic health surveys (DHS), and integrated biobehavioral surveillance studies (IBBSS) conducted by large international non-governmental organizations. Governmental surveillance reports were searched, including EuroHIV surveillance, U.S. Centers for Disease Control, Australian Surveillance Reports, Public Health Agency of Canada, Pan American Health Organization reports, and structured government-sponsored surveillance assessments from Asia. Expert researchers in the field were contacted to identify unpublished or in-press data not identified through other search methods though data were only included if the studies met all inclusion and exclusion criteria.

Inclusion/Exclusion Criteria

Studies of any design were included that measured the prevalence and/or incidence of HIV among female sex workers, even if sex workers were not the main focus of the study. Studies were accepted if clear descriptions of HIV testing methods were included such as laboratory derived HIV status using biologic samples from blood, urine, or oral specimens. Only studies from countries defined as low or middle income based on the World Bank Atlas Method including all countries with a gross national income per capita of equal to or less than \$12,275. To be included, clear descriptions of the sampling, HIV testing, and analytic methodologies were required with sources including peer-reviewed journals and non-peer reviewed publications meeting other criteria and available online in the public domain. Studies published in English, French, Spanish, or Portuguese were included.

Studies were excluded if the sample size of female sex workers was less than 50 in a larger study of sex workers or where the total sample size was less than 50 in studies that only included female sex workers. In addition, studies that only included self-reported HIV status rather than biological testing were excluded from the analysis.

Screening and Data Extraction

The search criteria described above resulted in 19,180 citations, of which 2,240 were unique records (Figure 2.1). All titles were originally screened by two independent reviewers to include those that potentially included HIV prevalence data, were not included in duplicate, and originated from low or middle income countries. If either author found a title to be relevant, the abstract was reviewed. Two independent reviewers examined the abstracts of the 415 remaining articles and retained those that either clearly met the inclusion criteria or for whom the full text of the article had to be reviewed before a final decision about inclusion could be made. If either author found an article to be relevant, a full-text copy was obtained. Full text review was completed by two independent reviewers. Subsequently, data were extracted by two trained coders using standardized data extraction forms that included details about study design, methods of recruitment, location, sample size, period of study, reported HIV prevalence and/or incidence among female sex workers, HIV prevalence among comparison groups (if provided), and confidence intervals. Coders showed high (90%) agreement, with discrepancies resolved through referral to a third senior study team member. Methodological quality of each study was assessed via evaluation of sampling and recruitment methods, response rates, data reporting, and information on unmeasured biases and confounders.

Meta-Analysis

For each country, HIV prevalence data among sex workers was pooled and weighted by sample size. The prevalence for the general population was calculated using the 2009 UNAIDS to assess the number of women, aged 15 years or older, living with HIV in each country as the numerator. The denominator to assess general population prevalence among women was assessed two ways; first, the US Census Bureau International Division was used to assess the total number of women who are 15 and older and also the total number of reproductive age women, or those between the ages of 15 and 49. The meta-analysis represents the increased odds of being HIV seropositive for female sex workers as compared to all women. The meta-analysis was completed with the Mantel-Haenzel method with a random-effects model with the assumption that the HIV prevalence in one country was independent of the HIV prevalence in other countries. A standard correction of 0.5 is added to all zero cells by the statistical package used (STATA v11, College Station, Texas). Heterogeneity testing was completed using the DerSimonian and Laird's Q test (Takkouche, Cadarso-Suarez et al. 1999). The data are presented both in the form of forest plots including the odds ratio, its 95% CI, and the relative weight of any particular study in estimating the summary odds ratio for all countries.

Meta-analyses were also completed on subgroups of countries including by prevalence level and region. The following categorization schema used the prevalence among reproductive age adults or those aged 15–49 years as including very low prevalence, <0.5% of adults living with HIV; low prevalence, 0.5–1.0%; medium prevalence 1.1–5%; and high prevalence as over 5% of adults living with HIV (Stover, Bertozzi et al. 2006). A similar approach was used for systematic review of HIV among men who have sex with men in Low and Middle Income Countries (Baral, Sifakis et al. 2007).

Sensitivity Analyses

As a sensitivity analysis, the meta-analysis was completed using the two different aforementioned calculated background rates. There was not a statistically significant difference observed in this analysis between estimates calculated through these two methods. However, since women above the age of 49 contribute relatively few infections in most low and middle income countries, it was deemed more conservative to use the background rate calculated with the numerator as those women 15+ and the denominator of those 15–49. As of 2009, UNAIDS did not produce estimates of number of people living with HIV for Afghanistan, Laos, and Albania and thus these countries were excluded from the meta-analysis.

Figure 2.1   Systematic Review of HIV among Sex Workers: Search Results

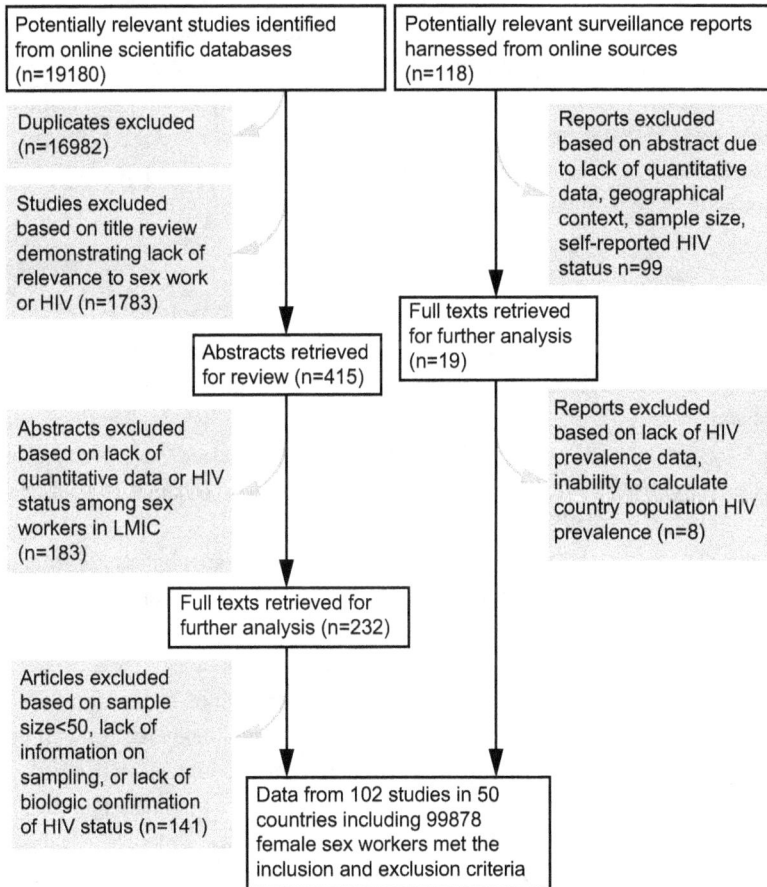

Potentially relevant studies identified from online scientific databases (n=19180)

Potentially relevant surveillance reports harnessed from online sources (n=118)

Duplicates excluded (n=16982)

Reports excluded based on abstract due to lack of quantitative data, geographical context, sample size, self-reported HIV status n=99

Studies excluded based on title review demonstrating lack of relevance to sex work or HIV (n=1783)

Abstracts retrieved for review (n=415)

Full texts retrieved for further analysis (n=19)

Abstracts excluded based on lack of quantitative data or HIV status among sex workers in LMIC (n=183)

Reports excluded based on lack of HIV prevalence data, inability to calculate country population HIV prevalence (n=8)

Full texts retrieved for further analysis (n=232)

Articles excluded based on sample size<50, lack of information on sampling, or lack of biologic confirmation of HIV status (n=141)

Data from 102 studies in 50 countries including 99878 female sex workers met the inclusion and exclusion criteria

Source: Authors.

To quantify the number of infections among reproductive age women attributable to infections among female sex workers, estimates of the prevalence of female sex workers by country and region characterized primarily by

Vandepitte et al from 2006 unless more recent data were available were used (Vandepitte, Lyerla et al. 2006; Ahoyo, Alary et al. 2007; Talbott 2007; Zhang, Wang et al. 2007; Emmanuel, Blanchard et al. 2010; Vuylsteke, Vandenhoudt et al. 2010). Where an estimate of the total number of female sex workers by country was available this estimate was utilized; otherwise a regional estimate was used. In each case, the lowest estimate in the range provided was used to be conservative. The estimates of the proportion of cases among women attributable to female sex workers by country are provided in Table 2.1. The meta-analysis was completed with these estimates and globally there was not a statistically significantly different magnitude in the relationship. However, in China, India, Malaysia, Egypt, and Rwanda there were statistically significant increases in the odds of being infected with HIV among female sex workers as compared to other reproductive age women. To be conservative, the odds ratios reported refer to the comparison of female sex workers to that of all reproductive age women, including female sex workers.

Results

Data from 102 studies including 91 articles and 11 surveillance reports representing 99,878 female sex workers across 50 countries met inclusion and exclusion criteria for the systematic review: 14 countries in Asia, 4 countries in the Eastern Europe (EE) region, 11 countries in Latin America/Caribbean region (LAC), 5 countries in the Middle East/North Africa (MENA), and 16 countries in Sub-Saharan Africa (SSA).

Table 2.1 shows the summary statistics, including odds ratios, aggregate sample sizes, average prevalence of HIV among female sex workers, background HIV prevalence among women as well as the respective prevalence level. The overall HIV prevalence among sex workers in all regions was 11.8% (95% CI 11.6–12.0) with significant variation by region reflective of background rates of HIV. Table 2.1 provides a summary of the data available by region with the highest prevalence in SSA among 21421 women from 16 countries with a pooled prevalence of 36.9%, followed by Eastern Europe with a prevalence of 10.9% among 3037 women in 4 countries, then Latin America and the Caribbean with a pooled prevalence of 6.1% among 10237 women in 11 countries, 64,224 women from 14 countries in Asia with a pooled prevalence of 5.2%; the lowest rate was found in the MENA with a pooled prevalence of 1.7% among 959 women in 5 countries.

Table 2.1 also provides a summary of the sub-group analysis by region and by prevalence level. The overall observed estimate for the odds ratio for a female sex workers to be living with HIV as compared to all reproductive age women in low and middle income countries is 13.5 (95% CI 10.0–18.1). The highest odds ratio (OR) associated with female sex workers was observed in Asia with an OR of 29.2 (22.2–38.4), followed by Sub-Saharan Africa with an OR of 12.4 (95% CI 8.9–17.2), and the lowest in Latin America and the Caribbean with an OR of 12.0 (95% CI 7.3–19.7). Grouping the 21 countries with very low or low prevalence included 69729 women with an overall prevalence of 5.1% (95% CI 4.9–5.3) and an OR of 24.5 (95% CI 19.1–31.3). Medium and high HIV prevalence countries included 26 countries with a prevalence of 30.7% (95% CI 30.2–31.3) among 28075 women and an OR of 11.6 (95% CI 9.1–14.8). Figure 2 represents a Forest plot of the results of the country-level comparisons of HIV risk among female sex workers to that of the general population, the pooled estimate, and the relative weight of each country's results to the pooled estimate. Figure 3 provides a visual representation of these data by categorizing the HIV prevalence in each low and middle income country among female sex workers as well as the pooled regional HIV prevalence among female sex workers along with regional sample sizes.

Table 2.1   Meta-Analyses of Aggregate Country Data Comparing HIV Prevalence among Female Sex Workers and Reproductive Age Women in Low and Middle Income Countries with Data on Female Sex Workers HIV Prevalence, 2007–11

Country	Sample size	Prevalence among female sex workers (95% CI)	Female populationn prevalence	OR (95% CI)	Prev. level[a]	% Female HIV infections among female sex workers	References
Asia							
Afghanistan	544	0.2% (0–0.5)	N/A	–	–	–	Todd, Nasir et al. 2010
Bangladesh	9383	0.2% (0.1–0.3)	0.00%	47.8 (30.8–74.3)	VL	9.5	Programme 2008
Cambodia	160	23.1% (16.6–29.7)	0.86%	34.8 (24.–50.3)	L	8.1	Couture, Sansothy et al. 2011
China	18773	3.0% (2.8–3.3)	0.06%	50.0 (46.0–54.4)	VL	48.6	Lau, Tsui et al. 2007; Xu, Wang et al. 2008; Li, Lin et al. 2009; Lu, Jia et al. 2009; Wang, Chen et al. 2009; Hong, Xu et al. 2010; Li, Wang et al. 2010; Li, Detels et al. 2010; Xu, Wang et al. 2010; Jin, Chan et al. 2011; Wang, Brown et al. 2011; Xu, Brown et al. 2011
India	13386	13.7% (13.1–14.3)	0.29%	54.3 (51.7–57.0)	VL	23.49	Mehendale, Gupte et al. 2007; Talsania, Dinesh et al. 2007; Ramesh, Moses et al. 2008; Sarkar, Bal et al. 2008; Shahmanesh, Cowan et al. 2009; Shethwala, Mulla et al. 2009; Wayal, Cowan et al. 2011
Indonesia	7482	4.9% (4.4–5.4)	0.14%	38.0 (34.2–42.2)	VL	14.5	Magnani, Riono et al. 2010; Silitonga, Davies et al. 2011
Lao PDR	1422	0.5% (0.1–0.9)	–	–	–	–	Center for HIV/AIDS/STI (CHAS) 2009
Malaysia	552	10.7% (8.1–13.3)	0.15%	81.2 (62.0–106.5)	VL	65.4	Malaysian AIDS Council 2009
Mongolia	931	0.0% (0.0–0.0)	0.02%	2.4 (0.2–39.1)	VL	0.0	Enkhbold, Tugsdelger et al. 2007; Hagan and Dulmaa 2007; Davaalkham, Unenchimeg et al. 2009

(continued next page)

Table 2.1 *(continued)*

Country	Sample size	Prevalence among female sex workers (95% CI)	Female populationn prevalence	OR (95% CI)	Prev. level[a]	% Female HIV infections among female sex workers	References
Nepal	1687	8.3% (7.0–9.6)	0.26%	35.0 (29.4–41.6)	VL	64.4	Silverman, Dekcer et al. 2007), (Control 2008; Control 2008
Pakistan	5999	0.1% (0.0–0.1)	0.06%	0.8 (0.3–2.5)	VL	0.3	Bokhari, Nizamani et al. 2007; Hawkes, Collumbien et al. 2009) (Program 2008
Papua New Guinea	205	16.6% (11.5–21.7)	1.20%	16.1 (10.1–25.7)	M	5.6	Bruce, Bauai et al. 2010; Bruce, Bauai et al. 2011
Thailand	319	11.9% (8.4–15.5)	1.15%	11.6 (8.3–16.3)	M	2.1	Nhurod, Bollen et al. 2010
Vietnam	3381	6.5% (5.7–7.3)	0.32%	22.0 (19.2–25.2)	VL	4.1	Tuan, Fylkesnes et al. 2007; Vu Thuong, Van Nghia et al. 2007; Nguyen, Van Khuu et al. 2009
Eastern Europe							
Albania	92	1.1% (0.0–3.2)	–	–	–	–	Qyra, Basho et al. 2011
Estonia	433	8.1% (5.5–10.7)	0.95%	9.1 (6.5–12.9)	L	9.3	Uuskula, Fischer et al. 2008; Uuskula, Johnston et al. 2010
Georgia	234	0.4% (0.0–1.3)	0.13%	3.3 (0.5–23.8)	VL	2.3	Dershem, Tabatadze et al. 2007
Ukraine	2278	12.9% (11.5–14.3)	1.46%	10.0 (8.9–11.3)	M	3.6	International HIV/AIDS Alliance 2010
Latin America							
Argentina	625	3.2% (1.8–4.6)	0.34%	9.6 (6.1–15.0)	VL	1.9	Bautista, Pando et al. 2009

(continued next page)

Table 2.1 (continued)

Country	Sample size	Prevalence among female sex workers (95% CI)	Female populationn prevalence	OR (95% CI)	Prev. level[a]	% Female HIV infections among female sex workers	References
Brazil	90	6.7% (1.5–11.8)	0.47%	15.3 (6.7–34.9)	VL	10.0	Schuelter–Trevisol, Da Silva et al. 2007
Chile	626	0.0% (0.0–0.0)	0.27%	0.3 (0.02–4.6)	VL	0.0	Barrientos, Bozon et al. 2007
Guatemala	1110	4.4% (3.2–5.6)	0.58%	7.9 (5.9–10.5)	L	4. 6	Soto, Ghee et al. 2007; Lahuerta, Sabido et al. 2011
El Salvador	484	3.3% (1.7–4.9)	0.67%	5.1 (3.1–8.3)	L	3.0	Soto, Ghee et al. 2007
Guyana	450	27.6% (23.4–31.7)	1.48%	25.3 (20.5–31.2)	M	11.2	Persaud, Cox et al. 2008
Honduras	493	9.7% (7.1–12.4)	0.59%	18.1 (13.5–24.5)	L	9.9	Soto, Ghee et al. 2007
Jamaica	433	8.8% (6.1–11.4)	1.31%	7.3 (5.2–10.1)	M	4.0	Duncan, Gebre et al. 2010
Mexico	4743	6.2% (5.6–6.9)	0.19%	35.0 (31.1–39.4)	VL	19.8	Patterson, Semple et al. 2008; Ojeda, Strathdee et al. 2009; Loza 2010; Rusch, Brouwer et al. 2010; Sirotin, Strathdee et al. 2010; Strathdee, Lozada et al. 2011; Ulibarri, Strathdee et al. 2011
Nicaragua	460	2.2% (0.8–3.5)	0.13%	16.8 (8.9–31.4)	VL	9.9	Soto, Ghee et al. 2007
Paraguay	723	2.8% (1.6–4.0)	0.22%	12.8 (8.2–19.9)	VL	7.5	Aguayo, LagunaTorres et al. 2008
Middle East and North Africa							
Egypt, Arab Rep.	118	0.8% (0.0–2.5)	0.01%	73.2 (10.2–524.1)	VL	36.3	Ministry of Health and Population 2007

(continued next page)

Table 2.1 *(continued)*

Country	Sample size	Prevalence among female sex workers (95% CI)	Female populationn prevalence	OR (95% CI)	Prev. level[a]	% Female HIV infections among female sex workers	References
Lebanon	95	0.0% (0.0–0.0)	0.10%	5.4 (0.34–87.5)	VL	0.0	Mahfoud, Afifi et al. 2010
Somalia	237	5.5% (2.6–8.4)	0.67%	8.6 (4.9–15.0)	L	29.4	Kriitmaa, Testa et al. 2010
Sudan	321	0.9% (0.0–2.0)	1.32%	0.7 (0.2–2.2)	M	2.6	Abdelrahim 2010
Tunisia	188	0.0% (0.0–0.0)	0.03%	8.0 (0.5–128.7)	VL	0.0	Znazen, Frikha–Gargouri et al. 2010
Sub-Saharan Africa							
Benin	792	40.9% (37.5–44.3)	1.54%	44.2 (38.3–51.0)	M	15.9	Ahoyo, Alary et al. 2007; Lajoie, Massinga Loembe et al. 2010
Guinea	937	36.7% (33.6–39.8)	1.72%	33.1 (29.0–37.8)	M	2.5	Diallo, Alary et al. 2010
Cameroon	1005	29.5% (26.6–32.3)	7.0%	5.5 (4.8–6.3)	H	5.1	Mosoko, Macauley et al. 2009
Togo	1311	36.2% (33.6–38.8)	4.2%	12.7 (11.4–14.2)	M	76.7	Sobela, Pepin et al. 2009
Senegal	1656	19.9% (18.0–21.9)	1.04%	23.7 (21.0–26.7)	M	11.5	Wang, Hawes et al. 2007; Toure Kane, Diawara et al. 2009
Nigeria	3477	33.7% (32.1–35.3)	4.54%	10.7 (10.0–11.5)	M	4.5	Imade, Sagay et al. 2008; Nigerian Federal Ministry of and Fhi 2008; Sule, Adewumi et al. 2009
Congo, Dem. Rep.	1066	9.4% (7.6–11.1)	1.6%	6.4 (5.2–7.8)	VL	3.5	Gupta, Murphy et al. 2007; Vandepitte, Malele et al. 2007; Mwandagalirwa, Jackson et al. 2009)
Uganda	1027	37.2% (34.2–40.2)	8.51%	6.4 (5.6–7.2)	H	15.7	Vandepitte, Bukenya et al. 2011

(continued next page)

Table 2.1 *(continued)*

Country	Sample size	Prevalence among female sex workers (95% CI)	Female populationn prevalence	OR (95% CI)	Prev. level[a]	% Female HIV infections among female sex workers	References
Kenya	7544	45.1% (44.0–46.2)	7.72%	9.8 (9.4–10.3)	H	32.2	Chersich, Luchters et al. 2007; Hirbod, Kaul et al. 2008; Kimani, Kaul et al. 2008; Lacap, Huntington et al. 2008; Luchters, Chersich et al. 2008; Elst, Okuku et al. 2009; Luchters, Vanden Broeck et al. 2010; Tovanabutra, Sanders et al. 2010; McClelland, Richardson et al. 2011
Malawi	273	70.7% (65.3–76.1)	13.33%	15.7 (12.1–20.4)	H	12.7	National AIDS Commission of Malawi 2007
Rwanda	800	24.0% (21.0–27.0)	3.32%	9.2 (7.8–10.8)	M	26.0	Braunstein, Ingabire et al. 2011
South Africa	775	59.6% (56.2–63.1)	25.32%	4.4 (3.8–5.0)	H	5.7	van Loggerenberg, Mlisana et al. 2008
Zimbabwe	214	61.2% (54.7–67.7)	21.42%	5.8 (4.4–7.6)	H	6.9	Cowan, Pascoe et al. 2008
Mauritius	291	32.6% (27.3–38.0)	0.71%	67.4 (52.6–86.4)	L	9.1	Mauritius AIDS Unit 2010
Comoros	153	0.7% (0.0–1.9)	0.06%	11.3 (1.6–81.7)	VL	27.0	Dada, Milord et al. 2007
Madagascar	100	0.0% (0.0–0.0)	0.15%	3.4 (0.2–54.7)	VL	0.0	Harijaona, Ramambason et al. 2009
Pooled Estimate	99878	11.8% (11.6–12.0)	OR 13.5 (95% CI 10.0–18.1) degrees of freedom=46 Heterogeneity X2=7002.14, I2=99.3% Test of OR=1, z=17.60, p=0.000					

Source: Authors.

Note: Prev. = prevalence; CI = confidence interval; OR = odds ratio; – = not available.

a. Prevalence Level: VL–very low (<0.5%), L–low (0.5–1.0%), M–medium (1.1–5%), H–high (>5%).

Table 2.2 Subgroup Meta-analysis of Pooled OR for HIV Infection among Female Sex Workers Region and Prevalence Level Forest Plot Showing Meta-Analysis of Risk of HIV Infection among Female Sex Workers Compared to Women 15–49 in Low and Middle Income Countries, 2000–06

Region	Number of countries	Sample size of HIV positive female sex workers	Sample size of female sex workers	Pooled HIV prevalence (95% ci)	Background prevalence	Pooled odds ratios (95% CI)
Asia	14	3323	64224	5.2% (5.0–5.3)	0.18%	29.2 (22.2–38.4)
Eastern Europe	4	331	3037	10.9% (9.8–12.0)	0.20%	N/A
Latin America and the Caribbean	11	627	10237	6.1% (5.7–6.6)	0.38%	12.0 (7.3–19.7)
Middle East and North Africa	5	17	959	1.7% (0.94–2.60)	0.43%	N/A
Sub-Saharan Africa	16	7899	21421	36.9% (36.2–37.5)	7.42%	12.4 (8.9–17.2)
Very Low/Low Prev.	21	3561	69729	5.1% (4.9–5.3)	0.17%	24.5 (19.1–31.3)
Med./High Prev.	26	8627	28075	30.7% (30.2–31.3)	5.47%	11.6 (9.1–14.8)
Total[a]	50	12197	99878	11.8% (11.6–12.0)	13·5 (95% CI 10.0–18.1)	

Source: Authors.
Note: CI = Confidence Interval
a. Meta-Analysis of Prevalence does not include Afghanistan; Lao PDR; and Albania.

Figure 2.2   Forest Plot Showing Meta-Analysis of Risk of HIV Infection among Female Sex Workers Compared to Women 15–49 in Low and Middle Income Countries, 2000–06

Country	Weight	Odds ratio (95% CI)
Asia		
Bangladesh	2.34	47.82 (30.76 – 74.32)
Cambodia	2.38	34.84 (24.12 – 50.32)
China	2.46	50.04 (46.02 – 54.40)
India	2.47	54.27 (51.66 – 57.02)
Indonesia	2.46	37.99 (34.19 – 42.20)
Malaysia	2.42	81.22 (61.96 – 106.46)
Mongolia	0.77	2.44 (0.15 – 39.11)
Nepal	2.45	35.00 (29.42 – 41.63)
Pakistan	1.81	0.82 (0.26 – 2.54)
Papua New Guinea	2.38	16.43 (11.37 – 23.75)
Thailand	2.39	11.63 (8.29 – 16.32)
Vietnam	2.46	21.96 (19.15 – 25.18)
Eastern Europe		
Estonia	2.39	9.14 (6.45 – 12.93)
Georgia	1.18	3.34 (0.47 – 23.82)
Ukraine	2.46	10.03 (8.87 – 11.34)
Latin America and the Caribbean		
Argentina	2.34	9.59 (6.14 – 14.98)
Brazil	2.07	15.25 (6.66 – 34.91)
Chile	0.78	0.29 (0.02 – 4.64)
Guatemala	2.41	7.88 (5.92 – 10.50)
El Salvador	2.31	5.06 (3.07 – 8.33)
Guyana	2.44	25.26 (20.47 – 31.17)
Honduras	2.41	18.15 (13.47 – 24.46)
Jamaica	2.39	7.25 (5.19 – 10.12)
Mexico	2.45	35.04 (31.14 – 39.43)
Nicaragua	2.22	16.76 (8.94 – 31.40)
Paraguay	2.34	12.77 (8.18 – 19.93)
Middle East and North Africa		
Egypt, Arab Rep.	1.18	73.19 (10.22 – 524.12)
Lebanon	0.77	5.43 (0.34 – 87.48)
Somalia	2.27	8.59 (4.91 – 15.03)
Sudan	1.81	0.71 (0.23 – 2.20)
Tunisia	0.77	8.02 (0.50 – 128.72)
Sub-Saharan Africa		
Benin	2.46	44.20 (38.35 – 50.95)
Camaroon	2.46	5.51 (4.81 – 6.31)
Comoros	1.17	11.33 (1.57 – 81.71)
Congo, Dem. Rep.	2.44	6.37 (5.18 – 7.82)
Guinea	2.46	33.07 (28.95 – 37.79)
Kenya	2.47	9.83 (9.39 – 10.29)
Madagascar	0.77	3.40 (0.21 – 54.72)
Malawi	2.42	15.69 (12.09 – 20.36)
Mauritius	2.43	67.39 (52.58 – 86.37)
Nigeria	2.47	10.69 (9.96 – 11.46)
Rwanda	2.45	9.20 (7.82 – 10.82)
Senegal	2.46	23.69 (20.99 – 26.74)
South Africa	2.45	4.35 (3.77 – 5.03)
Togo	2.46	12.72 (11.36 – 14.24)
Uganda	2.46	6.37 (5.61 – 7.23)
Zimbabwe	2.42	5.79 (4.40 – 7.62)
Overall	100.00	13.49 (10.04 – 18.12)

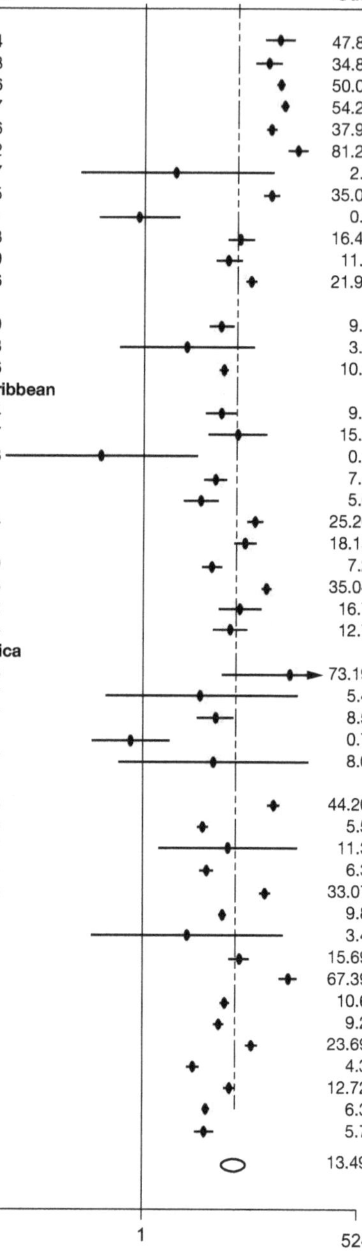

0.00191   1   524

Source: Authors.

Map 2.1   Map of HIV Prevalence among Female Sex Workers in Low and Middle Income Countries including Data from 2007–11 Categorized by HIV Prevalence and Pooled HIV Prevalence Estimates by Region

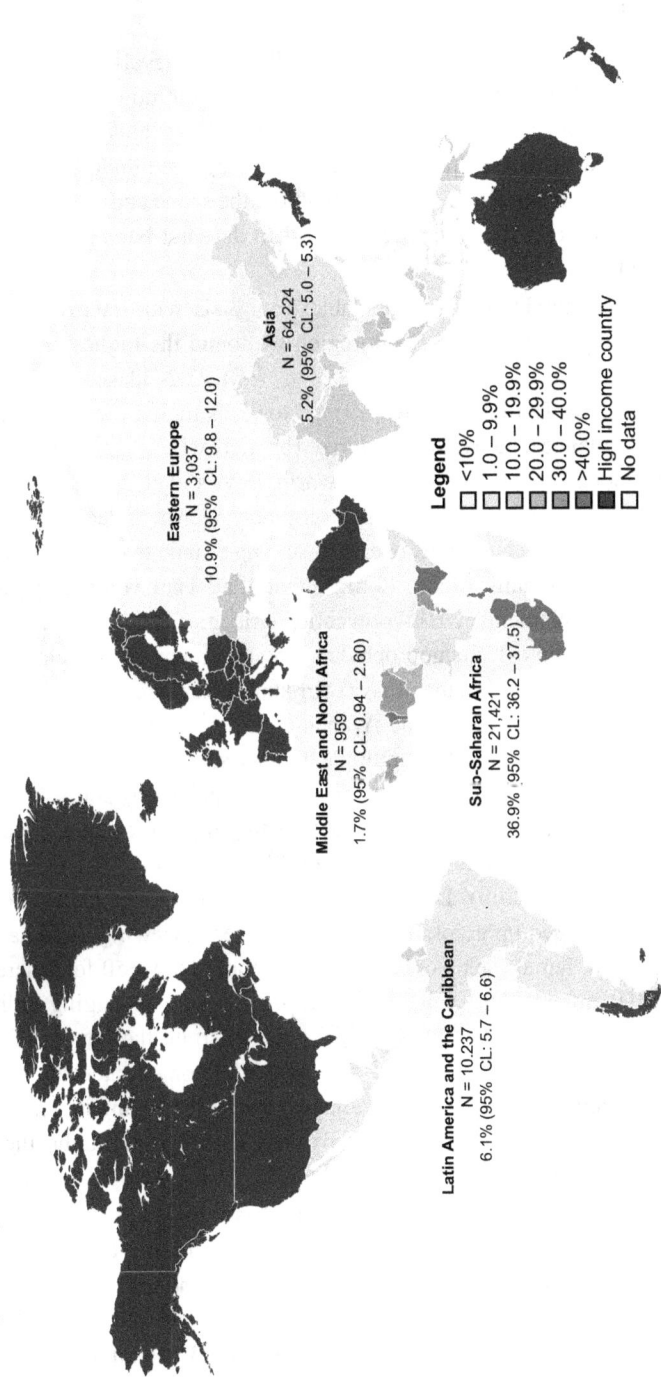

Eastern Europe
N = 3,037
10.9% (95% CL: 9.8 – 12.0)

Asia
N = 64.224
5.2% (95% CL: 5.0 – 5.3)

Middle East and North Africa
N = 959
1.7% (95% CL: 0.94 – 2.60)

Sub-Saharan Africa
N = 21,421
36.9% (95% CL: 36.2 – 37.5)

Latin America and the Caribbean
N = 10.237
6.1% (95% CL: 5.7 – 6.6)

Legend
<10%
1.0 – 9.9%
10.0 – 19.9%
20.0 – 29.9%
30.0 – 40.0%
>40.0%
High income country
No data

Source: Authors.

USAID funding over the need to sign the "Prostitution Pledge" which was mandated as part of the President's Emergency Plan for AIDS Relief (PEPFAR) in 2003 which would have limited the ability to do comprehensive surveillance and service provision for sex workers (Masenior and Beyrer 2007; Ditmore and Allman 2010). Consequently, Brazil has continued to invest in HIV prevention for female sex workers across the country (Kerrigan, Telles et al. 2008). In these analyses, Guyana is an anomaly in that female sex workers carry over a 25 times increased odds of HIV infection. These analyses highlight that the HIV epidemic among female sex workers in LAC is not over given that these women have more than ten times increased odds of being HIV positive than other women.

There was insufficient data to warrant meta-analyses in Eastern Europe and the Middle East and North Africa given that the majority of data in EE was derived from Ukraine and in MENA the studies combined included less than one thousand female sex workers. The studies that have been completed demonstrate that female sex workers exist and that the limited HIV in these settings is concentrated among these women. Given the importance of the parenteral transmission of HIV through injection drug use in EE, it is arguably important to characterize the synergies of the injecting drug user epidemics and those among female sex workers in this region to guide prevention.

While there is wide variation in the prevalence HIV across Western, Eastern, and Southern Africa, female sex workers have high HIV prevalence burdens in each of these regions (Table 2.1). Variation in the relative odds of infection among these women appears to be largely attributable to high background rates of HIV prevalence among all adults in hyper-endemic zones, particularly the African South. By UNAIDS criteria these countries have generalized epidemics because the HIV prevalence among reproductive age women (as measures in antenatal clinics) is above 1% (UNAIDS and WHO 2000). Using the system by Stover et all employed here, these prevalence levels correspond to medium and high prevalence HIV epidemics. Overall, even in the generalized epidemics of SSA female sex workers have approximately a 14 times increased odds of living with HIV as compared to all women. Similarly, in other medium and high HIV prevalence settings, or generalized HIV epidemics, the OR for HIV infection was 11.6 (95% CI 9.1–14.8) for female sex workers. These findings counter the notion that female sex workers are less relevant in generalized epidemics.

The largest body of data on the continent was available from Kenya where in 2010, the Kenyan National AIDS & STI Control Program (NASCOP) developed a set of National Guidelines for HIV/STI Programs for Sex Workers (NASCOP 2010). These guidelines were developed in response to the Kenya National

HIV Strategic Plan (KNASP III) 2009–2013 identifying that female sex workers were a most at risk population and that there are barriers that limit their access to health and social services because some of their work is both criminalized and stigmatized in society (NASCOP 2009). Encouragingly, there has been evidence of incidence rates decreasing among some female sex workers in Kenya, heralding decreasing in HIV incidence in the general population.

In Pakistan, Chile, and Sudan the OR for HIV associated with sex work suggested a trend towards this practice being protective though not statistically significant in any of these countries. Moreover, in Mongolia and Madagascar, the OR for HIV among female sex workers was also not statistically significantly increased. There is likely a combination of truth and artifact that accounts for these results. Non-probability samples of female sex workers may have under-estimated the actual HIV prevalence among female sex workers in the country. However, in each of these countries except for Sudan, the majority of prevalent HIV infections in 2009 are among men with risk factors including same-sex practices and injecting drug use(Baral, Sifakis et al. 2007; Beyrer, Baral et al. 2010; Mathers, Degenhardt et al. 2010; UNAIDS 2010). In Sudan, there are competing risk factors for HIV including migration and rape which may, in part, account for the results observed here(Supervie, Halima et al. 2010).

There are several limitations to this study. The focus on data from the last five years with inclusion criteria of January, 2007 excluded data from a number of countries. While this represents a limitation, the aim of this study was to characterize current burdens of HIV among female sex workers. Any pooling of data comes at the risk of masking intra- and inter-country variations in the risk status, including practices and HIV prevalence, and variations in the social contexts of female sex workers. This is especially true in countries such as India and China that have wide spatial variations in HIV prevalence and risk factors for HIV infection. Furthermore, these estimates are of limited generalizability given that the majority of studies were completed in urban settings, with female sex workers working in more rural settings, border areas and truck stops, underrepresented. The pooled estimates also mask differences between the various contexts in which sex work is practiced including establishment versus non-establishment based sex work or additional risk factors among sex workers including injecting drug use and migration. There is significant heterogeneity of the HIV prevalence results included in the meta-analysis as these are studies from different populations of female sex workers completed in different countries. To account for this, a random-effects model was used for the meta-analysis.

The comparison of HIV prevalence among female sex workers and rates among all women are conservative given that HIV infections are included in the estimates provided by UNAIDS for all reproductive age women. To address this, sensitivity analysis was completed removing infections among reproductive age women attributable to female sex workers and then completing the meta-analysis. The magnitude of the global pooled estimate did not change though it did in certain countries where a high proportion of HIV among women is attributable to sex work. While the pooled analysis is limited related to the heterogeneity estimates by country, it does have utility in demonstrating the continued disease burden among female sex workers, and their continued need for services. A recent report on the investment framework for the global AIDS response suggested that current levels of resource allocation for sex workers was adequate (Schwartlander, Stover et al. 2011). This analysis, contextualized by evidence that female sex workers living with HIV have more partners than other reproductive age women living with HIV and higher rates of STIs facilitating HIV transmission, suggests that more resources are needed to address these sub-epidemics (Brahmam, Kodavalla et al. 2008; Bautista, Pando et al. 2009; Chohan, Baeten et al. 2009; Kang, Liao et al. 2011).

This synthesis highlights that 50 countries out of 145 low and middle income countries have published data including a biological assessment of HIV prevalence among female sex workers in the last 5 years (World 2009). In other words, approximately two thirds of low and middle income countries (65.5%, n=95/145) do not have a current estimate of the burden of HIV among female sex workers. There are several potential explanations for these data gaps including social stigma, criminalization of sex work, and the aforementioned "Prostitution Pledge" which conflated the issue of sex work and human trafficking and markedly reduced research funding and investigator interest in this area (Masenior and Beyrer 2007).

These findings suggest an urgent need to scale up access to quality HIV prevention programming and services among female sex workers secondary to their heightened burden of disease and likelihood of onward transmission through high numbers of sexual partners as clients. Given the high burden of HIV among female sex workers and recent biomedical advances related to treatment as prevention it is also critical to improve linkages to anti-retroviral treatment and retention in care and ongoing prevention for female sex workers living with HIV (Cohen, Chen et al. 2011). The dramatically increased odds of living with HIV among sex workers merits continued research regarding the role of not only behavioral but also structural factors associated with HIV among female sex workers. Considerations of the legal and policy environments in which sex work operate, and the critical role of stigma, discrimination, and violence targeting female sex workers globally will be required to reduce the disproportionate disease burden among these women.

References

Abdelrahim, M. S. (2010). "HIV prevalence and risk behaviors of female sex workers in Khartoum, north Sudan. (Special Issue: Progress in HIV research in the Middle East and North Africa: new study methods, results, and implications for prevention and care.)." *AIDS* 24 (Supplement 2): S55–S60.

Aguayo, N., V. A. LagunaTorres, et al. (2008). "Epidemiological and molecular characteristics of HIV-1 infection among female commercial sex workers, men who have sex with men and people living with AIDS in Paraguay." *Revista da Sociedade Brasileira de Medicina Tropical* 41 (3): 225–231.

Ahoyo, A. B., M. Alary, et al. (2007). "Enquête de surveillance intégrée du VIH et des autres infections sexuellement transmissibles chez les travailleuses du sexe au Bénin en 2002." *Cahiers D'Études et De Recherche Francophone/ Santé* 17 (3): 143–151.

Ahoyo, A. B., M. Alary, et al. (2007). "Female sex workers in Benin, 2002. Behavioural survey and HIV and other STI screening." *Cahiers Sante* 17 (3): 143–151.

Ainsworth, M., C. Beyrer, et al. (2003). "AIDS and public policy: the lessons and challenges of "success" in Thailand." *Health Policy.* 64 (1): 13–37.

Baral, S., F. Sifakis, et al. (2007). "Elevated risk for HIV infection among men who have sex with men in low- and middle-income countries 2000–2006: a systematic review." *PLoS Med* 4(12): e339.

Barrientos, J. E., M. Bozon, et al. (2007). "HIV prevalence, AIDS knowledge, and condom use among female sex workers in Santiago, Chile." *Cadernos de Saude Publica* 23 (8): 1777–1784.

Bautista, C. T., M. A. Pando, et al. (2009). "Sexual practices, drug use behaviors, and prevalence of HIV, syphilis, hepatitis B and C, and HTLV-1/2 in immigrant and non-immigrant female sex workers in Argentina." *Journal of Immigrant and Minority Health* 11 (2): 99–104.

Beyrer, C., S. D. Baral, et al. (2010). "The expanding epidemics of HIV type 1 among men who have sex with men in low- and middle-income countries: diversity and consistency." *Epidemiol Rev* 32 (1): 137–151.

Bokhari, A., N. M. Nizamani, et al. (2007). "HIV risk in Karachi and Lahore, Pakistan: An emerging epidemic in injecting and commercial sex networks." *International Journal of STD and AIDS* 18 (7): 486–492.

Brahmam, G. N., V. Kodavalla, et al. (2008). "Sexual practices, HIV and sexually transmitted infections among self-identified men who have sex with men in four high HIV prevalence states of India." *AIDS* 22 Suppl 5: S45–57.

Braunstein, S. L., C. M. Ingabire, et al. (2011). "High human immunodeficiency virus incidence in a cohort of Rwandan female sex workers." *Sexually Transmitted Diseases* 38 (5): 385–394.

Bruce, E., L. Bauai, et al. (2011). "Effects of periodic presumptive treatment on three bacterial sexually transmissible infections and HIV among female sex workers in Port Moresby, Papua New Guinea." *Sexual Health* 8 (2): 222–228.

Bruce, E., L. Bauai, et al. (2010). "Knowledge, attitudes, practices and behaviour of female sex workers in Port Moresby, Papua New Guinea." *Sexual Health* 7 (1): 85–86.

Caceres, C. F. (2002). "HIV among gay and other men who have sex with men in Latin America and the Caribbean: A hidden epidemic?" *AIDS* 16 (SUPPL. 3): S23–S33.

Celentano, D. D., K. E. Nelson, et al. (1998). "Decreasing incidence of HIV and sexually transmitted diseases in young Thai men: evidence for success of the HIV/AIDS control and prevention program." *AIDS*. 12 (5): F29–F36.

Center for HIV/AIDS/STI (CHAS) (2009). *Integrated Behavioral Biological Surveillance, Laos*. Ministry of. Health. Vientiane, Family Health International.

Chersich, M. F., S. M. F. Luchters, et al. (2007). "Heavy episodic drinking among Kenyan female sex workers is associated with unsafe sex, sexual violence and sexually transmitted infections." *International Journal of STD & AIDS* 18 (11): 764–769.

Chohan, V., J. M. Baeten, et al. (2009). "A prospective study of risk factors for herpes simplex virus type 2 acquisition among high-risk HIV-1 seronegative women in Kenya." *Sexually Transmitted Infections* 85 (7): 489–492.

Cohen, M. S., Y. Q. Chen, et al. (2011). *"Prevention of HIV-1 infection with early antiretroviral therapy."* The New England journal of medicine 365(6): 493–505.

Control, N.-N. C. f. A. a. S. (2008). *Integrated Biological and Behavioral Surveillance Survey among Female Sex Workers in Kathmandu Valley: Round III*. F. H. International. Kathmandu, Ministry of Health and Population.

Control, N.-N. C. f. A. a. S. (2008). *Integrated Biological and Behavioral Surveillance Survey among Female Sex Workers Pokhara Valley: Round III*. Ministry of Health. and Populations. Kathmandu, Family Health International.

Couture, M. C., N. Sansothy, et al. (2011). "Young women engaged in sex work in Phnom Penh, Cambodia, have high incidence of HIV and sexually transmitted infections, and amphetamine-type stimulant use: New challenges to HIV prevention and risk." *Sexually Transmitted Diseases* 38 (1): 33–39.

Cowan, F. M., S. J. Pascoe, et al. (2008). "A randomised placebo-controlled trial to explore the effect of suppressive therapy with acyclovir on genital shedding of HIV-1 and herpes simplex virus type 2 among Zimbabwean sex workers." *Sexually Transmitted Infections* 84 (7): 548–553.

Dada, Y., F. Milord, et al. (2007). "The Indian Ocean paradox revisited: HIV and sexually transmitted infections in the Comoros." *International journal of STD & AIDS* 18 (9): 596–600.

Davaalkham, J., P. Unenchimeg, et al. (2009). "High-risk status of HIV-1 infection in the very low epidemic country, Mongolia, 2007." *International journal of STD & AIDS* 20 (6): 391–394.

Dershem, L., M. Tabatadze, et al. (2007). Characteristics, high-risk behaviors and knowledge of STI / HIV / AIDS, and STI / HIV prevalence of facility-based female sex workers in Batumi, Georgia: 2004–2006. *Report on two behavioral surveillance surveys with a biomarker component for the SHIP Project*. Tbilisi, Georgia: Save the Children.

Diallo, B. L., M. Alary, et al. (2010). "HIV epidemic among female sex workers in Guinea: Prevalence, associated risk factors, vulnerability and trend from 2001 to 2007." *Revue d'Epidemiologie et de Sante Publique* 58 (4): 245–254.

Ditmore, M. and D. Allman (2010). "Implications of PEPFAR's anti-prostitution pledge for HIV prevention among organizations working with sex workers." *HIV/AIDS Policy & Law Review* 15 (1): 63–64.

Duncan, J., Y. Gebre, et al. (2010). "HIV prevalence and related behaviors among sex workers in Jamaica." *Sexually Transmitted Diseases* 37 (5): 306–310.

Elst, E. M. v. d., H. S. Okuku, et al. (2009). *"Is audio computer-assisted self-interview (ACASI) useful in risk behaviour assessment of female and male sex workers, Mombasa, Kenya?"* PLoS ONE (May): e5340.

Emmanuel, F., J. Blanchard, et al. (2010). "The HIV/AIDS Surveillance Project mapping approach: An innovative approach for mapping and size estimation for groups at a higher risk of HIV in Pakistan." *AIDS* 24 (SUPPL. 2): S77–S84.

Enkhbold, S., S. Tugsdelger, et al. (2007). "HIV/AIDS related knowledge and risk behaviors among female sex workers in two major cities of Mongolia." *Nagoya Journal of Medical Science* 69 (3–4): 157–165.

Gupta, S. B., G. Murphy, et al. (2007). "Comparison of methods to detect recent HIV type 1 infection in cross-sectionally collected specimens from a cohort of female sex workers in the Dominican Republic." *AIDS Research and Human Retroviruses* 23 (12): 1475–1480.

Hagan, J. E. and N. Dulmaa (2007). "Risk factors and prevalence of HIV and sexually transmitted infections among low-income female commercial sex workers in Mongolia." *Sexually Transmitted Diseases* 34 (2): 83–87.

Harijaona, V., J. D. Ramambason, et al. (2009). "Prevalence of and risk factors for sexually-transmitted infections in hidden female sex workers." *Medecine et Maladies Infectieuses* 39 (12): 909–913.

Hawkes, S., M. Collumbien et al. (2009). "HIV and other sexually transmitted infections among men, transgenders and women selling sex in two cities in Pakistan: a cross-sectional prevalence survey." *Sexually Transmitted Infections* 85 Suppl 2: ii8–16.

Hirbod, T., R. Kaul, et al. (2008). "HIV-neutralizing immunoglobulin A and HIV-specific proliferation are independently associated with reduced HIV acquisition in Kenyan sex workers." *AIDS* 22 (6): 727–735.

Hong, H., G. Xu, et al. (2010). "Long-term follow-up of a comprehensive HIV and sexually transmitted infection prevention program for female sex workers in Ningbo, China." *International Journal of Gynecology & Obstetrics* 111 (2): 180–181.

Imade, G., A. Sagay, et al. (2008). "Prevalence of HIV and other sexually transmissible infections in relation to lemon or lime juice douching among female sex workers in Jos, Nigeria." *Sexual Health* 5 (1): 55–60.

International HIV/AIDS Alliance in Ukraine. (2010). Behavioral Monitoring and HIV infection prevalence among female sex workers as a component of second generation surveillance. *Analytic Report: based on results of 2009 survey among female sex workers.* Kyiv.

Jin, X., S. Chan, et al. (2011). "Prevalence and risk behaviours for Chlamydia trachomatis and Neisseria gonorrhoeae infection among female sex workers in an HIV/AIDS high-risk area." *International Journal of STD and AIDS* 22 (2): 80–84.

Kang, D., M. Liao, et al. (2011). *"Commercial sex venues, syphilis and methamphetamine use among female sex workers."* AIDS Care - Psychological and Socio-Medical Aspects of AIDS/HIV 23 (SUPPL. 1): 26–36.

Kerrigan, D., P. Telles, et al. (2008). "Community development and HIV/STI-related vulnerability among female sex workers in Rio de Janeiro, Brazil." *Health Education Research* 23(1): 137–145.

Kimani, J., R. Kaul, et al. (2008). "Reduced rates of HIV acquisition during unprotected sex by Kenyan female sex workers predating population declines in HIV prevalence." *AIDS* 22 (1): 131–137.

Kriitmaa, K., A. Testa, et al. (2010). "HIV prevalence and characteristics of sex work among female sex workers in Hargeisa, Somaliland, Somalia. (Special Issue: Progress in HIV research in the Middle East and North Africa: new study methods, results, and implications for prevention and care.)." *AIDS* 24 (Supplement 2): S61-S67.

Lacap, P. A., J. D. Huntington, et al. (2008). "Associations of human leukocyte antigen DRB with resistance or susceptibility to HIV-1 infection in the Pumwani Sex Worker Cohort." *AIDS* 22 (9): 1029–1038.

Laga, M., C. Galavotti, et al. (2010). "The importance of sex-worker interventions: the case of Avahan in India." *Sexually Transmitted Infections* 86 Suppl 1: i6–7.

Lahuerta, M., M. Sabido, et al. (2011). "Comparison of users of an HIV/syphilis screening community-based mobile van and traditional voluntary counselling and testing sites in Guatemala." *Sexually Transmitted Infections* 87 (2): 136–140.

Lajoie, J., M. Massinga Loembe, et al. (2010). "Blood soluble human leukocyte antigen G levels are associated with human immunodeficiency virus type 1 infection in Beninese commercial sex workers." *Human Immunology* 71 (2): 182–185.

Lau, J. T. F., H. Y. Tsui, et al. (2007). "Variations in condom use by locale: A comparison of mobile Chinese female sex workers in Hong Kong and Mainland China." *Archives of Sexual Behavior* 36 (6): 849–859.

Li, N., Z. Wang, et al. (2010). "HIV among plasma donors and other high-risk groups in Henan, China." *Journal of Acquired Immune Deficiency Syndromes* 53 Suppl 1: S41–47.

Li, Y., R. Detels, et al. (2010). "Prevalence of HIV and STIs and associated risk factors among female sex workers in Guangdong Province, China. (Special Issue: China meets new AIDS challenges.)." *Journal of Acquired Immune Deficiency Syndromes* 53 Su.

Li, Y., P. Lin, et al. (2009). "Prevalence of HIV infection and sexually transmitted diseases and associated risk factors among female sex workers in Guangdong province." *Disease Surveillance* 24 (8): 599–602.

Loza, O. (2010). *Factors associated with early initiation into sex work and sexually transmitted infections among female sex workers in two Mexico-U.S. border cities.* 70, ProQuest Information & Learning.

Lu, F., Y. Jia, et al. (2009). "Prevalence of HIV infection and predictors for syphilis infection among female sex workers in Southern China." *Southeast Asian Journal of Tropical Medicine and Public Health* 4 (2): 263–272.

Luchters, S., M. F. Chersich, et al. (2008). "Impact of five years of peer-mediated interventions on sexual behavior and sexually transmitted infections among female sex workers in Mombasa, Kenya." *BMC Public Health* 8(Journal Article): 143–143.

Luchters, S. M., D. Vanden Broeck, et al. (2010). "Association of HIV infection with distribution and viral load of HPV types in Kenya: a survey with 820 female sex workers." *BMC Infectious Diseases* 10: 18.

Magnani, R., P. Riono, et al. (2010). "Sexual risk behaviours, HIV and other sexually transmitted infections among female sex workers in Indonesia." *Sexually Transmitted Infections* 86 (5): 393–399.

Mahfoud, Z., R. Afifi, et al. (2010). "HIV/AIDS among female sex workers, injecting drug users and men who have sex with men in Lebanon: Results of the first biobehavioral surveys." *AIDS* 24 (SUPPL. 2): S45–S54.

Malaysian AIDS Council (2009). *Malaysia Integrated Bio-behavioural Surveillance (IBBS) Survey.* Kuala Lumpur.

Masenior, N. F. and C. Beyrer (2007). "The US anti-prostitution pledge: First Amendment challenges and public health priorities." *PLoS Medicine* 4 (7): e207.

Mathers, B. M., L. Degenhardt, et al. (2010). "HIV prevention, treatment, and care services for people who inject drugs: a systematic review of global, regional, and national coverage." *The Lancet* 375 (9719): 1014–1028.

Mauritius AIDS Unit (2010). *Integrated Behavioral and Biological Surveillance Survey among Female Sex Workers*, 2010. Ministry of Health Q. of Life. Port Louis, Mauritius.

McClelland, R. S., B. A. Richardson, et al. (2011). "Association between participant self-report and biological outcomes used to measure sexual risk behavior in human immunodeficiency virus-1-seropositive female sex workers in Mombasa, Kenya." *Sexually Transmitted Diseases* 38 (5): 429–433.

Mehendale, S. M., N. Gupte, et al. (2007). "Declining HIV incidence among patients attending sexually transmitted infection clinics in Pune, India." *Journal of Acquired Immune Deficiency Syndromes* 45 (5): 564–569.

Ministry of Health and Population, N. A. P. (2007). *HIV/AIDS Biological & Behavioral Surveillance Survey.* Cairo, Egypt: Family Health International.

Mosoko, J. J., I. B. Macauley, et al. (2009). "Human immunodeficiency virus infection and associated factors among specific population subgroups in Cameroon." *AIDS Behavior* 13 (2): 277–287.

Mwandagalirwa, K., E. Jackson, et al. (2009). "Local differences in human immunodeficiency virus prevalence: a comparison of social venue patrons, antenatal patients, and sexually transmitted infection patients in eastern kinshasa." *Sexually Transmitted Diseases* 36 (7): 406–412.

NASCOP (2009). *Kenya National AIDS Strategic Plan 2010–2013 - Delivering on Universal Access to Services.* Office of the President. Nairobi, Kenya.

NASCOP (2010). *National Guidelines for HIV/STI Programs for Sex Workers.* MOPHS. Nairobi, Kenya.

National AIDS Commission of Malawi (2007). *Biological and Behavioral Surveillance Survey.* Lilongwe. Family Health International.

Nguyen, T. V., N. Van Khuu, et al. (2009). "Correlation Between HIV and Sexual Behavior, Drug Use, Trichomoniasis and Candidiasis Among Female Sex Workers in a Mekong Delta Province of Vietnam." *AIDS and Behavior* 13 (5): 873–880.

Nhurod, P., L. J. M. Bollen, et al. (2010). "Access to HIV testing for sex workers in Bangkok, Thailand: a high prevalence of HIV among street-based sex workers." *Southeast Asian Journal of Tropical Medicine and Public Health* 41 (1): 153–162.

Nigerian Federal Ministry of Health and Fhi (2008). *Integrated Biological and Behavioural Surveillance Survey.* Nigeria.

Ojeda, V. D., S. A. Strathdee, et al. (2009). "Associations between migrant status and sexually transmitted infections among female sex workers in Tijuana, Mexico." *Sexually Transmitted Infections* 85 (6): 420–426.

Patterson, T. L., S. J. Semple, et al. (2008). "Prevalence and correlates of HIV infection among female sex workers in 2 Mexico-US border cities." *Journal of Infectious Diseases* 197 (5): 728–732.

Persaud, N., F. Cox, et al. (2008). Behavioral Surveillance Survey/Guyana: Out-of-school Youth, In-school Youth, Female Sex Workers, Men Who Have Sex with Men, Employees of the Sugar Industry and Members of the Uniformed Services. *F. H. International.* Georgetown, Ministry of Health.

Program, N. A. C. (2008). *HIV Second Generation Surveillance in Pakistan: National Report Round II.* C.-P. H. A. S. Project. Islamabad.

Programme, N. A. S. (2008). *National HIV Serological Surveillance, Bangladesh: 8th Round Technical Report.* Ministry of Health and. F. W. Directorate General of Health Services. Dhaka, Government of the People's Republic of Bangladesh.

Qyra, S., M. Basho, et al. (2011). "Behavioral risk factors and prevalence of HIV and other STI among female sex workers in Tirana, Albania." *New Microbiologica* 34 (1): 105–108.

Ramesh, B. M., S. Moses, et al. (2008). "Determinants of HIV prevalence among female sex workers in four south Indian states: analysis of cross-sectional surveys in twenty-three districts. (Special Issue: Characterizing the Indian HIV epidemic and assessing large-scale prevention efforts - Avahan.)." *AIDS* 22 (Supplement 5): S35–S44.

Rojanapithayakorn, W. and R. Hanenberg (1996). "The 100% condom program in Thailand." *AIDS* 10 (1): 1–7.

Rusch, M. L. A., K. C. Brouwer, et al. (2010). "Distribution of sexually transmitted diseases and risk factors by work locations among female sex workers in Tijuana, Mexico." *Sexually Transmitted Diseases* 37 (10): 608–614.

Sarkar, K., B. Bal, et al. (2008). "Sex-trafficking, violence, negotiating skill, and HIV infection in brothel-based sex workers of eastern India, adjoining Nepal, Bhutan, and Bangladesh." *Journal of Health, Population and Nutrition* 26 (2): 223–231.

Schuelter-Trevisol, F., M. V. Da Silva, et al. (2007). "HIV genotyping among female sex workers in the State of Santa Catarina." *Revista da Sociedade Brasileira de Medicina Tropical* 40 (3): 259–263.

Schwartlander, B., J. Stover, et al. (2011). "Towards an improved investment approach for an effective response to HIV/AIDS." *The Lancet* 377 (9782): 2031–2041.

Shahmanesh, M., F. Cowan, et al. (2009). "The burden and determinants of HIV and sexually transmitted infections in a population-based sample of female sex workers in Goa, India." *Sexually Transmitted Infections* 85 (1): 50–59.

Shethwala, N. D., S. A. Mulla, et al. (2009). "Sexually transmitted infections and reproductive tract infections in female sex workers." *Indian Journal of Pathology and Microbiology* 52 (2): 198–199.

Silitonga, N., S. C. Davies, et al. (2011). "Prevalence over time and risk factors for sexually transmissible infections among newly-arrived female sex workers in Timika, Indonesia." *Sexual Health* 8 (1): 61–64.

Silverman, J. G., M. R. Dekcer, et al. (2007). "HIV prevalence and predictors of infection in sex-trafficked Nepalese girls and women." *Journal of the American Medical Association* 298 (5): 536–542.

Sirotin, N., S. A. Strathdee, et al. (2010). "A comparison of registered and unregistered female sex workers in Tijuana, Mexico." *Public Health Reports* 125 (SUPPL. 4): 101–109.

Sobela, F., J. Pepin, et al. (2009). "A tale of two countries: HIV among core groups in Togo." *Journal of Acquired Immune Deficiency Syndromes* 51 (2): 216–223.

Soto, R. J., A. E. Ghee, et al. (2007). "Sentinel surveillance of sexually transmitted infections/ HIV and risk behaviors in vulnerable populations in 5 Central American countries." *Journal of Acquired Immune Deficiency Syndromes* 46 (1): 101–111.

Stover, J., S. Bertozzi, et al. (2006). "The global impact of scaling up HIV/AIDS prevention programs in low- and middle-income countries." *Science* 311 (5766): 1474–1476.

Strathdee, S. A., R. Lozada, et al. (2011). "Social and structural factors associated with HIV infection among female sex workers who inject drugs in the Mexico-US border region." *PLoS ONE* 6 (4): e19048–e19048.

Sule, W. F., M. O. Adewumi, et al. (2009). "Human immunodeficiency virus (HIV) specific antibodies among married pregnant women and female commercial sex workers attending voluntary counseling and HIV testing (HCT) centre in Abuja, Nigeria." *African Journal of Biotechnology* 8 (6): 941–948.

Supervie, V., Y. Halima, et al. (2010). "Assessing the impact of mass rape on the incidence of HIV in conflict-affected countries." *AIDS* 24 (18): 2841–2847.

Swendeman, D., B. Ishika, et al. (2009). "Empowering sex workers in India to reduce vulnerability to HIV and sexually transmitted diseases." *Social Science & Medicine* 69 (8): 1157–1166.

Takkouche, B., C. Cadarso-Suarez, et al. (1999). "Evaluation of old and new tests of heterogeneity in epidemiologic meta-analysis." *American Journal of Epidemiology* 150 (2): 206–215.

Talbott, J. R. (2007). "Size matters: the number of prostitutes and the global HIV/AIDS pandemic." *PLoS ONE* 2(6): e543.

Talsania, N. J., R. Dinesh, et al. (2007). "STI/HIV prevalence in Sakhi Swasthya Abhiyan, Jyotisangh, Ahmedabad: a clinico-epidemiological study." *Indian Journal of Sexually Transmitted Diseases* 28 (1): 15–18.

Todd, C. S., A. Nasir, et al. (2010). "HIV, hepatitis B, and hepatitis C prevalence and associated risk behaviors among female sex workers in three Afghan cities. (Special Issue: Progress in HIV research in the Middle East and North Africa: new study methods, results, and implications for prevention and care.)." *AIDS* 24 (Supplement 2): S69–S75.

Toure Kane, C., S. Diawara, et al. (2009). "Concentrated and linked epidemics of both HSV-2 and HIV-1/HIV-2 infections in Senegal: Public health impacts of the spread of HIV." *International Journal of STD and AIDS* 20(11): 793–796.

Tovanabutra, S., E. J. Sanders, et al. (2010). "Evaluation of HIV type 1 strains in men having sex with men and in female sex workers in Mombasa, Kenya." *AIDS Research and Human Retroviruses* 26(2): 123–131.

Tuan, N. A., K. Fylkesnes, et al. (2007). "Human immunodeficiency virus (HIV) infection patterns and risk behaviours in different population groups and provinces in Viet Nam." *Bulletin of the World Health Organization* 85 (1): 35–41.

Ulibarri, M. D., S. A. Strathdee, et al. (2011). "Injection drug use as a mediator between client-perpetrated abuse and HIV status among female sex workers in two Mexico-US border cities." *AIDS and Behavior* 1 (1): 179–185.

UNAIDS (2009). UNAIDS *Guidance Note on HIV and Sex Work*. Geneva.

UNAIDS (2010). UNAIDS *Report on the Global AIDS Epidemic: 2010*. Geneva.

UNAIDS (2011). *Global HIV/AIDS Response: Epidemic update and health sector progress towards Universal Access*. Geneva.

UNAIDS and WHO (2000). *Guidelines for Second Generation HIV Surveillance*. Geneva.

Uuskula, A., K. Fischer, et al. (2008). "A study on HIV and hepatitis C virus among commercial sex workers in Tallinn." *Sexually Transmitted Infections* 84 (3): 189–191.

Uuskula, A., L. G. Johnston, et al. (2010). "Evaluating recruitment among female sex workers and injecting drug users at risk for HIV using respondent-driven sampling in Estonia." *Journal of Urban Health: Bulletin of the New York Academy of Medicine* 87 (2): 304–317.

van Loggerenberg, F., K. Mlisana, et al. (2008). "Establishing a Cohort at High Risk of HIV Infection in South Africa: Challenges and Experiences of the CAPRISA 002 Acute Infection Study." *PLoS ONE* 3 (4): e1954–e1954.

Vandepitte, J., J. Bukenya, et al. (2011). "HIV and other sexually transmitted infections in a cohort of women involved in high-risk sexual behavior in Kampala, Uganda." *Sexually Transmitted Diseases* 38 (4): 316–323.

Vandepitte, J., R. Lyerla, et al. (2006). "Estimates of the number of female sex workers in different regions of the world." *Sexually Transmitted Infections* 82 Suppl 3: iii: 18–25.

Vandepitte, J. M., F. Malele, et al. (2007). "HIV and other sexually transmitted infections among female sex workers in Kinshasa, Democratic Republic of Congo, in 2002." *Sexually Transmitted Diseases* 34(4): 203–208.

Vu Thuong, N., K. Van Nghia, et al. (2007). "Impact of a community sexually transmitted infection/HIV intervention project on female sex workers in five border provinces of Vietnam." *Sexually Transmitted Infections* 83 (5): 376–382.

Vuylsteke, B., H. Vandenhoudt, et al. (2010). "Capture recapture for estimating the size of the female sex worker population in three cities in Cote d'Ivoire and in Kisumu, western Kenya." *Tropical Medicine & International Health* 15 (12): 1537–1543.

Wang, C., S. E. Hawes, et al. (2007). *Sexually Transmitted Infections* 83 (7): 534–540.

Wang, H., K. S. Brown, et al. (2011). "Knowledge of hiv seropositivity is a predictor for initiation of illicit drug use: Incidence of drug use initiation among female sex workers in a high hiv-prevalence area of china." *Drug and Alcohol Dependence.*

Wang, H., R. Y. Chen, et al. (2009). "Prevalence and predictors of HIV infection among female sex workers in Kaiyuan City, Yunnan Province, China." *International Journal of Infectious Diseases* 13 (2): 162–169.

Wayal, S., F. Cowan, et al. (2011). "Contraceptive practices, sexual and reproductive health needs of HIV-positive and negative female sex workers in Goa, India." *Sexually Transmitted Infections* 87 (1): 58–64.

World Bank. (2009). *Gross national income per capita 2008*, Atlas method and PPP. Geneva.

Xu, J., K. Brown, et al. (2011). "Factors associated with HIV testing history and HIV-test result follow-up among female sex workers in two cities in Yunnan, China." *Sexually Transmitted Diseases* 38 (2): 89–95.

Xu, J., H. Wang, et al. (2010). "Application of the BED capture enzyme immunoassay for HIV incidence estimation among female sex workers in Kaiyuan City, China, 2006–2007." *International Journal of Infectious Diseases* 14 (7): e608–e612.

Xu, J., N. Wang, et al. (2008). "HIV and STIs in clients and female sex workers in mining regions of Gejiu City, China." *Sexually Transmitted Diseases* 35 (6): 558–565.

Zhang, D., L. Wang, et al. (2007). "Advantages and challenges of using census and multiplier methods to estimate the number of female sex workers in a Chinese city." *AIDS Care - Psychological and Socio-Medical Aspects of AIDS/HIV* 19 (1): 17–19.

Znazen, A., O. Frikha-Gargouri, et al. (2010). "Sexually transmitted infections among female sex workers in Tunisia: High prevalence of Chlamydia trachomatis." *Sexually Transmitted Infections* 86 (7): 500–505.

CHAPTER 3

Country Case Studies on Sex Work and HIV Prevention

In this chapter we present eight country case studies to provide greater depth on the diverse typologies, contexts, risks, and epidemiology of sex work and HIV across geographic regions.

Case study countries have been selected to ensure representation from the geographic regions of Eastern Europe, South and Southeast Asia, Latin America and the Caribbean, and Sub-Saharan Africa, as well as diverse HIV epidemic scenarios. The eight countries selected include: Benin, Nigeria and Kenya; India and Thailand; the Dominican Republic and Brazil; and Ukraine.

These descriptive pieces include attention to diversity across male, female, and transgender populations as well as sex work environments such as brothels, bars, and the street. Considerable attention is placed on the legal, policy and socio-economic context of sex work in each country.

Documentation of differential HIV risk patterns and conditions among sex workers and their clients within a given context, as well as, an analysis of differing social and structural barriers related to accessing HIV prevention, treatment and care services are provided in each case study. We report HIV prevention intervention coverage data for sex workers per setting as available.

These case studies draw on the public health and social science peer-reviewed literatures, the grey literature related to sex work and HIV prevention for a given country, input from NSWP members, and additional consultations with sex worker representatives from these countries.

Later in this report, we conduct additional comparative analyses examining further the socio-political and historical depth the experiences of Brazil, India and Thailand, and the role of sex worker leadership in effectively responding to HIV among sex workers in those settings.

Benin

Introduction

Key Themes

- There is evidence of a disproportionate burden of HIV among sex workers in Benin in comparison to the general population of adults
- While still elevated, the HIV prevalence among sex workers has steadily declined over the last decade
- Interventions targeting female sex workers and their male clients have been implemented in several "hot spots" in the country
- To date, there are no reported HIV prevention interventions with male or transgender sex workers in Benin

The Republic of Benin gained independence from France on August 1, 1960 and transitioned to a constitutional democratic multiparty government in 1990. Approximately 9 million people live in the small coastal West African nation. French is the official language; however, multiple local languages are spoken, including Fon and Yoruba which are the most often spoken in southern Benin while Baatonum and Fula are most often spoken in the northern Benin. The capital of Benin is Porto-Novo, but the seat of government is located in the country's largest city of Cotonou. The economy is highly dependent upon agriculture. Benin is a low income country with a per capita Gross Domestic Product (GDP) of $745 and a growth rate of 3.8%. It ranked 137 out of 193 countries for GDP according to the World Bank in 2010. Despite some growth, the economy of Benin remains underdeveloped and ranks low (134 out of 169 countries) on the 2010 UNDP Human Development Index (U.S. Department of State 2010).

Historical Perspectives and Trends of the HIV Epidemic

The first case of AIDS in Benin was documented in 1985 and the numbers slowly increased after that. However, sentinel surveillance data from 2002–2010 indicate a stabilization of the epidemic in the general population at about 1.2% (Cherabi, Greenall et al. 2011). The PNLS (Programme National de

Lutte contre le SIDA, i.e. National AIDS Program) was created in 1987 within the Ministry of Health. Between 1987 and 2001, the government developed and implemented a short-term plan (1987–1988) and two medium-term plans (1989–1993 and 1994–1998), before completing its first full strategic plan for the 2000–2005 period (Le Comité National de Lutte contre le Sida (CNLS) 2010). This plan included the establishment in 2002 of the National Committee to Fight against AIDS (CNLS), the decision- and policy-making institution responsible for coordination and promotion of a multi-sector response to HIV and STIs in Benin. The Committee is chaired by the head of state and includes government ministries; networks of national nongovernmental organizations (NGOs); international NGOs; people living with HIV (PLHIV); religious and traditional leaders; the private sector; and development partners. CNLS has decentralized units at the department, commune, arrondissement, and village levels.

The most recent National AIDS Strategic plan covers 2006–2010. The National Strategic Framework covers 2007–2011 and was based on previously conducted needs assessments (CNLS Bénin). Funding for implementation of the strategic plan was awarded on April 5, 2007 by the World Bank for 35 million USD (The Global Fund). In 2009 Benin spent 28 million USD on HIV. 45.2% was from domestic public sources, 9.4% was from bilateral international sources, 25.8% was from the Global Fund to Fight AIDS, Tuberculosis, and Malaria (GFATM), 11.7% was from the UN, and 3.5% was from other multilaterals; 4.3% was from other international sources (UNAIDS). Benin scored 4 out of 5 for civil society involvement on the United Nations General Assembly Special Session (UNGASS) indicator for National Composite Policy Index in 2010 and reported implementing risk reduction services for female sex workers. Benin reported that they have not implemented risk reduction activities among men who have sex with men, including male sex workers, due to lack of reliable statistical data on this group and lack of specialized interventions for effective prevention (UNAIDS).

On 14 October 2010, the European Union (EU), the Government of Benin and the Joint United Nations Programme on HIV/AIDS (UNAIDS), signed a Memorandum of Understanding (MOU) on a Technical Support Plan to enhance coordination of the AIDS response in Benin and improve the implementation of the Global Fund grants. This MOU is intended to address effective allocation of existing financial resources, strengthen coordination, and improve coverage of prevention of mother-to-child transmission services. Benin has received 70 million USD for HIV programming from the Global Fund to Fight AIDS, TB and Malaria, with another 60 million USD planned for round 9. UNAIDS will facilitate the coordination, as well as resource mobilization to ensure the implementation of the technical support plan and the EU has approved 500,000 USD to support implementation of the technical support plan over three years, 70 % of the total need.

Currently, UNAIDS estimates that 60,000 [CI: 52,000–69,000] people are living with HIV in Benin and 3,300 new infections occur annually (UNAIDS, 2009). It has an adult (15–49 years) prevalence of 1.2%, and women carry the largest burden of HIV infection at 1.5% compared to 0.8% among men. Approximately 5,000 children under age 15 are living with HIV compared to 55,000 adults aged 15 and older (UNAIDS 2009).

Sex workers and their clients are disproportionally affected by HIV (UNAIDS 2009). A systematic review of the peer reviewed literature found one journal article on HIV prevalence among sex workers in Benin, and it described an HIV prevalence of 46% in 2002. In a more recent unpublished surveillance survey done in 2008, 26.5 % (CI 23.8–29.2%) of sex workers were found to be HIV positive. Estimated HIV prevalence among clients of sex workers was 3.7% (PNLS 2009). HIV prevalence among truck drivers was 1.5%, with drivers over age 30 years being the most likely to be infected (2.6%).

There are substantial regional differences in prevalence, with a more than nine-fold variation (from 0.4% to 3.8%) in different regions based on antenatal clinic sentinel surveillance. HIV prevalence is highest in urban areas compared to rural ones. The 2006 Benin Demographic and Health Survey found the lowest prevalence in the regions of Collines and Alibori (0.0–0.5%). HIV prevalence was highest in Couffo and Donga (greater than 2%). According to 2008 survey data reported in the 2010 UNGASS report, substantial differences in seroprevalence exist among sex workers by region as well. Donga has the highest HIV prevalence among sex workers (40%) whereas Atacora has the lowest (13%).

Benin began providing antiretroviral treatment (ART) in 2002 with three sites in Cotonou. As of 2009, it had 68 treatment sites throughout the country; and 15,401 people were receiving antiretroviral therapy by the end of that year. Of those on ART, 6,468 (42%) were men and 8,933 (58%) were women. Overall 53% of people needing ART by WHO 2010 guidelines were on ART in 2009 (72% by 2006 WHO guidelines).

Scope, Typology, and Context of Sex Work

For the purposes of surveillance studies, the National AIDS Program (NAP) in Benin identifies sex workers as women of at least 15 years of age who either sell sex openly or in a clandestine manner (PNLS 2009). The former are found in brothels, bars, hotels, and other specific sites, while the latter are those who do not have a fixed site, but who are found on or near certain roads, public places, hotels, restaurants, etc.

In 2008, a total of 13,619 sex workers (37.6% who are open and 62.4% who practice clandestinely) operating out of 2,901 sex work sites or "hot spots" were identified through the mapping exercise conducted by the National AIDS Program. According to the study's findings, most sex work sites (93%) are found in urban areas. Half of sex workers (49.9%) are between the ages of 20 and 29, and 10.9% were less than 20 years old (PNLS 2009).

Map 3.1   Geographical Distribution of HIV Prevalence among Female Sex Workers in Benin

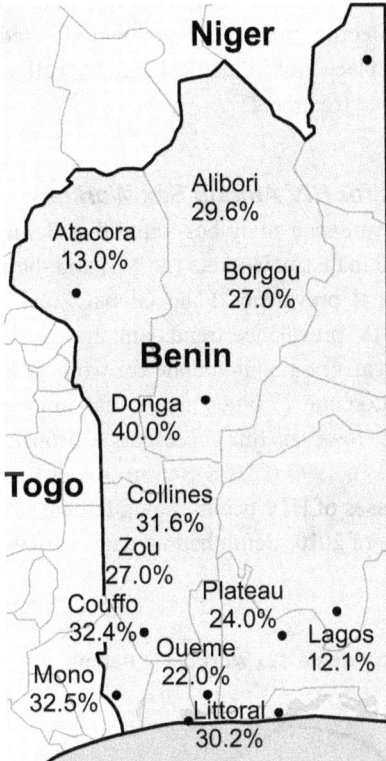

Source: Authors (developed from references HIV epidemiologic studies).

The average reported time selling sex was five years. Overt sex workers saw an average of four clients on the last day they worked before the study was conducted, while clandestine sex workers saw an average of two clients. 64.5% of sex workers had at least six sexual encounters with partners that were not clients during the 30 days before the study was conducted.

Many sex workers in Benin arrived from nearby countries. 31.5% were Togolese, 30.3% were Beninese, and 19.8% were Nigerian. The rest were from either Ghana or Burkina Faso. Nearly half of sex workers (45.2%) listened to the radio everyday or several times a week and 36.7% watched television. (*Le Comité National de Lutte contre le Sida* (CNLS) 2010)

Legal and Policy Issues

There is no specific legal statute banning sex work in Benin, but sex workers may be legally censored under laws about disrupting public order (personal communication, USAID Benin). Those who facilitate sex work and individuals who profit financially from it, including brothel owners, face penalties including imprisonment of six months to two years and fines of 400,000 to four million CFA (approximately 890 USD to 8,900 USD) depending on the severity of the offense.

In their 2010 report to UNAIDS, Benin reported having non-discrimination laws or regulations which specify protections for young people, injecting drug users, men who have sex with men, sex workers, prison inmates, and migrants / mobile populations (UNAIDS). This refers specifically to Law No. 2005–31 passed in April 10, 2006 on the prevention, care and control HIV / AIDS in Benin. The law includes provisions protecting people infected and affected by HIV from discrimination in the workplace and in medical care as well as providing the right to HIV information and treatment.

Epidemiology of and Risks Factors for HIV Among Sex Workers

As described above, the most recent surveillance study has found that Benin has an elevated HIV prevalence among female sex workers (26.5%) and their clients (3.7%) compared to 1.2% national prevalence (The Global Fund ; PNLS 2009). Figure 3.1 presents the HIV prevalence trends among female sex workers from 1986 to 2008. HIV prevalence among female sex workers is 20 times higher than the general population and 13 times higher than among women presenting at antenatal clinics. However, this represents a drop in reported prevalence from a peak of 55% in 1999 (CNLS Bénin). According to a 2009 modeling study, 32% of new cases of HIV occur among female sex workers (Guedeme, Ekanmian et al.). As of 2010, Benin had no data on male sex workers or transgender sex workers.

Figure 3.1   HIV Prevalence Trends among Female Sex Workers in Benin

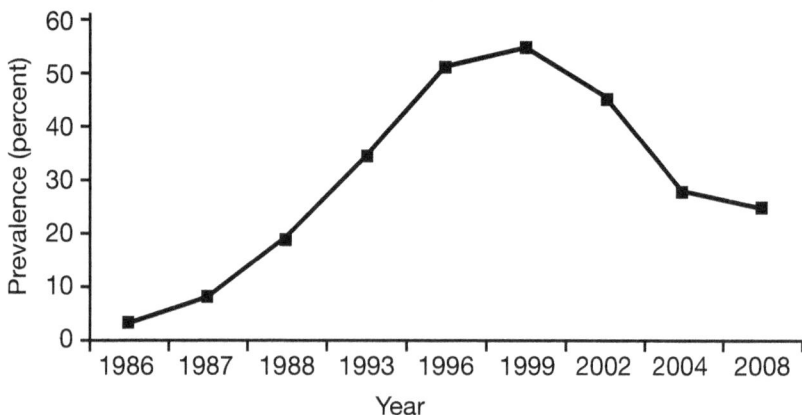

Source: PNLS Surveillance Reports, documented in *National AIDS Strategy 2006–10 Benin & ESDG* 2010.

According to Benin's most recent report on UNGASS indicators (UNAIDS), in 2009, 60% of sex workers correctly identified ways of preventing sexual transmission of HIV and also rejected major misconceptions about HIV transmission. Fifty-six percent of female sex workers were reached with HIV prevention programs, defined by UNAIDS as both knowing where to get an HIV test and having been given condoms in the preceding 12 months. In 2009, 85% of female sex workers had received an HIV test in the last 12 months and knew their results. (UNAIDS).

In the most recent national surveillance studies, 2,986 people across the country were interviewed including 1,082 female sex workers, 1,117 truckers and 787 sex worker clients (PNLS 2009). Thirty-two percent of female sex workers used condoms consistently with their intimate partners during the 30 days before study in 2008. Approximately, eight out of ten (79.7%) of sex workers used condoms with their clients on the last day they worked before the 2008 study compared to 82.8% in 2005. During the 30 days before the 2008 study, 61.9% of sex workers used a condom every time they had sex with a client compared to 68.3% of sex workers in 2005. Finally, 72.4% of sex workers in 2005 and 55.3% in 2008 used a condom every time they had sex with a client during the previous seven days of work. The decline in condom use has been attributed to the loss of a long-running program, Project SIDA, described below in the section on HIV prevention and treatment interventions.

In 2008, 44.3% of sex workers use lubricants to facilitate sex and avoid friction. The most commonly used products were Vaseline (37.3%), glycerin (12%), K-Y Gel (28.3%), and honey (1.2%). Use of the female condom was very limited. 71.4% of sex workers report knowing of the female condom, but only 20.6% had ever used one. The main reasons cited for not using the female condom were as follows: do not know how (50.7%), not practical (23.4%), not available (13.0%), and very expensive (1.1%).

Clients and Partners of Sex Workers. While targeted studies have demonstrated that sex workers in Benin are less likely to use condoms with their intimate partners than with their clients, interventions and data collection have focused on sex workers and their clients (PNLS 2009; PSI Benin 2009). Among married men, the proportion who admitted have sex with a sex worker was 19.6% in face-to-face interviews and 41.6% by anonymous voting box. Among unmarried men, 13% admitted to sex with a sex worker during the face-to-face interview and 25.5% did so by voting box (Minani, Alary et al. 2009). According to the 2008 Second Generation study, approximately 14.2% of clients of sex workers were uncircumcised. 84.5% of them reported using condoms during their last sexual encounter with a sex worker. Thirty of the 761 clients tested positive for HIV, thus HIV prevalence is estimated to be 3.9% among this group.

Stigma, Discrimination, and Violence. While gender based violence is believed to be widespread, there is little data on violence against women in Benin. We were unable to find specific data on stigma, discrimination, or violence against sex workers.

Substance Use. According to the most recent report from CNLS, 19.1% of sex workers have never consumed alcohol, while 15.3% drank alcohol frequently. The study also showed that 8.8% of sex workers in 2009 used drugs compared to the 3.2% who used drugs in 2005. Among clients, one-fourth drank alcohol frequently and 16.7% of drank daily. One-fifth of them have used drugs. (Le Comité National de Lutte contre le Sida (CNLS) 2010).

HIV Prevention and Treatment Interventions for Sex Workers

From 1993 to 2006, the Canadian International Development Agency (CIDA) funded an HIV/STI preventive intervention project entitled Project SIDA-3 in Benin. It was first implemented in Cotonou. This intervention initially targeted female sex workers, and included routine STI screening, condom promotion, as well as activities aiming at capacity building, community development and empowerment. In 2000, after a study demonstrated high HIV prevalence and high sexual risk behavior among clients and regular partners of female sex workers in Cotonou, a pilot intervention targeting these men was set up. During the pilot, approximately 15,000 individual contacts were made with men at sex work sites where leaflets and condoms were distributed. During the period of the pilot intervention, 625 men visited the STI clinic. In 2001–2002, interventions targeting both female sex workers and clients were progressively scaled up to five other cities in Benin (Porto-Novo, Abomey-Bohicon, Parakou, Kandi, Malanville). Approximately 70% of all female sex workers enumerated in Benin in 2004 live in the six cities where the intervention was implemented. (Lowndes, Alary et al. 2007; PNLS 2009).

Male client interventions included the following: Male peer outreach workers approached male clients at sex work venues mainly at night to provide HIV/STI education and condom demonstrations. A free and confidential STI clinic for men was established near the main sex work areas in Cotonou, and men were offered physical exams, STI screening and treatment, and risk reduction counseling. Data was collected by the male peer outreach workers during the pilot phase, and after a positive one-year evaluation, the intervention was progressively scaled up. Subsequent longitudinal data was collected via IBBS. About 300–400 clients took part in each round of the IBBS across the country, except in Cotonou in 2002 where 600 clients participated. From 1998–2005, consistent condom use with female sex workers increased from

39% (n=404) to 86.2% (n=313), prevalence of gonorrhea decreased from 5.4% to 1.6%, yet there was no significant change in prevalence of Chlamydia (2.6–3.2%) or HIV (8.4 to 6.9%) (Lowndes, Alary et al. 2007). The closure of Project SIDA in 2006 and subsequent financial fluctuations have had negative repercussions for prevention programs for sex workers and clients. An analysis of HIV spending in 2009 showed that funding for programs sex workers was decreased, and the majority of resources were allocated to interventions for the general population (Cherabi, Greenall et al. 2011).

USAID has supported the Beninese Association for Social Marketing (ABMS) and PSI International in efforts to prevent sexually transmitted diseases and AIDS in Benin. ABMS has traditionally focused on condom distribution and social marketing as well as health communication strategies. ABMS also manages voluntary counseling and testing services and STI treatment programs. PSI uses social marketing to promote syndromic treatment of STIs using pre-packaged standard therapy that typically includes antimicrobial medication, male condoms, partner referral cards, and information on the STI itself. It developed a mobile counseling and testing model in October 2008 as part of a national scale up of testing activities. In January 2011, ABMS became a PSI affiliate (PSI Benin). PSI/ABMS has trained peer educators to teach sex workers and their clients about HIV/STIs and how to prevent transmission (Agbemavo March 2011). ABMS has supported PNLS in establishing an HIV care and treatment clinic for sex workers in Cotonou. ABMS also has two partner clinics that offer the same services in cities with high concentrations of sex workers (Parakou and Malanville).

In September 2009, ABMS/PSI conducted an evaluation of their condom promotions activities, comparing data from 2007 to 2009 (PSI Benin 2009). In 2007, they found that the greatest predictor of condom use was condom availability. In 2009, they found that the program had succeeded in increasing the availability of condoms among female sex workers and in increasing their perception of the reliability of the Prudence Plus brand. Social support for condom use from elders and peers to use condoms was also strengthened. However, in 2009, despite condom promotion activities, the proportion of female sex workers consistently using condoms with intimate partners had not risen significantly (47.6% to 53.5%, p>0.05). This low use of condoms with intimate partners was in contrast to the 80% of sex workers who reported using a condom with their last client (PNLS 2009).

During 2008, 2,280 peer educators were trained by 57 NGOs spread throughout the country. With support from GFATM, these NGOs and community groups have carried out activities to raise awareness among sex workers as well as youth and adolescents, refugees, truck drivers and men in uniform. In 2009, PMLS funded the implementation of 20 sub-projects initiated by NGOs for sex workers in all regions. In addition, 17 NGOs selected by the NAP were supported by the PMLS 2 as part of a contract to provide services for sex workers (Cherabi, Greenall et al. 2011).

The most developed programs for HIV/STI prevention are STI reference centers. STI management for sex workers and their partners, clients of sex workers and truck drivers is carried out in health facilities called Special Needs Services and are installed in all departments with a concentration in large cities as well as several "hot spots" such as Cotonou, Porto-Novo, Sèmè-Kpodji, Bohicon, Malanville, Kandi, Parakou, Hillacondji, etc. A mathematical modeling exercise conducted in 2009 (Cherabi, Greenall et al. 2011) demonstrated that interventions with sex workers in Benin have prevented approximately 63% of new infections in sex workers and 51% of new infections among women in the general population over the previous 15 years.

A longitudinal cohort study conducted from 2008–2010 in Cotonou, compared antiretroviral therapy outcomes among 53 female sex workers recruited at the Dispensaire IST (a medical center dedicated since 1989 to routine check-up and STI treatment among female sex workers) and 318 "general population" patients from the Centre de Traitement Ambulatoire du Centre National Hospitalier Universitaire de Cotonou (a reference center for HIV treatment in Benin) (Agbemavo 2011). Female sex workers in this study were less educated and more likely to be migrants compared to the general population. Despite better stage of disease at initiation of therapy, female sex workers had higher crude mortality, less virologic suppression, and lower CD4 count recovery—all attributable to poorer adherence. The authors asserted that greater mobility among female sex workers (motivated by shifting demand for sex work and need to avoidance harassment by police and others) led to greater difficulty with adherence. They concluded that efforts to improve response to antiretroviral therapy among female sex workers should target factors impacting adherence. In addition, little is known in general about the number of sex workers that have access to HIV treatment.

Recently, 1.9 million dollars from the Institutes for Health Research in Canada was granted to Laval University for a study entitled "Sex Work, marginalization and health: research approach to health equity in the context of prostitution in Benin." The research is funded through 2016 to develop, implement, and evaluate interventions to prevent HIV and promote sexual and reproductive health among female sex workers. The project aims to take a health equity approach and involve female sex workers, their clients, intimate partners, site owners, health officers, military, and police. In the first phase of the project, as many as 150 qualitative interviews will be conducted. This data will be used to develop quantitative instruments and to inform interventions.

Sex Worker Rights Organizations

The Network of Sex Work Projects (NSWP) is an international membership organization whose members include sex work networks and organizations from all global regions; however the website does not list any networks located in Benin (http://www.nswp.org/members/africa). The African Sex Worker Alliance (ASWA) works to build an enabling human rights environment for sex workers, and it works through a network of partner organizations across Africa. Limited funding currently restricts the group's activities to Southern and Eastern Africa (http://www.africansexworkeralliance.org). In fact, no donor funding has gone to support the development of sex worker led organizations in Benin. Funding to enhance the ability of the current sex worker organizations such as AWSA to expand and organize in Benin would help to ensure that research and interventions are led by the expressed needs of sex workers in Benin.

Gaps in Research and Practice

Benin was among the first countries in the West and Central Africa region to benefit from CIDA resources targeted to HIV prevention and referral programs for sex work and clients. Similarly, World Bank resources, allocated through the MAP project, invested in programs for sex workers and clients. However, resources allocated to sex work programs are mostly from international assistance, which has resulted in discontinuity of funds and disruption of HIV prevention services for the sex work community as donor funding and priorities shift over time. There has been no investment by these international donors in community led approaches to HIV prevention among sex workers in Benin. Important HIV prevention programs for sex workers continue to exist in Benin, but the number of programs and the coordination of programs have declined over the last few years. The impact of this decrease in services is evident from the change in behavioral indicators between 2005 and 2008.

In 2009, NASA estimated that only 0.6 % of HIV and AIDS resources were allocated to HIV prevention programs for sex workers in Benin, despite the fact that the HIV prevalence among the sex work population was twenty times higher than in the general population. While currently GFATM resources fund HIV prevention programs for sex workers, it is crucial that internal public resources be allocated to ensure sustainability and coordination of implementation over time.

In general, stigma, discrimination and violence are important factors in the vulnerability of sex workers to HIV. Unfortunately, Benin does not have data on the prevalence of discrimination or violence against sex workers. It will be important to better understand these factors in order to address them appropriately in the context of HIV prevention programs. Lack of data on male sex workers or transgender sex workers has hampered the ability to determine if prevention interventions are needed among those groups. Gathering such data should be a priority.

For female sex workers living with HIV, limited data suggest adherence to antiretroviral therapy may be a challenge due to their need for mobility related to finding work and to avoiding police harassment. Gaps remain in knowledge on the best models for providing HIV care and treatment for mobile populations of female sex workers. Identifying interventions that address barriers to adherence among female sex workers is a pressing need.

Brazil

Introduction

Key Themes

- Brazil's "solidarity and citizenship" approach to HIV prevention which has promoted the human and labor rights of sex workers has been a key element in keeping the country's overall HIV prevalence low
- Stigma and discrimination persists among sex workers and is one of the primary barriers to access to services, prevention and advocacy actions
- Successful interventions among sex workers in Brazil have been those that adopt a rights based, community building approach and actions to decrease sex work related stigma

Brazil is the largest and most populated country in Latin America with a population of over 190 million (IBGE 2010) and is considered one of most important emerging economies in the world (Brainard and Martinez-Diaz 2009). It is also widely recognized for its "solidarity and citizenship" approach to HIV prevention and treatment (Berkman, Garcia et al. 2005) and long-standing, and at times politically controversial, commitment to working in partnership with sex worker rights organizations (Hinchberger 2005).

The political context in which HIV emerged distinguished the broad, and rights based nature of the civil society and government response (Grangeiro, Silva et al. 2009; Parker 2009). When the first cases of AIDS were reported in the 1980s, the country was amidst a social, economic, and political transformation as part of a redemocratization process after two decades of military dictatorship. The National AIDS Program was established alongside the country's universal health care system in the late 1980s, and from very early in the Program's existence, representatives of vulnerable population groups, including sex workers, were invited to participate in designing prevention actions for their peers. Prevention actions remained primarily focused on these groups throughout the 1980s, until 1993 when Brazil entered into a loan agreement with the World Bank (AIDS I 1994–1998) that expanded their prevention actions and increasingly focused on the relationship between poverty and HIV in addition to access to ART treatment (Parker 2009). In 1996, the country began offering anti-retroviral treatment through the public health system and in 1998, Brazil entered into a second four year loan agreement with the World Bank, that continued the solidarity and human rights focus of earlier projects and instituted the policy that all prevention projects would be implemented directly by non-governmental organizations.

In 1992, the World Bank had projected that 1.2 million people would be living with HIV in Brazil by 2000 (Ministry of Health 2001). However the close partnership with civil society organizations and commitment to decreasing stigma and discrimination, combined with universal access to ART treatment, are the three components that most mark what has been celebrated as the "Brazilian Response to HIV and AIDS" that has been attributed to helping to maintain the country's prevalence rates low and keeping the number of people living with HIV at just over half over what was originally predicted by the World Bank (Bastos, Kerrigan et al. 2001; Berkman, Garcia et al. 2005; Okie 2006; Nunn 2009). At the same time, the number of HIV prevention projects implemented within a human rights framework for sex workers has greatly reduced since 2008, and the structure of the the the HIV/AIDS program in the Ministry of Health, public health system, and funding mechanisms for NGOs has also changed substantially in the country. The majority of empirical research available primarily refers to the time periods from the late 1990s to mid 2000s, and more research is needed to understand worrisome signs indicated in recent case studies and critical analysis that the quality and breadth of government policies and programs is not the same as in the past, and that such recent structural changes of government policies and programs have contributed to reduced actions and influence of sex worker rights NGOs, barriers to sex workers' access to health and social services, and the persistence of stigma and discrimination (Pimenta, Correa et al 2010; Correa and Olivar in press). The current context contributed to the recent decision by the Brazilian Prostitute Network to increasingly advocate for partnerships with government offices outside of the Ministry of Health as a way to reduce the frequent association of sex work with disease and draw attention to the broader need for policies that promote the human and labor rights of sex workers (Lenz 2011).

Historical Perspectives and Trends of the HIV Epidemic. There are an estimated 710,000 people, aged 15 years and older, living with HIV in Brazil (UNAIDS 2008). The government reports that the prevalence rate has stabilized around 0.6% in the general population since 2004 (Brazilian Ministry of Health 2010), although the most recent UNAIDS 2010 report indicates slight increases from 2008 to present, yet it has remained under 0.7% (UNAIDS 2010).

Map 3.2   Prevalence of HIV among Sex Workers: Data from Select Epidemiologic Studies in Brazil

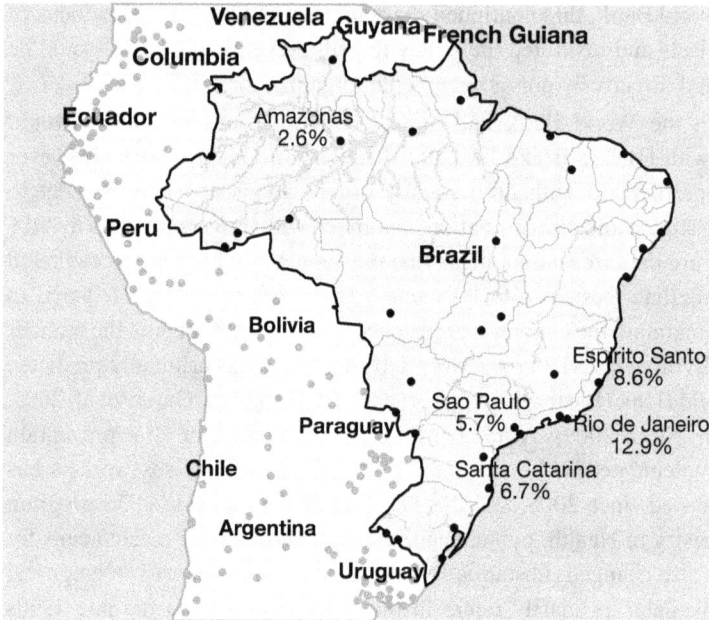

Source: Authors (data are from several studies implemented between 1996–2006).

When the epidemic emerged in the early 1980s, it was primarily concentrated among men who have sex with men and injection drug users (Barbosa Jr., Szwarcwald et al. 2009). In the 1990s, the spread of HIV increased among the heterosexual population, most notably among young women, yet overall the transmission rate of the epidemic is seen to have slowed down since the mid 1990s, a tendency attributed to prevention and treatment programs, and the introduction of HAART therapy in 1996 (Fonseca and Bastos 2007). The prevalence of HIV among men remains higher at 0.8%, as compared with 0.4% for women (Szwarcwald, Barbosa et al. 2008), yet the differences between the sexes has diminished over time: in 1989, the ratio of male AIDS cases to females was 3.7/1 and in 2009, it was 1.2/1 (Ministry of Health 2010a). There are also regional differences within Brazil. The country is divided into 5 macro-regions—South, Southeast, North, Northeast, and Mid-west, and the highest percentage of AIDS cases has remained in the Southeastern (59.3%) and Southern (19.2%) regions over time (in part because of these regions are Brazil's most populous). In all of these regions, incidence rates have increased in municipalities of 50,000 inhabitants or less (Ministry of Health 2010b), and increasingly affected poorer populations since the mid 1990s, reflecting the broader gender, race, class, and sexuality inequalities in Brazil society (Parker and Camargo Jr 2000; Szwarcwald, Barbosa Jr. et al. 2005; Fonseca and Bastos 2007).

Data are from several studies implemented between 1996–2006. Estimates from Espirito Santo are from data collected between 1994–96; the remaining studies were conducted between 2003–2006. Studies are further described in a review by Malta et al (2010)

Three studies commissioned by the Brazilian government using Respondent Driven Sampling (RDS) provide the most recent estimates of HIV prevalence among men who have sex with men (10.5%) (Ministry of Health 2010b), female sex workers (4.8%) (Szwarcwald, Souza Junior et al. 2011) and illicit drug users (5.9%) (Ministry of Health 2010b). HIV prevalence was calculated based only on the 10 cities (N=2,523) included in each study and therefore cannot be considered as nationally representative, in addition to methodological limitations of RDS that affected the geographical and population coverage in some cities where it was applied (Toledo, Codeco et al. 2011). While not comparable, the 4.8% HIV prevalence among female sex workers is lower than the 6.1% HIV prevalence found in the last study commissioned by the Ministry of Health in 2000 with 2,712 women to evaluate prevention actions in 3 regions of the country (Ministry of Health 2004).

Male and *travesti*[1] sex workers have also been the focus on HIV related research in Brazil, although in comparison with female sex workers, there are very few published studies or available government data on HIV prevalence among these populations. Both men who have sex with men and transgender groups are included within the same men who have sex with men category in Brazil's national reporting system implemented throughout the public counseling and testing services. Combining these populations presents challenges for understanding trends of the two groups which have very different profiles and vulnerability to HIV infection (Parker 1999). However, the few published studies that exist indicate that HIV prevalence among both groups is much higher than the Ministry of Health's HIV prevalence estimate for men who have sex with men of 10.5% (Ministry of Health 2010). One of the earliest published studies, which also surveyed female sex workers, was conducted in Rio de Janeiro and Minas Gerais with a small number of homosexual (N=11) and bisexual (N=6) male sex workers, and found HIV prevalences of 45% and 32% respectively (Cortes, Detels et al. 1989). A cross sectional study conducted with 530 male and *travesti* sex workers recruited by their peers from 1992–1998 in Sao Paulo found an HIV prevalence of 22% among male sex workers and 40% among *travesti* sex workers (Grandi et al 2000). A three-year cohort study with 647 men who have sex with men in Rio Janeiro from 1994–1998 reported higher incidence rates among male sex workers and *travesti*s than men who have sex with men who did not report commercial sex or identifying as *travestis* (Sutmoller, Penna et al. 2002). A qualitative and quantitative study conducted with 100 *travestis* in Rio de Janeiro as part of a larger intervention study looking at drug use and HIV from 1994–1997 found 48% HIV prevalence among *travestis* (Inciardi 2000). Finally, a RDS study conducted with 658 men who have sex with men in Campinas, Sao Paulo from 2005–2006 found that male and *travesti* sex workers had a combined HIV prevalence of 14% as compared to 6% among men who have sex with men who did not report selling sex (Tun et al 2008).

Scope, Typology, and Context of Sex Work

The social and cultural context of female, male, and *travesti* sex work in Brazil is complex and reflects the heterogeneity of the country in terms of its gender, race, class, and geographical distinctions. Here, a brief overview is provided, with references to texts that provide more details. While far from homogenous in terms of their backgrounds and extent to which they identify as *profissionais do sexo* (sex professionals), female sex work is a more visible presence in public spaces, the media, and research on sex work as opposed to *travestis*, and to an even greater extent, male sex workers. There is no national estimate of the number of male and *travesti* sex workers, and the only estimate for the number of female sex workers comes from a study conducted in 2005 which estimated that of Brazil's total population of over 190 million, 500,000 women, or approximately 1% of the female population between 15 and 49, are involved in sex work (Szwarcwald, Barbosa Jr. et al. 2005).

Figure 3.2   Trends in HIV Prevalence among the General Adult Population and Female, Male, and Travesti Sex Workers

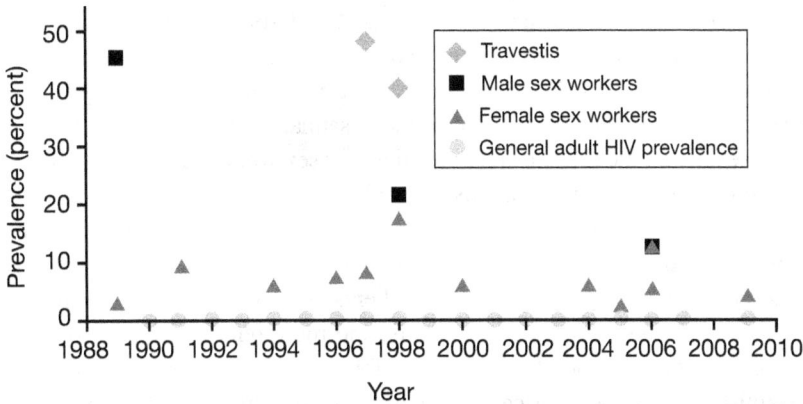

Sources: General Adult HIV Prevalence from UNAIDS 2008 and 2009 Country Reports. Female sex worker estimates for 1991, 1994, 1996–2000 from UNAIDS 2008 Country Epidemiological Report and are median prevalence rates from non-representative studies in urban areas. The 2000 and 2009 are pooled HIV prevalence from two studies commissioned by the Ministry of Health and reported in the 2010 UNGASS report, and 2004, 2005 and 2006 are from a meta-analysis (Malta et al. 2010). The travesti and male sex work data from 1998 is from a cross-sectional study carried out from 1992–1998 among male sex workers and travestis in Sao Paulo (Grandi et al. 2000). The travesti prevalence from 1997 is from a Rio de Janeiro study (Inciardi 2000), and male sex work prevalence in 2006 is from an RDS study in Campinas, Sao Paulo and includes both male and travesti sex workers (Tun et al. 2008). Data from 1989 is drawn from a seriologic survey conducted in Rio de Janeiro and Minas Gerais in 1987 (Cortes et al. 1989).

Research and interventions have tended to group male and *travesti* sex workers under the umbrella of "male prostitution", although there are important distinctions between the two groups (see Parker 1992; Larvie 1999). Male sex workers who dress as men, have predominantly male clients, and generally assume an active sexual role with their clients, are referred to as *michês* (hustlers) or *garotos de programa* (rent boys). In contrast, the clients of *travestis* tend to identify as heterosexual, and often seek them out due to their femininity combined with their psychical ability to engage in both penetrative and receptive sex. It is important to note that the term *travesti* is not synonymous with sex worker, many *travestis* engage in sex work as a result of the difficulty in finding other work due to stigma, discrimination and the high level of social vulnerability of the population in terms of education and class (Grandi, Goihman et al. 2000; Inciardi 2000; Pelucio 2009; Cortez, Boer et al. 2010; Garcia and Lehman 2011).

Common forms of sex work. Sex work in Brazil exists in a variety of forms and modalities that vary depending on the social and cultural context, and gender of the sex worker and their clients. Yet despite its heterogeneity, the types of spaces within which sex work occurs are fairly consistent, and include the street, hotels, bars, through internet/print media ads, and more formal establishments, such as a brothels, sauna, or private clubs. In each of these spaces, the types of relationships that sex workers have with owners or agents range from no relationship at all (i.e., completely independent), to working under agreements with strict rules and regulations of their time and movement. In cases where any type of work agreement exists, sex workers generally earn money from dates with clients, and owners primarily earn off the sale of drinks, entry fees for clients, and room rentals—in part to avoid being prosecuted under Brazilian law for managing a sex establishment. Establishments vary in price and exclusivity, and are generally considered to be the hardest to access both for prevention activities, research, and sex worker organizations as opposed to sex workers who work independently on the street or in bars (Pimenta, Correa et al. 2009; Olivar 2011). A recent body of ethnographic research has highlighted how in tourist settings, sexual, gender, and racial subjectivities affect the price charged for services, types of affective relationships formed between sex workers and tourists and sex worker organizing (Silva and Blanchette 2005; Piscitelli 2007; Mitchell 2011; Mitchell 2012; Williams Forthcoming).

Legal and Policy Issues

The legal and policy issues surrounding sex work in Brazil can be divided into two categories: those that deal with federal, state and municipal laws on sex work, and policy issues more specifically tied to the politics of AIDS funding.

The sale of sex for money is not illegal in Brazil provided the sex worker is over 18, however commercial activities associated with sex work (such as owning a brothel or pimping) are illegal. In 2002, due to pressure from Brazil's strong sex worker movement, "sex worker" was included as an official occupation in the Brazilian Occupation Classification of the Ministry of Labor, thereby entitling sex workers to social security and other work benefits. However, sex workers' labor rights are restricted due to the illegality of sex work businesses (Simões 2010). In 2003, in consultation with the National Prostitute's Network, a federal law was proposed to the Brazilian legislature to regulate the profession as labor and remove the penal codes associated with it. The law was not passed, yet its passage remains one of the main goals of the Brazilian Prostitute's Network. Additionally, changes in the international policy environment in terms of increased attention and investment in anti-trafficking campaigns combined with growing religious influence in Brazil have highlighted contradictions within state policy in terms of prostitution and human rights discourses, and the conflation of sex work and voluntary migration with trafficking in some laws and political discourses (Blanchette and Silva 2012) (Piscitelli 2008; Pimenta, Correa et al. 2009).

Policy issues that impact HIV funding in Brazil have placed the country in the spotlight in several occasions. The most notable being in June of 2005, when a policy directive from USAID mandated that all recipient organizations have a "policy explicitly opposing prostitution" (USAID 2005). At the time, a multi-million dollar HIV prevention project, The Elos Program, was being implemented in collaboration with over 30 NGOs comprised of sex workers, men who have sex with men, and *travestis* as part of a bilateral agreement between USAID and the Brazilian Ministry of Health. In a decision made in partnership with the Brazilian Network of Prostitutes, the country's government was the only one to take a strong political stance and refuse to sign what came to be known as the 'prostitution pledge' in contractual agreements, thereby rejecting over $40 million dollars of funding for HIV prevention (Hinchberger 2005; Leite 2010). The government did implement national level projects with *travesti* and female sex workers soon after, but the USAID policy prevented the scale-up of actions originally planned and negatively impacted the overall funding available to NGOs working with vulnerable population groups. More detail about current interventions with sex workers is discussed in detail below.

Epidemiology of and Risks Factors for HIV Among Sex Workers

The most commonly found factors associated with HIV and STI prevalence among female, male, and *travesti* sex workers include co-infection with other STIs, injecting drug use, time spent in sex work, and social and demographic factors such as earnings and education. Among female sex workers, factors associated with HIV prevalence in multivariate analysis of the RDS study in 10 cities, included the period of time spent in sex work (OR 1.020; 95% CI 1.013–1.067), price charged for sex (lower the price, higher the prevalence rate) (OR 0.713; 95% CI 0.522–0.970), other STIs (syphilis scars [OR 2.186; 95%CI 1.064–4.488]) and willingness to waive condom use at the client's request (OR 3.735; 95% CI 1.449–9.661) (Damacena, Szwarcwald et al. 2011). In the Ministry of Health's evaluation of sex worker interventions, positive HIV test results were correlated with injection drug use (OR 6.77; CI 3.44–13.17), testing positive for syphilis (OR 3.56; 95% CI 2.00–6.29) and Hepatitis C co-infection (OR 11.26; 95%CI 7.28–17.40). Increased age, length of time in profession, and decreased education and income were also associated with HIV infection (Ministry of Health 2004).

In general, knowledge of HIV prevention methods and condom use with clients tends to be high among female sex workers, although studies have found that structural factors and exposure to HIV prevention interventions affect both. In the study conducted by the Ministry of Health, evaluating HIV prevention programs found that women who were not reached through the Ministry's programs had significantly lower knowledge of transmission methods, with some indicating that HIV could be transmitted through mosquito bites (33.8%) or the toilet seat (23.4%) (Ministry of Health 2004). Across studies, condom use with paying clients is much higher than non-paying regular partners (Ministry of Health 2004; Kerrigan, Telles et al. 2008; Lippman, Donini et al. 2010). Consistent condom use with clients was found to be associated with income, time in the profession, and exposure to HIV prevention interventions (Ministry of Health 2004). Social environmental factors have also been significantly associated with condom use in studies conducted with female sex workers in Rio de Janeiro (Kerrigan, Telles et al. 2008) and Corumba (Lippman, Donini et al 2010). Multi-variate analysis of baseline data conducted among 434 sex workers in Rio de Janeiro demonstrated that social cohesion and mutual aid (OR 1.30; 95% CI 1.02–1.66), possession of government documents/access to resources (OR 1.36 (95% CI 1.11–1.65), and participation in a community organizations (OR 1.56; 95% CI 1.04–2.34) were significantly associated with consistent condom use with clients in the last four months (Kerrigan et al 2008). Among female sex workers in Corumba, increased social cohesion was inversely associated with the number of unprotected sex acts in the previous week (IRR = 0.80; p<0.01), and women's participation in social networks was associated with a decrease in the frequency of unprotected sex acts (IRR =0.83; p=.04) (Lippman, Donini et al 2010).

Among male and *travesti* sex workers in Sao Paulo, HIV infection was significantly associated with oral sex (p=0.010), receptive anal sex (p<0.001), working in sex work for three years or longer (p<0.001), injected drug use (p<0.001), and a history of prior syphilis (p<0.001) (Grandi et al 2000). In the study with 100 *travesti* sex workers in Rio de Janeiro, age (OR 5.267; 95% CI: 1.51–18.3), education (OR .174; 95%CI:0.04–0.81), drug injection history (OR 11.68; 95% CI: 1.07–128.12), and unprotected insertive anal sex (OR 8.67; 95% CI: 1.21–62.2) were all significant predictors of HIV infection. In the study comparing male and *travesti* sex workers with men who have sex with men who did not report sex work, men who have sex with men and *travesti* sex workers more often reported unprotected receptive (22.4% v. 4.6%) and unprotected insertive anal intercourse with more than two male partners in the last two months (20.5% v. 5.0%) (Tun, Mello et al. 2008). Male sex workers were also more likely to report unprotected vaginal intercourse with women in the last two months (22.7% v 3.6%) (Tun, Mello et al. 2008). A multi-variate analysis of protective behaviors demonstrated that male sex workers' access to social and material resources was associated with a decrease in frequency of unprotected sex acts in the past week (IRR =0.15; p = 0.01) (Lippman, Donini et al. 2010).

Clients and partners of sex workers. There are no published studies in the international literature of HIV prevalence among male clients and partners of sex workers, although a study in 2005 estimated that approximately 4.6% of the Brazilian male population between 15–49 are clients of sex workers (Szwarcwald, Barbosa Jr. et al. 2005). A study conducted with Brazilian army conscripts from 1997–2002 found that over the five year period, between 16–17% reported having had at least one paid partner, and reported condom use with their paid partner to be 68.8%, 67.0%, and 77.9% respectively for each year studied (Szwarcwald, Carvalho et al. 2005).

Violence, stigma, and discrimination. Historical research has documented stigmatizing attitudes and policies towards sex work in Brazil since the mid 19th century (Rago 1991; Lenz 2011). Ethnographic and qualitative research has noted the permanence of stigmatizing attitudes in contemporary discourses surrounding sex work and quantitative studies have found these issues to be closely related to sex worker's vulnerability to HIV and STI infection (Santos et al 2006; Pimenta, Correa et al. 2009), in addition to being linked to lower levels of participation in HIV prevention actions and sex worker organizing (Kerrigan et al. 2008; Murray et al. 2010; Mitchell 2011). While there is little research looking specifically at the issue of violence among female sex workers, the Ministry of Health evaluations have highlighted the persistence of police violence against sex workers (Camara 2008) and several quantitative studies have found significant associations between violence and HIV. In the RDS study conducted with 2,523 female sex workers in ten Brazilian cities, ever being physically forced to have sexual intercourse was significantly associated with HIV prevalence among female sex workers in the bivariate analysis (OR 1.73; 95% CI 1.002–3.030) (Damacena, Szwarcwald et al. 2011). A study in Rio de Janeiro found that 15.8 percent of sex workers had experienced violence related to being a sex worker in the last four months and that having experienced violence in the last four months was significantly associated with lower odds of consistent condom use (OR 0.37; 95% CI 0.17–0.81) (Kerrigan et al. 2008). In 2008, the National Network of Prostitutes printed a report systematizing the most recurring rights violations experienced by sex workers at their national meeting, citing police violence, extortion, harassment and violence from drug dealers, expulsion from public spaces, workplace violations ranging from excessive fines to restricting access to emergency medical care, and verbal and physical violence from pedestrians as frequent occurrences across regions (Rede Brasileira de Prostitutas 2009).

High levels of violence have been found in studies among male and travesti sex workers. A cross-sectional study using RDS with 106 male and travesti sex workers in Campinas found that 83.3% had experienced what the study termed as "psychological abuse due to homophobia", 48.5% had experienced "physical abuse related to homophobia", and 16.5% had experienced "abuse from the police due to homophobia" in the past year (Tun et al. 2008). The same study found that men who have sex with men reporting practicing sex work were significantly more likely to experience psychological (80.9% compared to 58.4%) and physical abuse (48.2% as compared to 15.2%) when compared to men who did not practice sex work (Tun et al. 2008). A study of 45 travesti sex workers and 41 male sex workers found that travesti sex workers were more likely to report physical aggression by clients (Cortez et al. 2011). In a study implemented by members of the national network of travestis, ANTRA (National Association of Travestis), as part of a project funded through the Ministry of Health, of the 663 travestis interviewed in 35 Brazilian cities, 71% reported experiencing verbal abuse and 52% reported physical violence at some point in their lives (Menezes, Brito et al. 2010).

Substance use. In broad terms, alcohol use is common among female, male, and travesti sex workers, and use of drugs such as cocaine and crack is much lower, although more associated with unsafe sexual behavior and HIV infection. Among female sex workers interviewed in the Ministry of Health 2000–2001 evaluation, alcohol was the most commonly reported substance used (64.2%), followed by a much smaller percentage of marijuana (16.7%), and even smaller percentage reporting cocaine use (12.8%) and crack (4.4%) (Ministry of Health 2004). In an RDS study conducted with men who have sex with men in the state of Sao Paulo, 55% of those involved in sex work reported using drugs in the past six months, a percentage that was significantly higher than the rate reported by non-sex workers (Tun, Mello et al. 2008). A cross-sectional epidemiological study of HIV among male and travesti sex workers in Sao Paulo reported a prevalence of drug use among 57.6% of travestis and 60.4% of male hustlers enrolled in the study; of these, 8.3% of travestis and 10.4% of male hustlers injected drugs (Grandi, Goihman et al. 2000). In a study with 100 travestis in Rio de Janeiro interviewed as part of a larger study and intervention focused on HIV prevention among drug users and travestis (Inciardi 2000), 91% reported ever using alcohol, 61.0% using marijuana, and 76.0% using cocaine. A total of 12% reported ever injecting drugs, and this was highly correlated to HIV infection (OR 11.682; 95% CI: 1.07–128.12) (Inciardi 2000). While the percentages of injecting drug use have been found to be low among female, male and travesti sex workers, injecting drug users has also been found to be significantly associated with HIV infection in two of the aforementioned studies (Ministry of Health 2004; Grandi et al. 2000) and qualitative work has confirmed a relationship between crack cocaine use and sexual risk behaviors, in addition to physical and sexual violence among female sex workers (Malta et al 2010).

HIV Prevention Interventions for Sex Workers

HIV prevention interventions implemented with sex workers through the Ministry of Health have involved a rights based approach, and especially in interventions implemented up until 2010, included components focused on strengthening the organizational capacity of sex worker organizations. Evaluations and results of the Ministry of Health's national level projects have not yet been published in international peer-reviewed journals, yet information is available through the Ministry's publications and a few systematic evaluations commissioned by the government.

Common, successful interventions. National level HIV prevention interventions with sex workers in Brazil date back to 1989 when the government implemented the project, "Previna" designed for female, travesti, and male sex workers. Sex worker leaders were invited to participate in the design of the project, due in large part to sex worker activism against being cast as a "risk group" or "vectors" early in the HIV epidemic and their expressed demands to be seen as protagonists and equal partners in HIV prevention efforts (Ministry of Health 2002). "Previna" employed a peer education approach, included trainings for the emerging organizations of sex workers and local HIV and AIDS programs, and developed specific materials for male, female, and travesti sex workers. Under the first World Bank loan AIDS I, (1994–1998), the government began to expand its actions with sex workers through Previna II, and the number of sex worker organizations in Brazil began to grow, along with the strength of the female sex worker and travesti movement. Under the second World Bank loan, AIDS II (1998–2002), the government transferred the majority of its money for prevention actions directly to NGOs, who they perceived as being more effective in reaching the sex worker population on a local level.

Beginning in 2000, the government began to decentralize the HIV/AIDS program to give more autonomy to local and state programs, and also started the "Esquina da Noite," project (Night Street Corner), for female sex workers and "Tulipa" for *travestis*. Both projects sought to strengthen the female sex worker and *travesti* and transsexual movements respectively by funding projects through regional NGO networks. All of the projects implemented during this time continued peer-education and free condom distribution, yet also employed a human rights approach, focused on empowerment, leadership training, raising self-esteem, labor rights of sex workers, and fighting stigma and discrimination (Ministry of Health 2002). The broadening of the focus also meant increased investment and importance placed on strengthening the organizational capacity of sex worker and *travesti* NGOs both to implement HIV prevention projects and advocate for the human and labor rights of sex workers—largely as a result of increasing evidence of the relationship between stigma and discrimination and the lack of citizenship rights and HIV vulnerability. Emblematic of this approach is the 2002, Ministry of Health national campaign entitled, "Without Shame, Girl", that was designed in partnership with the National Network of Prostitutes, and in 2004, the campaign, "*Travesti* is Respect", formulated and disseminated in partnership with ANTRA (Brazil's National Association of Travestis and Transsexuals).

In 2004, through a bilateral agreement with USAID, the Elos Program funded eight projects with female sex workers, two with male sex workers, and two projects with *travestis* until the implementation of the "prostitution pledge" in 2005. The National AIDS Program continued prevention activities with sex workers through the national level project, "Without Shame" from 2006–2008, which was led by one of the oldest and most prominent sex worker NGOs in Brazil, "Davida", based out of Rio de Janeiro. The project was focused on building the capacity of sex worker organizations, the strength of the network, and the leadership skills of sex workers (Camara 2008). Around this same time, Davida received unprecedented national and international media attention for a clothing line they founded as a sustainability strategy amidst the funding crises. Called, Daspu (Of the Whores), five collections with provocative and playful designs promoting the rights of sex workers were produced in partnership with professional designers and more than 300 sex workers, activists, and celebrities modeled in dozens of fashion shows in clubs, conferences, and primetime television under the motto of "Daspu: Fashion without Shame" (Lenz 2008; Leite 2010). The use of the word, "whore" in the name of Daspu is illustrative of the approach of Davida, and the Brazilian Network of Prostitutes in reappropriating terms like "whore" and "prostitute" as ways to more directly challenge and change the stigma associated with them and frame sex work both as a sexual and labor right (Lenz 2011). Also of note and emblematic of the way in which cultural forms have been used for activism are the theatre and cultural activities implemented by the sex worker organization, GEMPAC in Belem, Para and Radio Zona, in Salvador, Bahia. Radio Zona was founded by APROSBA, an organization of sex workers in Salvador in 2006 both to reach out to sex workers in Salvador, and to dispel negative stereotypes associated with sex workers and promote the dignity of the profession (Williams forthcoming). Radio Zona is the first radio station founded by sex workers in the world, and like Daspu, has received international attention for its innovation and success.

In 2009, the Ministry of Health financed an HIV prevention project implemented on a national scale and led by APROCE, a sex worker organization in Fortaleza, Ceara (in the Northeast of Brazil). The project was implemented with six additional NGOs throughout Brazil's five regions and sought to establish an additional national network to promote and expand access to information and advocacy best practices in terms of STI and HIV prevention, and to strength organizations that work with sex workers, with a focus on implementing the Ministry of Health's Integrated Plan to Confront the Feminization of the AIDS and STD Epidemic.

The most recent national level project with the *travesti* community is "TRANSpondo Barreiras" (Removing Barriers). Implemented for two years by the Ministry of Health and in direct partnership with the institutions that make up the national network of *travestis*, ANTRA, the project reached Brazil's five regions and received technical support from an international NGO with an office in Brazil. It was designed in accordance with the objectives of the Affirmative Plan for Travestis and the National Plan Confront the Feminization of the AIDS and STD Epidemic (due to the inclusion of transsexuals in the program's actions) (www.transpondott.com.br). The strategies and activities developed in the period from 2008–2010 were focused on health promotion, STI and HIV prevention, defense of human rights, strengthening advocacy actions, and the positive visibility of the national movement of *travestis*.

While male sex workers were included in the Ministry's early prevention programs, there have been noticeably less projects and NGOs dedicated to them than female and *travesti* sex workers. Only three projects with male sex workers have been featured in international literature, one, called *Pegação* (slang similar to cruising), implemented and directed by the late sex worker activist Paulo Longo in Rio de Janeiro (Longo 1998; Larvie 1999) and another project implemented by the Brazilian Interdisciplinary AIDS Association (ABIA), with young male sex workers focused on collective mobilization and sexual health promotion as part of their ongoing activities with men who have sex with men implemented since the early 1990s (Munoz-Laboy, de Almeida et al. 2004). In the South of Brazil, two NGOs in Porto Alegre, GAPA and NUANCES have also worked in HIV prevention projects with male sex workers and *travestis* since the early 1990s, and have been featured in ethnographic work (Klein 1999).

In 2010, the Ministry of Health and World Bank agreed upon a new loan of US$200 million (AIDS-SUS) to support prevention actions that is focused on increasing access to prevention actions among vulnerable population groups and improving health governance (World Bank 2011). These actions are likely to be guided by two national level plans of particular importance for female, male and *travesti* sex workers implemented in 2009: The Affirmative Plan for Prostitutes that, after national level consultations, was included in the Ministry of Health's Integrated Plan to Confront the Feminization of the AIDS and STD Epidemic in 2009, and the National Plan to Confront AIDS and STDS among men who have sex with men, Gays, and Travestis.

Coverage and access to HIV prevention services. It is difficult to assess the coverage of prevention programs due to the lack of population estimates for male and travesti sex workers and the available data on interventions with female sex workers. The coverage data that does exist is limited, and often does not effectively measure HIV prevention "reach". The 2010 UNGASS report for Brazil, for example, reports data from the 2009 RDS study indicating that 57% of the female sex workers interviewed knew where they could be tested for HIV and 77.2% had received free condoms in the last 12 months (Ministry of Health 2010). Of these women, 47% were considered as being "reached" by prevention programs in that they knew where to be tested for HIV and had received free condoms. There is a notable difference between receiving condoms once in the past twelve months and the more comprehensive interventions implemented with sex workers described above. As such, the UNGASS coverage indicators should be interpreted within this limitation.

Facilitators and barriers to accessing prevention programs have been assessed through quantitative and qualitative studies, which all emphasize the role of stigma and social vulnerabilities, especially related to poverty, race, gender, and age, as the primary barriers to access to services (Ministry of Health 2004; Santos, Silva et al. 2006; Kerrigan, Telles et al. 2008; Pimenta, Correa et al. 2009; Murray, Lippman et al. 2010). In all of these studies, it is clear that real barriers to accessing services exist, despite the presence of policies that are considered as progressive in other settings. In a case study of the Brazilian response to HIV/AIDS among sex workers in Porto Alegre and Rio de Janeiro conducted in 2008–2009 (Pimenta, Correa et al 2010), interviews with a limited number of sex workers in each site found that while sex workers in Porto Alegre reported more access to health and prevention services than women in Rio de Janeiro, the quality of services and access to prevention materials in both cities was low. In interviews, health officials noted that in recent years, government attention, and investment, has diminished with sex workers and shifted more to other groups such as men who have sex with men, and that the scale and extent to which the government developed prevention actions with sex workers was perceived as being related to the strength and presence of sex worker organizations (Pimenta, Correa et al 2010). The evaluation of the national "Without Shame" project noted that although the project strengthened communication among the national network of prostitutes, low organizational technical capacity and a lack of sustainability of actions remained key concerns of the participating NGOs at the end of the project's implementation (Camara 2008).

The evaluation of a project that incorporated the community development model of Sonagachi into a peer education based program in Rio de Janeiro found that while mutual aid and social cohesion were significantly associated with consistent condom use, internalized stigma and social vulnerabilities limited participation in the community development activities (Kerrigan et al 2008). Sex workers reporting to be less comfortable with their profession (OR 0.61, 96% CI=0.38–0.97), and who supported two or more people through sex work (OR 0.38; 95% CI 0.33–0.87), were significantly less likely to report participating in an activity with other sex workers in the previous four months (Kerrigan et al 2008). Limited participation in the intervention activities also contributed to the lack of impact in terms of behavioral outcomes in the follow-up survey applied at the end of the 18-month intervention (Kerrigan et al 2008).

The barriers for male and travesti sex workers are similar to those experienced by female sex workers in terms of stigma and social vulnerabilities, yet distinct when it comes to access to services and NGOs. For male sex workers, the diversity and heterogeneity of the population, in terms of where and how they work, their social and professional networks, the extent to which they identify as sex workers, and their stated sexual and gender orientations make them distinct from each other despite similar sexual risks and, thus, an especially difficult population to quantify and reach through prevention actions (see Parker 1992; Longo 1998; Mitchell 2011). An evaluation of Pegação identified listening to the needs of the male sex workers, self-esteem, and forming long term contact and emotional bonds between the outreach workers and boys contacted through the program as important factors to the program's perceived success among male sex workers in the Rio de Janeiro (Longo 1998). A more recent prevention program in Rio built on several of these lessons, and targeted young male sex workers more generally through interventions with young men who have sex with men, participatory methodologies that place the youth as protagonists in the design and implementation of prevention programs for their peers, and focus less on their identities as sex workers, and more on the common structural factors, such as being from the lower, working classes and often having little access to government services, that place them at increased risk for HIV infection (Munoz-Laboy et al 2004).

In terms of spending on HIV and AIDS in Brazil, decentralization of the Ministry of Health has made it more difficult to accurately measure how much is being spent on prevention actions with female, male and travesti sex workers on the local and state level where many of the prevention actions supported through the government are implemented. In the Ministry of Health's 2010 report to UNGASS, in 2008 (the most recent year for which detailed information is available), 6.7% (R$76 million[2]) of the R$1.14 billion total budget spent on HIV and AIDS went to prevention, and of this, R$35,820 went specifically to programs with sex workers and their clients and R$99,500 went to programs for men who have sex with men (Ministry of Health 2010). However it is important to emphasize that the UNGASS estimate does not take into account all prevention activities, such as the HIV rapid test, blood bank actions, and mother-to child transmission—and that the Ministry spent nearly R$30 million on communication and R$10 million on community mobilization—programs that also encompass sex workers although detailed information about how much of this money was spent on these populations is not available.

Available impact evaluation data. Studies evaluating interventions, such as the Ministry of Health's 2004 study and those looking more closely at the effects of a social-environmental interventions (Lippman et al 2010), have demonstrated positive effects of educational interventions that combined peer education with community building. In the Ministry of Health's evaluation of eight educational intervention projects with sex workers, significant differences in consistent condom use with clients were observed between women participating in the interventions and those in the control group who were not exposed to any intervention (OR 1.86, 95% CI: 1.57–2.20). Differences were also observed in the number reporting condom use with steady partners (OR 1.67, 95% CI: 1.37–2.03), reporting being tested for HIV (OR 1.69; 95% CI:1.44–1.98), and having a gynecological exam in the last year (OR 1.55; 95% CI: 1.32– 1.82) (Ministry of Health 2004).

The *Encontros* study followed 420 male, female, and *travesti* sex workers on the Brazilian border of Bolivia from 2003–2005 to evaluate the effect of a multi-level intervention on STI incidence and condom use (Lippman et al 2010; Murray et al 2010). The project combined a social mobilization component that included community-building activities with peer education and improved clinical care. While participation in the community activities was at first difficult due to the stigma surrounding sex work and a reluctance of women to identity as sex workers, qualitative work found that involving community members not involved in sex work in project activities and using cultural and social activities led to broadening participation and the eventual founding of a sex worker NGO (Murray, Lippman, et al. 2010). The cohort study documented greater odds of reporting consistent condom use with regular clients among sex workers actively engaged in the intervention (OR 1.9; 95% CI: 1.1–3.3), and the odds of incident STI were reduced for those actively participating in intervention activities as opposed to those who did not, although this difference was not significant (OR:0.46; 95% CI 0.2–1.3) (Lippman, Chinaglia, et al 2012).

Aside from the small number of male and *travesti* sex workers included in the *Encontros* study, only two additional studies, both from Rio de Janeiro, were found evaluating HIV prevention interventions with male or *travesti* sex workers. The first study, a six month qualitative evaluation commissioned by the WHO of the *Pegação* program in 1992 found that homophobia was both one of the primary factors structuring the organization of male sex work and the principal obstacle to effective HIV prevention programs with this population (Larvie 1999). Specifically, the evaluation team found that male sex workers' perceived risk to HIV as being related to their identification with 'risk groups' and partner choice (i.e. choosing partners they did not perceive as being gay or promiscuous). In practice, this meant that both men who did not identify as gay or sex workers and those who reported choosing partners they perceived as being 'safe' considered themselves as being at lower risk for HIV (Larvie 1999). In another Rio de Janeiro study evaluating a basic education and testing/counseling intervention with 100 *travestis*, the project staff was only able to relocate and re-interview 39 of those included in the baseline and no changes in sexual behaviors were found (Inciardi 2000).

Sex Worker Rights Organizations

There are a variety of diverse organizations that work with sex workers in Brazil. The most visible and oldest network in the country is The Brazilian Network of Prostitutes—a national network of 32 organizations founded in 1987 amidst the popular movements that emerged during the country's redemocratization after two decades of dictatorship. Initially founded to address police violence and human rights abuses, the focus of the network shifted in the late 1980s with the emergence of the HIV epidemic. In addition to the aforementioned projects through the Ministry of Health, the Network has also been active in organizing international, regional, and national meetings on sex work, HIV and human rights. They position sex work as a sexual right, and their key issues include fighting stigma and discrimination, violence, access to sexual and reproductive health services, and continued advocacy for the complete decriminalization and regulation of sex work. They circulate a newspaper called Beijo da Rua first published in 1988, still being distributed throughout

Brazil in press and online (www.beijodarua.com.br). The network is currently led by a group of sex worker organizations including NEP in Porto Alegre and GEMPAC in Belem—both considered to be two of the strongest and currently most active sex worker NGOs in the country. While STIs and HIV are recognized as important issues, the Network has increasingly advocated for human and labor rights to take priority over AIDS specific actions, as these are seen as fundamental to improving the citizenship status and quality of life of sex workers (Leite 2010). In addition to the Brazilian Prostitute's Network, there is also the National Federation of Sex Workers, based out of Fortaleza in the Northeast, that brings together a group of sex worker NGOs throughout the country that have political positions distinct from those of the Prostitute's Network. The Federation was the network that most recently implemented an HIV prevention project on a national level with support from the Ministry of Health.

The first organization of *travestis* in Brazil, ASTRAL (Association of *Travestis* and *Liberados*) was founded in 1992 in Rio de Janeiro. In 1993 and 1994, ASTRAL organized the first two National Encounters of *Travesis* and *Liberados* that Work in AIDS Prevention—ENTLAIDS. In its first years, ENTLAIDS focused on mobilizing regional *travesti* leaders. At the time, ASTRAL and the *Grupo Esperança* in Curitiba (a city in the state of Parana, in the south of Brazil), were the only NGOs led by *travestis* in Brazil. The number of *travesti* leaders and NGOs expanded, and in the third ENTLAIDS, a national network of *travestis* and transsexuals was created and named RENATA–*Rede Nacional de Travestis*. The network's primary actions and political platform was centered upon HIV prevention, citizenship, the recognition and regulation of sex work as a profession, access to health services, human rights, violence and education (Simpson and Baby n/d). National meetings were held annually, and in 2002, the name of the group was changed to ANTRA–*Articulação Nacional de Travestis e Transexuais*. The *Grupo Esperança* in Curitiba was the first NGO to direct ANTRA, and it was later led by the most visible and politically strong NGOs of *travesti*es in Brazil, ATRAC (*Associação de Travestis de Ceara*–Ceara Association of *Travestis*), located in Fortaleza, and currently, by ATRAS (*Associação de Travestis de Salvador*—Salvador Association of *Travestis*). Tulipa and Transpondo Barreiras, both projects financed by the Ministry of Health and mentioned above, were extremely important for the expansion and strengthening of the movement in the 2000s as they promoted actions focused on HIV prevention, leadership training, and the promotion of citizenship and rights in Brazil's five regions. Currently ANTRA is made up of 123 non-governmental institutions and aims to promote the human rights of the *travesti* community, raise awareness around violence, stigma, and discrimination, implement STI and HIV prevention activities and advocate for actions that improve the quality of life of people living with HIV (Simpson and Baby n/d).

Currently, there is no national network dedicated exclusively to male sex workers. There is one NGO for male sex workers in the Amazonas state, and NGOs dedicated to LGBT rights have historically implemented HIV prevention actions with the population through either specific projects or larger prevention initiatives. In August 2010, the Ministry of Health organized the First National Prevention Meeting with Male Sex Workers (ENTRASEX) in Brasilia as part of actions to reach the goals of the National Plan for Gays, men who have sex with men, and Travestis with the aim of promoting space for male sex workers, government officials, and NGO activists to reflect and identify strategies for HIV prevention and human, sexual, and labor rights for male sex workers. Twenty-five representatives from LGBT NGOs in 23 cities throughout Brazil participated, giving some scope of the number of groups that work with the population.

Gaps in Research and Practice

Current research and reports in Brazil included in this case study highlight a gap between the existence of national level policies developed in a human rights perspective and the reality of the way in which these policies are often implemented to varying degrees dependent on the local social-political context. For sex worker organizations, one of the most pressing current gaps is in terms of funding and sustainability, both for interventions and for research evaluating the political, social and cultural contexts within which HIV prevention interventions with sex workers are implemented on a local level. Currently many sex worker rights organizations are surviving on a small amount of funding from local and state AIDS Programs and unable to implement a full range of prevention and advocacy actions. There is a particular need for projects with a human and labor rights focus. Such projects should follow the recommendations made in the National Consultation on STD/AIDS, Human Rights and Prostitution in 2008 (Consulta 2008), take an inter-sectorial approach and be designed in accordance with the social, cultural, and political context in which sex workers live and work. These projects should recognize regional diversities, the continued existence of internalized stigma among sex workers, persistence of stigma and discrimination in public health facilities, and address labor issues, such as working conditions and the need for the complete decriminalization and regulation of the profession. Investment in programs drawing on cultural forms and social events for activism, similar to the approaches employed by the *Encontros* project, *Daspu* and *Radio Zona* would be particularly important for reducing stigma on a broader scale, and reaching populations not reached by the peer education approach—although the sustainability of such initiatives has been varied. In 2012–13, the Department of STDs/Aids and Viral Hepatitis will fund a qualitative formative research project to explore current social, political, and cultural contexts of sex work, human rights, and HIV in several Brazilian municipalities as a way to contribute to strengthening the government's response in these areas.

A second large gap is the level of information available regarding male sex workers from both a research and intervention perspective. More research on the connection between violence and HIV vulnerability are needed for all sex workers and for *travesti* and male sex workers in particular, while epidemiological studies are also needed for more accurate estimates of population size and prevalence to inform the planning of appropriate prevention programs. ANTRA has been advocating for the government to include a "*travesti*" category in their public health reporting system which would provide national level information regarding AIDS incidence among the population. Brazil's national public health reporting system (SINAN) also only tracks AIDS cases, making it more difficult to track prevalence trends, and also does not include "sex work" as an exposure category. Finally, more investment in rigorous evaluations of HIV prevention interventions among sex workers would also contribute to documenting elements of the Brazilian response to HIV that have been effective and would be informative for expanding prevention actions both within the country and in other similar contexts.

Dominican Republic

Introduction

Key Themes

- The Dominican Republic (DR) has a long-standing, internationally recognized, community-led response to HIV among female sex workers.
- HIV prevalence has stabilized and declined in the DR among the general population and among female sex workers since the mid-1990s.
- Higher HIV prevalence has been documented among female sex workers in geographic areas of the country where HIV interventions have not been widely implemented.
- The HIV prevention needs of male and transgender sex workers and those of the male sexual partners of sex workers merit additional attention.

The Dominican Republic is a country of approximately 10 million people (World Bank, 2011) located in the Caribbean on the island of Hispaniola, neighboring Haiti. The Caribbean region has the highest HIV prevalence outside of sub-Saharan Africa (UNAIDS, 2010a). Unprotected sex between men and women, particularly in the context of paid sex, has been cited by UNAIDS as the main mode of HIV transmission in the Caribbean region (UNAIDS, 2010a).

Historical perspectives and trends of the HIV epidemic in the DR. The first case of HIV was documented in the Dominican Republic in 1983. Early in the epidemic the majority of reported HIV cases in the Dominican Republic were documented among men. In 1984, for example, the male to female ratio of HIV cases was 7:1. These dynamics have shifted significantly over the years, whereas the current male to female ratio is now 1:1 and the majority of HIV transmission is associated with heterosexual sex (UNAIDS, 2010).

In 1987 the Dominican government established a national agency to address the growing HIV epidemic in the country (*Dirección de Control de las Infecciones de Transmisión Sexual y SIDA* (DIGECITSS, formerly PROCETS) and local non-governmental organizations working with vulnerable populations such as female sex workers such as the *Centro de Orientación e Investigación Integral* (COIN) worked hand in hand with the government as implementing partners for community-based HIV prevention efforts including peer education and condom distribution. Governmental HIV prevention efforts in the Dominican Republic are coordinated by a multisectoral Presidential Commission now called the *Consejo Nacional para el VIH y el SIDA* (CONAVIHSIDA) which was first established in 2001 and formerly named COPRESIDA (Kerrigan, 2009).

Mathematical modeling efforts conducted in the early 1990s suggested that the Dominican Republic was headed for a generalized HIV epidemic with an overall HIV prevalence of over 5 percent (Kerrigan, 2009). Instead, HIV prevalence in the Dominican Republic stabilized from the mid 1990's onward with gradual declines in prevalence in recent years. These shifts are thought to reflect the results of successful HIV prevention campaigns and behavior change programs implemented mostly in large, urban areas across the country targeting HIV risk behaviors among both the general population and vulnerable populations. These interventions aimed at reducing the numbers of sexual partners among men and increasing consistent condom use in the context of female sex work (Halperin et al, 2009).

The most recent Demographic Health Survey (DHS) HIV seroprevalence survey conducted in 2007 documented HIV prevalence of 0.8 percent (CESDEM, 2008), while UNAIDS estimates 1.1 percent of the population is infected with HIV (UNAIDS, 2008). There are approximately 60,000 persons living with HIV (PLHIV) (UNAIDS, 2008). Current estimates of the level of anti-retroviral therapy (ART) coverage among PLHIV receiving treatment at government-sponsored clinics with CD4 counts at or below 200 in the Dominican Republic is approximately 60 percent (USAID, 2012).

Official reports suggest that the primary form of HIV transmission in the Dominican Republic is heterosexual transmission accounting for 76 percent of HIV infections nationally (USAID, 2011). Some have suggested that the current male to female AIDS case ratio (1:1) is incongruent with a largely heterosexual HIV epidemic and some authors have indicated that there is most likely significant under-reporting of AIDS cases among men who have sex with men in the Dominican Republic due to stigma and discrimination associated with homosexuality and bisexuality (Halperin et al, 2009; Rojas et al, 2011). Recent Modes of Transmission mathematical modeling analyses indicate that a significant percent (33.3%) of future HIV infections will be concentrated among men who have sex with men in the Dominican Republic, greater than any other sub-group included in the analysis (UNAIDS, 2010b). This analysis does not however indicate how much of these new HIV infections in the Dominican Republic may involve male sex workers or transgender persons.

The prevalence of HIV infection in the Dominican Republic has remained concentrated among vulnerable populations since the beginning of the epidemic. According to findings from the most recent integrated bio-behavioral surveillance survey (IBBSS) conducted in the Dominican Republic in 2008, the overall HIV prevalence among female sex workers is 4.8%, ranging from 3.3–6.4% depending on geographic location and the parallel intensity of interventions across regions. This is compared with an overall HIV prevalence of 6.1% among men who have sex with men and 8.0% among drug users, that latter of whom have not historically received significant attention for HIV prevention activities as compared to female sex workers and men who have sex with men where community organizations have more actively implemented HIV prevention activities. Additionally, other socially vulnerable groups include batey or sugar cane workers, many of whom are of Haitian descent, among whom HIV prevalence ranges from 3.2 to 4.7% (COPRESIDA, 2009).

Scope, Typology and Context of Sex Work

The local NGO, COIN, has estimated the number of female sex workers at 72,000 (COIN, 2008). There is no specific size estimation available for the numbers of male and transgender sex workers in the country, however, extensive ethnographic work conducted with these populations indicates that there are considerable numbers of both in large urban centers and tourist areas throughout the Dominican Republic (Padilla, 2008; Padilla et al, 2011). It is also important to note that a large number of Dominican women work as sex workers outside of the Dominican Republic, including many countries in Western Europe and other islands within the Caribbean (COIN, 2008).

Common forms of sex work. While historically, the majority of sex work in the Dominican Republic was establishment-based, COIN now estimates that 60 percent of female sex workers work independently, from streets, parks, and beaches, with the remaining 40 percent working from establishments such as brothels, bars, discos, liquor stores, and car washes. Among these establishments, indirect establishments are the more common. Indirect establishments are those where woman, for example, works as a waitress or exotic dancer and sell sex in addition to those roles and non-sex work related income (Kerrigan et al, 2003; Moreno and Kerrigan, 2000). Brothels, *casas de cita*, and other direct forms of sex establishments still exist but with time have become significantly less common in the Dominican Republic (Kerrigan et al, 2001).

Another differentiating factor between direct and indirect sex establishments in the Dominican Republic is whether the client pays a *salida* or quota to the sex establishment to go out and have sex with a woman who works there. Increasingly, establishments which do not have a *salida* and where the sex worker herself negotiates the terms of exchange directly with a client, such as car wash, liquor stores, *centro cerveceros* and *colmados*, have become more popular in the Dominican Republic (Kerrigan et al, 2001). Independent sex work exchanges, without a third party or sex establishment, coordinated through social media sites via the internet, and, cell phones and pagers, are also becoming increasingly common in the Dominican Republic (Personal communication, COIN, 2011).

Street-based sex work also exists in the DR. In Santo Domingo, the capital, street-based sex workers tend to be of lower socio-economic levels and include a significant Haitian population, and are often at heightened vulnerability to HIV due to the social conditions within which they work in public spaces (Moreno and Kerrigan, 2000). Street or non-establishment-based sex work is also popular in spaces near public beaches in tourist areas of the country (Padilla, 2007).

In both qualitative and quantitative studies conducted to date, female sex workers in the Dominican Republic tend to be relatively young women with low levels of education, limited economic opportunities and often have at least one child. Local clients of female sex workers in the Dominican Republic range in socio-economic status and background. Brothels, for example, attract higher income Dominican men and tourists willing to pay hundreds of dollars a date or a night, as compared to factory workers and moto-taxi drivers in lower end local bars (Kerrigan et al, 2003; Barrington et al, 2009).

Tourism, one of the largest sectors of the Dominican economy (World Bank, 2011) has been closely linked to sex work in the DR. Sex tourism takes on many forms ranging from sex for money between local staff members and foreign and domestic patrons within "all-inclusive" resorts to street-based sex work on public beaches, bars and discos in high-volume tourism areas such as Boca Chica near Santo Domingo, Puerto Plata in the Northeast and La Romana and Punta Cana in the East. Sex tourism in the Dominican Republic includes both foreign men seeking Dominican women and men, respectively, as well as, to a lesser extent, foreign women seeking Dominican men (Padilla, 2008). The majority of tourists in the Dominican Republic are from Europe and the United States (Padilla, 2010).

Ethnographic work in the context of both female and male sex work within tourist areas of the Dominican Republic has documented the important inter-play between migration, tourism and HIV, whereas many of the men and women who sell sex in tourist areas are migrating from other parts of the country to sell sex. Often times, sexual relationships formed between local sex workers from the Dominican Republic and foreign tourists have an important affective element and continue over long periods of time, with what have been termed "romance tourism" partnerships where both the clients and SWs may travel to and from the Dominican Republic as a part of an ongoing "trans-national" relationship (Padilla et al, 2008; Brennan, 2004; Cabezas, 2009).

Map 3.3   HIV Prevalence per Region among Female Sex Workers in the Dominican Republic

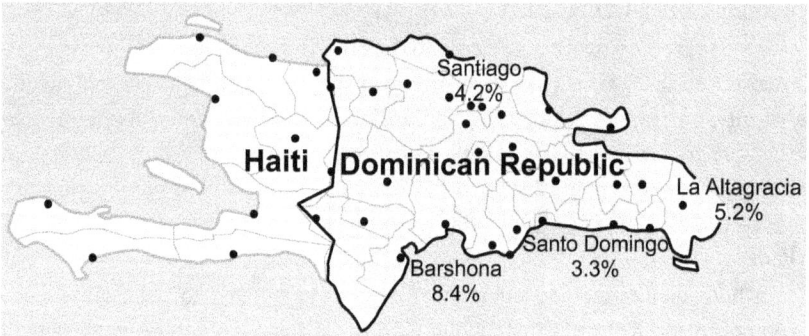

Source: Authors (developed from references HIV epidemiologic studies).

The role of steady partnerships and trust and intimacy within the context of sex work in the Dominican Republic is not limited to tourist settings by any means. In much of the research conducted on sex work to date, female sex workers have had a relatively low numbers of paying clients per week, but a high numbers of regular paying partners (Murray et al, 2007). Additional qualitative research has documented the ways in which many female sex workers specifically seek to develop regular paying partnerships which some hope will become non-commercial relationships over time (Kerrigan et al, 2001; Cabezas, 2009). Several papers have documented the manner in which the regular, intimate nature of these relationships lead to decreased consistent condom use and increased risk for HIV among both female and male sex workers in the Dominican Republic (Murray et al, 2007; Padilla et al, 2008).

Important work has also been conducted on the context of male and transgender sex workers in the Dominican Republic (Padilla et al, 2008; Thanel et al, 2009; Padilla et al, 2011). An ethnographic study of male sex workers in the greater Santo Domingo and Boca Chica documented a nuanced typology of different types of male sex workers depending on their client type (male, female, or both) as well as their performance of masculine roles within the context of sexual relationships with clients (Padilla et al, 2008). Based on the research available to date, most male SWs in the Dominican Republic do not identify as gay and report having sex with both men and women, outside of the context of sex work, indicating the importance of bisexuality in this setting (Padilla et al, 2008). Recent ethnographic research with both male and transgender sex workers in the Eastern part of the Dominican Republic has documented high levels of discrimination among these groups both from clients, police and the general public, and the critical need for increased HIV prevention programming, which has traditionally focused on female sex workers (Thanel et al, 2009; Padilla et al, 2011). No HIV surveillance efforts have specifically targeted male or transgender sex workers in the Dominican Republic to date (COPRESIDA, 2009).

Legal and Policy Issues

Sex work or the exchange of sex for money in the Dominican Republic is not explicitly illegal for persons over 18 years of age. Child prostitution is explicitly illegal as is profiting from another person's involvement in sex work (Codigo Penal, 2007).

Sex workers working in entertainment establishments are required under the Dominican public health code to attend monthly STI screenings and carry a health card provided at public health clinics demonstrating their attendance and screening results, although these requirements are often not followed (Kerrigan, 2006). Motels located near bars or discos or associated with sex work in the Dominican Republic, for example those along major highways, are mandated by law to have two condoms in every room for each new set of guests (UNFPA, 2010).

Recently, a new law was proposed in the Dominican Republic to introduce tolerance zones where entertainment businesses including sex work establishments would be forced to relocate themselves to a specific area of a given city. This law has not been passed to date and was objected to by sex worker rights groups and non-governmental organizations working on HIV prevention in the country as it would potentially lead to greater levels of violence and stigma and discrimination towards sex workers (Pantaleon, 2011).

Epidemiology of and Risks Factors for HIV Among Sex Workers

According to the most recent surveillance conducted in the Dominican Republic in 2008 the overall prevalence of HIV among sex workers is 4.8 percent, ranging from 3.3 percent in Santo Domingo, where intensive intervention activities have been conducted over the past two decades, to 6.4 percent in regions with limited to no interventions. Prior government sponsored sentinel surveillance systems among female sex workers as well as other groups such as pregnant women and STI clinic patients are not currently active. Currently periodic, every few years, bio-behavioral surveillance coordinated by the Dominican government with support from the U.S. Centers for Disease Control and Prevention (CDC) is being conducted in the country among female sex workers (COPRESIDA, 2009). Limited quantitative research and HIV-related surveillance has been conducted with male or transgender sex workers in the DR. The one known HIV prevalence assessment conducted among "gigolos", understood to be male sex workers, in the mid-1990s documented HIV prevalence at 6.5 percent among this population group (Tabet et al, 1996). No HIV surveillance efforts have ever specifically focused on the clients of sex workers in the DR.

Figure 3.3   Trends in HIV Prevalence among Female Sex Workers in Santo Domingo, 1991–2004

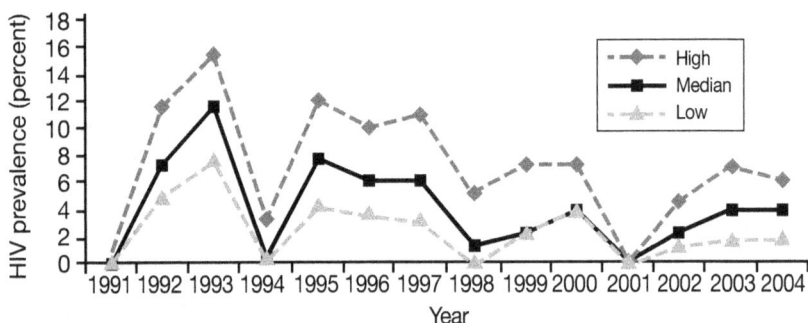

Source: Adapted from Halperin et al. 2009.

Analyses based on prior sentinel surveillance work conducted in Santo Domingo, where significant intervention work has taken place among female sex workers over the last two decades, demonstrated a significant downward trend in HIV prevalence between 1991 and 2004—from approximately seven to three percent during that time period. Important reductions in HIV prevalence among female sex workers from other cities where NGOs implementing HIV prevention activities were active such as Puerto Plata and La Romana have also been documented, including a decline from 12.5 percent in 1996 to 4.1 in 2006 in La Romana. However, as indicated earlier HIV prevalence has not declined significantly where interventions were not as common such as Barahona in the Southwestern region of the country (Halperin et al, 2009).

The only HIV incidence data currently available among female sex workers from the Dominican Republic is from an HIV Vaccine Trial Network (HVTN) feasibility trial (903) conducted in Santo Domingo among approximately 200 female sex workers. This study documented HIV incidence of less than one percent (Djomand et al, 2008).

Consistent condom use among female sex workers exposed to HIV prevention activities is generally high. In the most recent surveillance, for example, condom use at last sex with most recent client ranged from 64–94 percent across the four participating cities. These rates were lowest in Barahona were HIV prevalence was found to be the highest (8.4) and where minimal intervention work has been implemented. Consistent condom use with regular clients is much lower than with new clients, ranging from 33–81 percent across the four bio-behavioral surveillance sites wide range. Condom use with non-paying partners was documented at less than 10 percent across all sites (COPRESIDA, 2009). A study conducted among female sex workers in Santo Domingo and their regular paying male partners demonstrated the role of relationship intimacy as a significant factor associated with decreased consistent condom use in the context of those ongoing relationships (Murray et al, 2007).

HIV-related knowledge is generally considered to be high among female sex workers in the Dominican Republic receiving prevention interventions as is self-efficacy to use a condom with paying clients (Kerrigan et al, 2003). In the most recent bio-behavioral surveillance survey, sex worker knowledge of HIV transmission surpassed 90% on most indicators, with the exception of the variable concerning whether they could be infected by HIV by a regular partner, where approximately 70% responded incorrectly to this indicator (UNAIDS 2010c). This finding, combined with the lower rates of condom use with regular partners, indicates the need for new strategies to effectively communicate risks associated with regular partnerships among sex workers. Other factors found to be significantly associated with consistent condom use among female sex workers in past surveys include environmental-structural support for condom use on the part of the establishment and government including access to condoms, STI screening and social support from colleagues including both sex workers, owner-managers and other sex establishment employees. Additionally, women working as female sex workers in establishments of higher socio-economic status (SES) have been found to use condoms more consistently than those working in lower SES establishments (Kerrigan et al, 2003; Murray et al, 2007).

Clients and Partners of Sex Workers. Relatively limited information is available from clients or regular partners of sex workers in the DR. A few studies have been conducted, however, among the male, paying and non-paying regular partners of female sex workers in the DR. These studies indicate that consistent condom use between these partners and female sex workers is significantly lower than with new clients. Both surveys, conducted in Santo Domingo and La Romana, respectively, documented 60 percent consistent condom use (Kerrigan et al, 2003; Barrington et al, 2009). These studies also indicate that the sexual networks of female sex workers and their male partners are often similar in size. Whereas, the median number of sexual partners among both female sex workers and their regular, paying partners in Santo Domingo was found to be 3.0 during the last three months (Kerrigan et al, 2003). This finding reinforces the idea that female sex workers in the Dominican Republic often have a relatively low number of sexual partners compared to SWs from other settings, but a higher proportion of regular, paying partners, where condom use is less consistent (Murray et al, 2007).

Limited information is available regarding clients and protective behaviors among male and transgender sex workers. However, among a sample of 168 male sex workers participating in an ethnographic study from the greater Santo Domingo area reported consistent condom use was high with new clients (82%), but very low (14%) between male sex workers and their regular clients. This same study also reported high levels of bisexuality among participating male sex workers with almost all participants reporting both male and female recent sexual partners and only 3% of participants identifying themselves as gay or homosexual (Padilla et al, 2008).

Violence, Stigma, and Discrimination. Despite the fact that sex work is not illegal in the DR, sex workers, particularly street-based or sex workers based in public areas such as parks or beaches often report facing harassment from police and law enforcement officials or being arrested under the guise of public loitering laws (MODEMU & Murray, 2001). Sex worker reports of violence and mistreatment from clients has also been well documented as has the violation of labor rights among sex workers based in entertainment establishments such as bars and discos where they should receive a set monthly salary and benefits such as vacation and pensions by law in addition to sex work related income (MODEMU & Murray, 2001).

Substance Use. Substance use plays an important role within the context of sex work in the DR. For example, most sex establishments such as bars and liquor stores in the Dominican Republic make the majority of their money selling alcohol. Because sex workers generally drink with their clients, many female sex workers report drinking five or more drinks a night, and cite alcohol use as an impediment to condom use if they or their client has had too much to drink (Kerrigan, et al 2003; Barrington et al, 2009).

In addition to alcohol, the use of illicit drugs has reportedly increased among sex workers and their clients in the Dominican Republic in recent years and is cited by sex workers as a major concern with regard to their ability to protect themselves from HIV and in relation to violence and mistreatment from clients who consume such drugs (Kerrigan, 2001). In the most recent IBBSS, approximately 20 percent of female sex workers in Santo Domingo reported previous drug use, while almost 50 percent of female sex workers in Barahona reported prior drug use, the city with the highest HIV prevalence. The most common drugs reportedly consumed were crack cocaine and marijuana (COPRESIDA, 2009).

HIV Prevention Interventions for Sex Workers

The Dominican Republic has been recognized as a country with significant innovation in terms of its HIV prevention programming within the context of female sex work including efforts that emphasize environmental-structural interventions such as community solidarity and mobilization and supportive government policy (Kerrigan, 2006). However, important challenges exist with regard to the country's ability to address the health, human rights, and HIV prevention, treatment and care needs of sex workers in a comprehensive and sustainable manner given the size, geographic distribution, and diversity of sex work in the DR.

Common, successful interventions. Community-led education, condom distribution and referrals to HIV/STI clinical screening and treatment services have been implemented in the Dominican Republic since the late 1980s, coordinated by two non-governmental organizations, COIN covering the greater Santo Domingo area and parts of the Eastern region of the country, and CEPROSH covering the North and parts of the Southwestern region of the country. The approach of both COIN and CEPROSH has been based on Freirian principles of the promotion of critical consciousness and the philosophy of face-to-face education among equals. This peer-led strategy is named *Avancemos* or "We Shall Overcome" in the Dominican Republic and has emphasized not only information regarding HIV and STIs, but the promotion of self-esteem and human rights including the labor-related rights of sex workers. Street theater led by SWs has also been conducted over the years to engage clients in HIV prevention. In the mid-1990s MODEMU or the *Movimiento de Mujeres Unidas* a sex worker led organization was formed focusing on more of the political and economic issues facing sex workers, while collaborating with COIN and CEPROSH on HIV prevention outreach activities (Moreno and Kerrigan, 2000).

In the late 1990s, environmental-structural interventions began to develop among female sex workers in the Dominican Republic on the basis of extensive formative research (Kerrigan et al, 2001). A combined community-based solidarity and government policy HIV prevention model was developed and implemented in sex establishments in Santo Domingo and Puerto Plata. In both settings, a key intervention component was the development of *Compromiso Colectivo* or "Collective Commitment" formed among female sex workers, establishment owners, managers and staff as well as sex establishment clients with regard to the prevention of HIV in the context of sex work via community mobilization activities. The term and approach of "collective commitment" was developed on the basis of significant formative, qualitative research among sex workers and other stakeholders including government officials, establishment managers, clients and others (Kerrigan et al, 2011). Government policy and regulation was introduced in Puerto Plata to support female sex workers' access to HIV prevention services, including access to condoms, HIV prevention materials and STI screening and treatment (Kerrigan et al, 2006).

Coverage and Access to HIV Prevention Services. More intensive coverage of these efforts has been traditionally focused in Santo Domingo, Puerto Plata and La Romana and in particular among establishment-based sex workers. Over the years it has become clear that gaps in coverage exist not only among other regions of the country outside of those mentioned above, but also within these cities particularly among street-based sex workers and sex workers in less formal sex establishments and settings where the aforementioned salida does not take place and where the women may not identify as sex workers. Current coverage rates for female sex workers from the most recent UNGASS report from the Dominican Republic indicate that less than half or 44% of sex workers have been exposed to any type of HIV prevention message or educational activity while 67% report having been tested for HIV in the last year (UNAIDS 2010c).

There are no systematic interventions with male and transgender sex workers in the DR, although recent qualitative research conducted with both groups has highlighted the heightened levels of stigma and discrimination reported by both groups by the general public as well as clinical care facilities in the country and thus the need and importance of both HIV/STI prevention and human rights promotion with these populations. In response to these concerns, NGOs such as *Amigos Siempre Amigos* (ASA) and *Grupo Este Amor* have begun to conduct further assessments with these groups and COIN has opened a trans-friendly clinic in Santo Domingo which services transgender sex workers (Personal Communication, Rosario, 2011).

Since early in the HIV epidemic in the DR, the United States Agency for International Development (USAID) has played an important role in supporting HIV prevention activities among sex workers. Funding has generally flowed to COIN and CEPROSH, rather than MODEMU, for example, via U.S. NGOs with offices in Santo Domingo included Family Health International (FHI) and the Academy for International Development (AED), which have now merged into FHI360. The rationale for funding groups such as COIN and CEPROSH versus sex worker associations such as MODEMU has related to the greater management and financial capacity of these groups; however the "Prostitution Pledge" limits the use of United States Government funds for organizations that are not willing to explicitly denounce sex work. Currently, the PEPFAR program overall in the Dominican Republic has committed approximately 82 million dollars to HIV prevention, care and treatment services over a five-year period (USAID, 2011).

Activities funded include community-based, peer education on safer sex negotiation and sexual and reproductive health, promotion of HIV/ STI screening and management, condom social marketing, and community solidarity and government policy activities (Moreno and Kerrigan, 2000). Additional actors of import in terms of funding for HIV prevention among female sex workers in the Dominican Republic include the World Bank and the Global Fund, which have generally supported the Dominican government via its Presidential Commission of AIDS (COPRESIDA), which in turn has sub-contracted to COIN and CEPROSH to support activities among sex workers. The Global Fund for example has donated over 60 million dollars in funding to the Dominican Republic since 2004, largely to support ARTs (USAID, 2011). The William J. Clinton Foundation has also been an active donor in the DR, particularly in the area of access to treatment. Unfortunately, the level of expected funding to organizations supporting HIV prevention among SWs including COIN, CEPROSH and MODEMU in relation to female sex workers and ASA and *Este Amor* for male SWs has been limited in recent years and funds have tended to "get stuck" in intermediate governmental bodies rather than flowing the community level as imagined (Kerrigan et al, 2009). The American Foundation for AIDS Research (amfAR) has recently funded a community-based clinic for transgender persons including transgender sex workers in the Dominican Republic via the local NGO COIN based in Santo Domingo (Personal Communication, COIN, 2011).

Available Impact Evaluation Data. Pre-post Knowledge, Attitude, and Practice (KAP) surveys in Santo Domingo and Puerto Plata demonstrated significant increases in consistent condom use throughout the 1990s (CESDEM, 2000). In 2000, an impact evaluation of the *Compromiso Colectivo* intervention was conducted in Santo Domingo and Puerto Plata. While positive changes were seen in both cities, significantly greater gains took place in Puerto Plata where a combined, community-based solidarity and government policy model was implemented. Over the course of one year, a 40% reduction in STIs was documented (STI prevalence 28.8% to 16.3%; OR 0.50; 95% CI=0.32–0.78) and consistent condom use with regular paying and non-paying partners rose significantly (13.0% to 28.8%; OR 2.97; 95% CI 1.33, 6.66) (Kerrigan et al, 2006), the latter of which was a major gain given the historically low levels of consistent condom use among female sex workers and their regular paying and non-paying partners in the Dominican Republic and globally (Murray et al, 2007).

Both intervention models were also found to be cost-effective with the combined model significantly more cost-effective in terms of the number of HIV infections averted among sex workers and their partners. In Puerto Plata, where the combined community-based solidarity and government policy intervention was implemented 162 HIV infections were averted per 10,000 clients reached, yielding a cost per disability adjusted life year (DALY) saved of $457 (Sweat et al, 2006).

Sex Worker Rights Organizations

In 1994 as a result of the large peer-led network of SWs which had formed through COIN and CEPROSH, MODEMU or the Movimiento de Mujeres Unidas (Movement of United Women) held the first national organization for the promotion of sex workers rights and has had annual national congresses to unite and organize sex workers across the country since that time. Current MODEMU membership surpasses 6,000 female sex workers (Personal Communication, MODEMU, 2011). MODEMU has chapters in several cities within the Dominican Republic and serves not only as a programmatic partner with COIN and CEPROSH on HIV prevention efforts but also as a resource center for sex workers who have had their human or labor rights violated.

Additionally, MODEMU proactively advocates for the rights of sex workers and represents this constituency in political and public health forum both nationally and internationally. MODEMU has traditionally included mostly sex workers from establishments rather than street-based or other forms of sex work. Recently, an additional sex worker organization called COVIH has formed to represent the voices and needs of SWs living with HIV including issues of access to treatment, care and support. A transgender rights, community-based organization called TRANSA has recently formed in the Dominican Republic (Personal communication, COIN, 2011) and a small group of male sex workers has also recently developed (Personal Communication, MODEMU, 2011). Given restrictions in United States government funding, which has historically been the largest HIV prevention donor for the country, limited resources have been channeled directly to sex worker organizations in the Dominican Republic but rather have reached sex workers indirectly via local non-governmental organizations.

Gaps in Research and Practice

Current gaps in research in practice in the Dominican Republic in relation to sex work and HIV prevention include the need to further understand and address the diversity of types of sex work establishments and settings, including less formal, indirect sex work establishments and non-establishment based sex work; the expansion of evidence-based interventions to less intervened areas of the country where prevalence has not declined; systematic interventions with male and transgender sex workers particularly in tourist areas of the country; the differential needs of sex workers living with HIV; and the increasing role of substance use within the context of sex work in the Dominican Republic. Human rights and advocacy work continues to be critical particularly given the recent introduction of laws and policies which would segregate sex work into geographic tolerance zones further marginalizing sex workers and placing them at risk for greater stigma, discrimination and violence. Further engagement of clients and the regular paying and non-paying partners of sex workers is key to reducing HIV risk given the lower levels of consistent condom use with these partners.

Lastly, funding for sex worker interventions have been intermittent and lacking in robustness during recent years. Interventions demonstrated to be effective have not been scaled up as needed. The potential ramifications of this limited package of services approach for sex workers in select areas of the country and generally limited to female sex workers alone remains to be seen. However, this approach poses a potentially significant threat to the important reductions in HIV prevalence documented since the mid-1990s among female sex workers in areas receiving the innovative combined community-led, peer education and environmental-structural HIV prevention interventions led by joint efforts across governmental, non-governmental and community-based organization in the DR. While efforts to engage the male clients and regular partners of female sex workers have been initiated, none have been taken to scale or evaluated in terms of their impact on HIV-related outcomes in the DR. Lastly, given the importance of male sex workers and transgender populations in recent HIV-related mathematical modeling exercises focused on the distribution of future HIV infections across population groups in the DR, additional funding for HIV prevention and care among these groups is urgently needed.

India

Introduction

Key Themes

- India has multiple HIV epidemics largely among populations at heightened risk such as men who have sex with men, sex workers, transgender people and people who inject drugs
- There is great geographic diversity to India's epidemics, with greater concentration of HIV in the south and northeast states
- Empowerment-based HIV prevention interventions among sex workers have demonstrated efficacy on HIV related outcomes
- Although there are numerous NGOs and empowerment-based interventions that were spearheaded by female sex workers, sex workers remain marginalized and stigmatized throughout much of India

In the past two decades, India has experienced economic growth and progress in terms of human development. The economy has grown as high as 9% a year in 2006–2007 (UNICEF 2011) and the percentage of those living below poverty has fallen. However, entrenched poverty persists for millions who have not shared in the economic boom. In 2010, the gross national income per capita was $1,265 (Fund 2011; IMF 2011).

UNAIDS estimates 2.4 million people are living with HIV in India (UNAIDS 2008). India's HIV epidemic is primarily heterosexual, with women accounting for roughly 40% of adult infections (National AIDS Control Organization). The first cases of HIV in India were diagnosed in 1986 in a study of female sex workers (N=102) in Chennai, in which 10% tested positive for HIV (Simoes, Babu et al. 1987).

In response, the Government established the National AIDS Control Programme (NACP) in 1987 with the charge of developing a surveillance system, blood screening, and health education programs in high-risk areas. NACP evolved into the National AIDS Control Organization (NACO), established by the Indian Government in 1992 with major support by the World Bank (NACO). NACO manages the national surveillance system, which is the primary source of HIV prevalence data. Over time, the surveillance system has expanded to include 295 districts in which there were 1,134 sentinel sites in 2007; this includes 646 sites among the general population and 488 sites among population groups including female sex workers, men who have sex with men, injection drug users, migrants, and truckers (Chandrasekaran, Dallabetta et al. 2006). Additionally, HIV prevalence data is derived from a population based survey, the National Family Health Survey (IIPS), the last of which, NFHS-3, was conducted in 2005–2006. NFHS-3 sampled over 100,000 15–49 year old women and 15–54 year old men in six high prevalence states (IIPS 2007).

Recently there have been significant fluctuations in the estimates of the number of people infected with HIV in India. In 2006, NACO estimated that there were over 5.1 million reproductive age adults infected with HIV, based on anonymous testing data from public prenatal and STI clinics (Steinbrook 2007). But this estimate was reduced to approximately 2.5 million (range: 2.0–3.1 million) in the summer of 2007 based on information from 400 additional sentinel surveillance sites and the implementation of a comprehensive population survey. The Indian HIV epidemic is difficult to categorize given its size, the mobility of high-risk populations, geographic diversity, and heterogeneity of risk factors. These estimates are largely driven by the disproportionately high HIV rates among groups at heightened risk such as: female sex workers (5.1%); IDUs (7.2%); men who have sex with men (7.4%), and STI clinic attendees (3.6%) (National AIDS Control Organization 2008). Nationally, the adult HIV prevalence has declined from 0.41% in 2000 to 0.31% in 2009. NACO's HIV estimates for 2008–2009 indicate an overall reduction in HIV prevalence and incidence, although variations exist across states. In 2009, Manipur had the highest estimated adult prevalence of 1.4%, followed by Andhra Pradesh (0.90%), Mizoran (0.81%), Nagaland (0.78%), and Karnataka (0.63%) (National AIDS Control Organization 2008).

Scope, Typology, and Context of Sex Work
It is estimated that 1.1% of the female Indian population are sex workers (NACO). There is a complex typology of female sex workers in India, which,

as in any context, is important in understanding the nature and level of female sex workers' HIV risk. Female sex work typologies are dynamic, influenced by economic, legal, and social factors, and are critical in both understanding and intervening upon HIV among female sex workers in a given context (Chatterjee 2006). In the literature, there are a range of categorizations of sex work related to the mode of organization or management, the venue in which sex is solicited (e.g., street based), or the venue in which sex is conducted (e.g., apartment) (Cornish 2004; Blanchard, OíNeil et al. 2005; Halli, Ramesh et al. 2006; Buzdugan, Halli et al. 2009).

In an effort to provide clarity to the literature, Buzdugan and colleagues developed three typologies of place of sex work solicitation, the place where sex was conducted, and a combination of the two for direct sex work venues (Buzdugan, Halli et al. 2009). Data were derived from behavioral and biological assessments among female sex workers (N=2,312) conducted in five districts in Karnataka. The most common places of sex solicitation were: street (52%); rented or owned homes (34%); and brothels (11%). The most common places where sex occurred included: owned or rented homes (43%); lodges (24%); brothels (12%); rented rooms (11%); and the street (10%). Street-based referred to public spaces such as markets, train stations, or parks. Home solicitations are either traditional *Devadasis*, which are common to Karnataka where brothels are rare, or in female sex workers' homes (Jayasree 2004). Public spaces such as parks and street markets were similarly found to be the predominant location for client solicitation in a cross-sectional study of female sex workers (N=10,096) in 23 districts in the four high prevalence southern states of Tamil Nadu, Maharashtra, Andhra Pradesh, and Karnataka (Brahmam, Kodavalla et al. 2008). In this study, over half of participants primarily solicited clients in public spaces such as parks and street markets, while 18% primarily operated from homes and 16% worked from indoor venues such as brothels, lodges, or *dabhas* (Ramesh, Moses et al. 2008).

The level of female sex workers' autonomy and HIV risk is dependent upon the context in which sex work is conducted. Street-based female sex workers are often self managed as they solicit their own clients and work independently from third parties, the need for whom has largely been eliminated by the nearly 100% coverage of mobile phones. After women establish clients from the above-mentioned venues, they develop their own client list and conduct business via mobile phone while continuing to solicit new business from street-based venues.

The difference in where sex work is conducted is based on a range of factors, primary of which is the sex workers' economic profile. Low-income sex workers generally conduct business "on the street, while middle class or "family girls" conduct business within their homes. This economic profile often extends to that of clients, with lower income clients soliciting less expensive sex workers on the street and more middle class clients being able to afford to rent rooms in lodges for sex work (Buzdugan, Halli et al. 2009).

HIV risk behavior and infection has been found to vary significantly across these sex work solicitation and sex venues (Buzdugan, Halli et al. 2009). Buzdugan and colleagues found that female sex workers who solicited in the street and had sex in lodges had high prevalence of HIV (30%) and STI (27%) prevalence, a relatively high client volume of 51 clients per month, and the highest mean number of unprotected sexual contacts, 11 per month. Brothel-based female sex workers had the highest HIV prevalence (34%) and client volume, 94 clients per month, but the lowest mean number of unprotected sexual contacts of 1.4 per month. Ramesh and colleagues similarly demonstrated that context of sex work was associated with HIV, with brothel-and street-based female sex workers having higher HIV prevalence compared to those who conducted sex work in their homes (Ramesh, Moses et al. 2008).

In contrast to extensive research on female sex workers in the context of the Indian HIV epidemic, relatively little research focus has been placed on male sex workers. An understanding of the prevalence of HIV among male sex workers has often been captured to date within studies of HIV among men who have sex with men and transgendered populations. For example, of men who have sex with men and transgendered persons studies in epidemiologic assessments, 11% and 96%, respectively, have reported involvement in sex work (Hernandez, Lindan et al. 2006; Setia, Lindan et al. 2006; Shinde, Setia et al. 2009). These individuals are categorized by behaviors and level of "outness" and include self identified gay men (*kothis* who are anal receptive, *panthis* who are anal insertive) men who do not identify as gay but have sex with men, and a third gender, *hijras*, that is similar to the western notion of male-to-female transgenders (Brahmam, Kodavalla et al. 2008).

Several studies have indicated that sex work is common among men who have sex with men and among transgender people, including *hijras* in India. A small study of male sex workers (N=75) in suburban Mumbai reported an HIV prevalence of 17% in male sex workers and 41% in transgendered sex workers (Shinde, Setia et al. 2009). The large majority (87%) reported having had anal receptive intercourse in the past six months and 13% had never used a condom (Shinde, Setia et al. 2009). A cross sectional behavioral and HIV/STI seroprevalence study of men who have sex with men and transgendered persons in the four highest HIV prevalence states found that a large percentage of participants reported having "paying males partners" (40% in Maharashtra,

68% in Karnataka, 59% in Tamil Nadu, and 42% in Andhra Pradesh). Sex work varied by type of men who have sex with men and transgendered persons, with a significantly higher percentage of *kothis* reportedly ever having sold sex to men compared with other categories of self-identified men who have sex with men (20%–43%). Of all categories, *hijras* reported the greatest involvement in sex work (87%), and were largely dependent on sex work as their sole source of income. Consistent condom use was low among all partner types, with 4% of male sex workers reporting consistent condom use with regular female partners. HIV and STI prevalence was significantly higher among male sex workerss compared those who were not sex workers (14.5% vs. 10.8%, 17.5% vs. 11.2%, respectively). In tandem, these results indicate high levels of risk behaviors and HIV/STI prevalence among the range of male sex workerss, as well as their role in larger HIV transmission dynamics.

Legal and Policy Issues

In India, sex workers and others who profit from sex work (i.e., brothel owners) are restricted under the Immoral Traffic and Prevention Act (IPTA), which was first enacted in 1956 as the "Suppression of Immoral Traffic Act." This act was the Indian Government's ratification of the United Nations International Convention for the "Suppression of Traffic in Persons and the Exploitation of the Prostitution of Others." IPTA is the main statue addressing the criminalization of activities related to sex work and is based on the principle that sex work is exploitation and is incompatible with the dignity and self determination of those who engage in sex work (Jayasree 2004). The law's name conflates prostitution with trafficking, which is further confused by the fact that it does not define trafficking. Although the Indian Constitution guarantees the fundamental right of any person to conduct any trade, business, or profession, IPTA has effectively undermined sex workers' ability to claim protection under this.

The specific provisions IPTA criminalizes includes running a brothel, leasing to a sex worker, living on earnings derived from prostitution, procuring a person for prostitution, trafficking individuals for the purposes of prostitution, visiting a brothel, being found with a child in a brothel (even if the child is not engaged in prostitution), and conducting prostitution in the vicinity of a public space. Until 2009, soliciting for the purposes of prostitution was another offense often invoked against sex workers. Additionally, IPTA confers police with a wide range of enforcement powers. Police can enter and search premises based on simply suspicion of prostitution. Police can also remove any person on the premises where sex work is carried out, regardless of their age or consent or if the venue is a sex worker's home. Although IPTA contains provisions that could lead to the arrest of individuals who profit from sex work outside of sex workers, such brothel managers, 90% of those arrested under IPTA have been sex workers (Jayasree 2004). The majority of these arrests were for "solicitation in a public space." Many sex workers plead guilty in order to expedite the proceedings in order to minimize the expense of lawyers and earnings lost. Street-based sex workers are particularly vulnerable to being arrested for public solicitation and police harassment.

In March, 2011, the Lawyers Collective and the National Network of Sex Workers organized a meeting with Members of Parliament (MPs) in New Delhi, with over 200 attendants (National Network of Sex Workers and Unite 2011). The National Network of Sex Workers is a nationally representative body of female, male, and transgender sex workers from 10 states. The dialogue aimed to provide a forum for sex workers to inform MPs of the problems associated with the criminalization of sex work and to understand opportunities for raising policy debates to change IPTA. Sex workers shared a number of personal experiences that exemplified the "violence of the law," largely at the hands of the police. Such experiences included the common practice of police extorting money from sex workers and sexual favors, their challenges in renting homes because of the potential for landlords to be penalized, and how children of sex workers are penalized since they are being supported by earnings from sex work. Children of sex workers can further be penalized by not being allowed to study in local schools or not having contact with their mothers if they enter orphanages, thereby denying the right of motherhood to female sex workers and the right to having a mother to their children (Jayasree 2004).

Epidemiology of and Risks Factors for HIV Among Sex Workers

HIV prevalence estimates among female sex workers has varied by region and fluctuated over time. Among a pooled sample of seven studies ranging from 2007 to 2011, HIV among female sex workers (N=13,386) prevalence was 13.7%.(Baral et al., 2012) but this is not equally distributed across all geographic regions. Based on 2007–2008 National HIV Sentinel Surveillance conducted in 11,134 sites, 48 districts had greater than 5% HIV prevalence among female sex workers and eight female sex worker-specific sentinel surveillance sites (of 147) had 15% or higher prevalence among female sex workers in Pune, Mumbai, and Thane (NACO, 2008).

In 2007, the states with the highest HIV rates among female sex workers were: Maharashtra (17.9%); Andhra Pradesh (9.7%); Nagaland (8.9%); Mizoram (7.2%); Gujarat (6.5%); West Bengal (5.9%); and Karnataka (5.3%). There has been a decline in HIV prevalence among female sex workers in South Indian states, potentially indicating the impact of interventions targeting female sex workers. While rising trends in the Northeast, historically an epidemic that has characterized by injection drug use, suggest the diversity of and dynamic nature of the complex HIV landscape in India.

Map 3.4   Geographic Distribution of HIV Prevalence among Female Sex Workers in India

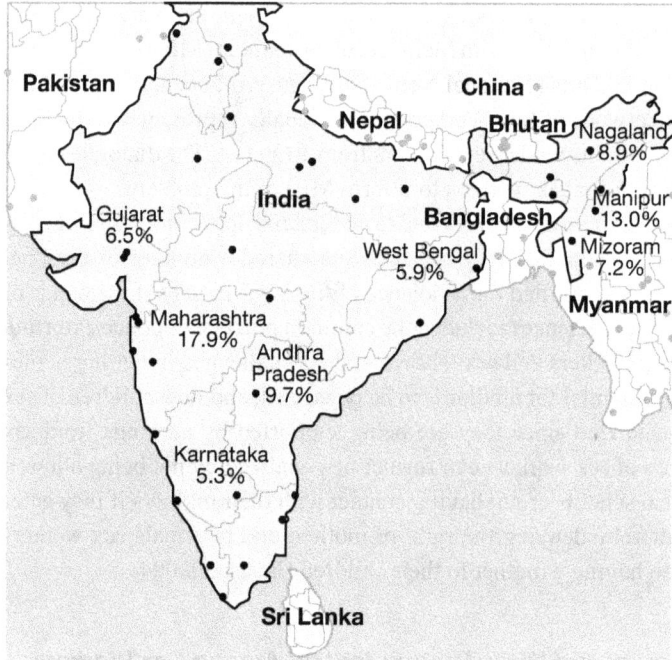

Source: Authors (developed from references HIV epidemiologic studies).

Risk of HIV infection among female sex workers is influenced by a number of individual, social, and structural environmental factors. In a study of female sex workers (N=6,648) in 13 districts of Andhra Pradesh, the median age was 27, 41% were married, 75% had no schooling, 53% were involved in no other work besides sex work (Dandona, Dandona et al. 2005). Twenty-four percent reported never having used a condom, with NGOs reported as the main source of condoms for 71% of female sex workers. In the presence of other variables, factors that were associated with no or inconsistent condom use during vaginal and anal sex included a lack of knowledge that HIV was preventable, lack of access to free condoms, not participating in a female sex workers support group, and selling sex on the street or home compared to in a brothel. The study indicates the importance of HIV prevention efforts, such as condom distribution and support groups, in reducing HIV among sex workers.

Figure 3.4   HIV Prevalence among the Adult Populations and Female Sex Workers by Region in India

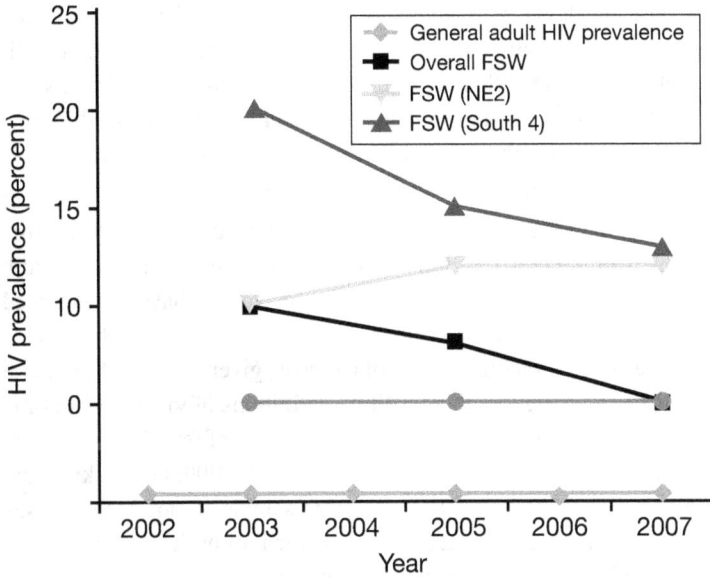

Source: NACA 2008. HIV Sentinel Surveillance and HIV Estimation in India, 2007.
Note: FSW = female sex worker.

Several large cross-sectional integrated behavioral and biological assessments from the Bill and Melinda Gates Foundation funded Avahan project provide estimates of HIV prevalence as well as associated risk factors among female sex workers. In the first such study of female sex workers (N=10,096) in Maharashtra, Andhra Pradesh, Karnataka, and Tamil Nadu, the overall HIV prevalence was 14.5% (Chandrasekaran, Dallabetta et al. 2008).

Clients and Partners of Sex Workers. The first large study of male clients (N=4,821) was a cross-sectional study and spanned 12 districts across Andhra Pradesh, Maharashtra, and Tamil Nadu as a part of the Avahan project. The study found that the mean age of first paying for sex was 21 years old, with 64% reporting that they also had regular non-paying female sexual partners. Close to two-thirds (61%) reported having sex with more than one female sex workers in the previous month, and 40% had sex with four or more female sex workers during this time. Consistent condom use with female sex workers ranged from 27%–58% across districts, while consistent condom use with regular female partners ranged from 0–16% across districts. Factors associated with inconsistent condom use with female sex workers were older age and being illiterate. HIV prevalence ranged from 2%–11%, with the highest reportedly in Maharashtra and the lowest prevalence estimates in Tamil Nadu. The study documents the frequency of sex with female sex workers as well as the relatively low level of condom use between clients and female sex workers, as well as with their primary non paying sexual partners. Additionally, HIV prevalence among male clients are relatively high across districts and consistent to those found among female sex worker populations in the same districts (NARI 2007), emphasizing the need of engaging this population in HIV prevention efforts that target female sex workers.

Violence, Stigma, and Discrimination. The prevalence of intimate partner violence against women is particularly high, with the National Family Health Survey (NFHS 3) reporting that 35% of married women have experienced physical violence from their husbands (Silverman, Decker et al. 2008). Female sex workers experience even higher rates of violence, given increased exposure by clients, police, and gang members. While definitions of violence and time periods vary, recent evidence suggests that 20% to 63% of female sex workers experience sexual violence (Shahmanesh, Cowan et al. 2009; Go, Srikrishnan et al. 2011; Swain, Saggurti et al. 2011). Among a sample of mobile female sex workers (N=5,498) interviewed in 22 districts in the four high HIV prevalence southern states, 20% reported being raped in the past year (Swain, Saggurti et al. 2011). In a study of female sex workers in rural Goa (N=326), 27% reported having been forced by a client to have unprotected sex in the past year. In a study of female sex workers (N=522) in Chennai, 63% reported having been raped by a partner in the past three months (Shahmanesh, Cowan et al. 2009; Go, Srikrishnan et al. 2011). In India, 70% of sex workers in a survey reported being beaten by the police and more than 80% had been arrested without evidence (Sangram 2002). Further, sex workers who are rounded up during police raids are often beaten and raped by corrupt police officials in exchange for their release or placed in institutions where they are sexually exploited or physically abused (Sangram 2002; Surtees 2003).

Sexual violence appears to confer HIV risk to female sex workers via a number of mechanisms. A handful of studies among Indian female sex workers have found that sexual violence is independently associated with a number of factors, including: inconsistent condom use; STI symptoms and infection; anal sex; physical violence; multiple forced pregnancy terminations, and suicide attempts.(Sarkar, Bal et al. 2008; Shahmanesh, Wayal et al. 2009;

Beattie, Bhattacharjee et al. 2010; Reed, Gupta et al. 2010; Swain, Saggurti et al. 2011). Among a robust sample of female sex workers from the four high prevalence states, Swain and colleagues found that among female sex workers inconsistent condom use was associated with experiences of sexual violence (AOR: 1.8; 95%CI: 14–2.3) and reporting STI symptoms (Swain, Saggurti et al. 2011). This small body of research demonstrates the extent of violence that female sex workers experience in both their home and work life. These findings echo a substantial body of research among women in India and elsewhere that implicate violence as a risk factor for sexually transmitted infections including HIV (Silverman, Decker et al. 2008; Weiss, Patel et al. 2008; Jewkes, Dunkle et al. 2010).

Although sex workers have been extremely successful in enhancing the human and labor rights of sex workers in India, sex work remains stigmatized. There are a number of factors that influence and/or may reduce the level of stigma and discrimination attached to sex work, with the level of empowerment among sex workers being one influential factor. For example, in the famous Sonagachi District of Kolkata, twenty years of community organizing among sex workers has effectively reduced stigma towards sex workers and their children, compared to areas in which sex workers are not organized or empowered. In one of the few studies of stigma among street-based female sex workers from Chennai, it was found that levels of perceived stigma from the community and stigma from one's family were lower if women had income from sources other than sex work. Additionally, access to health care was found to be associated with perceived community stigma, while heavier financial responsibility with one's family was associated with lower perceived family stigma among sex workers (Liu, Srikrishnan et al. 2011).

Substance Use. Similar to other contexts, the predominant substance used among Indian female sex workers and their clients is alcohol. Sexual risk behaviors, within and outside of the context of sex work, are heightened when alcohol is involved. In a study of migrant female sex workers (N=3,412) in the four high prevalence southern Indian states, nearly two-thirds of female sex workers and 90% of clients consumed alcohol in the past 30 days, with more than half of female sex workers and their clients reporting drinking prior to sex (Verma, Saggurti et al. 2010). Drinking alcohol prior to sex was associated with inconsistent condom use. As throughout the world, studies have documented the role of alcohol in escalating sexual violence and rape among Indian sex workers (Go et al., 2011; Kumar 2003). A study among Indian sex workers found that clients had been under the influence of alcohol in advance of violence, underscoring how alcohol functions as a facilitator for men's propensity towards and enactment of violence (Kumar 2003).

HIV Prevention Interventions for Sex Workers

Given the scope and geographic range of the HIV epidemic among female sex workers in India, there have been an extensive number of HIV prevention interventions targeting female sex workers since 1995. As of 2004, of the 835 government-supported targeted intervention programs for high-risk individuals in India, 199 (23.8%) target female sex workers (Dandona, Dandona et al. 2005). (Rao, Thomas et al. 2009). Indian sex workers have established some of the best examples in the world in terms of their holistic approach, empowerment and involvement of female sex workers, and sustainability. Sex worker community-led interventions among female sex workers have been successful in providing this environment by addressing issues such as lack of prevention information, access to condoms, and negotiating with brokers such as brothel owners (Basu, Jana et al. 2004). Sangram is an NGO based in the Sangli district, and works to further sex workers' human rights through advocacy and programming, including a sex worker initiated collective, VAMP, that has been conducting peer interventions for the past 15 years (http://www.sangram.org).

One of the largest and most successful sex worker organizations in India is the Durbar Mahila Samanwaya Committee (DMSC) in Kolkata (http://www.durbar.org). DMSC represents 65,000 male, female, and transgender sex workers with the mission of "identifying and challenging the underlying socio-structural factors that help perpetuate stigma material deprivation and social exclusion of sex-workers." Their explicit political objective is to "establish the rights of sex workers as workers." DMSC collective is sex worker-led and manages all intervention efforts with an emphasis on respect for sex workers; reliance on them to run programs; and recognition of their professional ability and agency. Through DMSC, a consumer co-operative society, Usha, was registered with the government, marking the first time that such a sex worker organization was registered in West Bengal. A number of programs are run through Usha, including a micro-credit program for sex workers, an alternative jobs program for retired sex workers, and a condom social marketing campaign.

The DMSC's Sonogachi Project is one of the best examples of a comprehensive empowerment approach and celebrates its 20th year of operation in 2012. The Sonagachi Project addresses multiple economic, social, and health needs of the 20,000 sex workers and their families, including, peer outreach, medical clinics, a support group for HIV-infected sex workers, banking cooperatives, a dance drama troupe, several schools for children of sex workers, sex worker trainings in negotiation with clients and brokers (i.e., brothel owners), and advocacy for reproductive health rights.(Ghose, Swendeman et al. 2008). It also provides community-level HIV and STI prevention and management within the context of an occupational health and safety standards public health approach

The relatively lower HIV estimate of 10% among female sex workers in Calcutta, compared to 50–90% during the late 1990s in Bombay, Delhi, and Chennai, is attributed to the success of Sonagachi (Gangakhedkar, Bentley et al. 1997; Basu, Jana et al. 2004). The project has been replicated in 49 sites throughout West Bengal where it has been shown to increase condom use. (Basu, Jana et al. 2004; Chakrabarty 2004) Early evaluations demonstrated Sonagachi's success. Between 1992 and 1995, condom use among sex workers rose from 27% to 82%. By 2001, it was 86% (Dutta, Mandel et al. 2002). HIV prevalence among sex workers in the area fell from 11% in 2001 to less than 4% by 2004 (UNAIDS 2005).

In 2003, the Bill and Melinda Gates Foundation funded the 'Avahan Initiative,' which aimed to build an HIV prevention model to scale in with the Indian HIV epidemic, controlling HIV spread in the higher prevalence states of India by concentrating prevention activities among high-risk groups in six high risk states (Tamil Nadu, Karnataka, Andhra Pradesh, Maharashtra, Nagaland, and Manipur) (Chandrasekaran, Dallabetta et al. 2008; Verma, Shekhar et al. 2010). Avahan aimed to impact the Indian HIV epidemic through high coverage across the communities hardest hit by HIV. Avahan targeted female sex workers, high-risk men who have sex with men, transgendered persons, and people who inject drugs. The core package included peer educator led behavior change communication, free clinical services to treat STIs, provision of condoms and needle exchange, and linkages to care. Female sex worker-related programs targeted female sex workers and their clients, in an effort to create an enabling environment for the adoption of safer sex practices. Community mobilization was used to implement these programs, and their effects were assessed through a series of district-level cross-sectional surveys assessing behavioral and biological endpoints (IBBA). The initiative resulted in the creation of an additional 274 community outreach settings in clinics in 77 districts. By December 2008, Avahan had reached 350,000 female sex workers and 100,000 men who have sex with mens through various programs (Chandrasekaran, Dallabetta et al. 2008). In meetings its broad agenda, Avahan has worked with hundreds of grassroots NGOs and thousands of peer educators. An initial impact assessment estimates that 100,178 HIV infections have been prevented at the population-level as a result of these efforts (Xu, Brown et al. 2011).

Coverage and Access to HIV Prevention Services. An estimated 53.1% of the female sex worker population in India has been reached by targeted

HIV interventions, compared to 74% of injection drug users and 78% of men who have sex with men (NACO 2010). Coverage has varied greatly by state with 10.2% of female sex workers reporting exposure to HIV prevention programs in Uttar Pradesh compared to 89.5% in Tamil Nadu (NACO 2010). One potential success of interventions targeting female sex workers may be reflected in the high levels of reported condom use among this population. Over 99% of female sex workers surveyed in Andhra Pradesh, Karnataka, and Maharashtra reported using a condom with their last paying client—(NACO 2010). However, given the HIV prevalence in these settings and the low levels of consistent condom use reported by clients of sex workers (NARI 2007), the potential limitations of these estimates must be noted. Notably, a smaller percentage of female sex workers in these same states reported consistent condom use with non-regular paying clients (Andhra Pradesh: 83%; Karnataka: 78%; Maharashtra: 74.6%) (NACO 2010). Levels of HIV testing, on the other hand, vary. The percentage of female sex workers who reported receiving an HIV test in the last 12 months and knowing their results ranged from 10.7% Uttar Pradesh to 74.1% in Andhra Pradesh. (NACO 2010) Misconceptions regarding transmission of HIV continue to be widespread. In each state surveyed, less than 50% of female sex workers were able to correctly identify ways of preventing sexual transmission of HIV and rejected major misconceptions about transmission. (NACO 2010)

Sex Worker Rights Organizations

India has a long-standing tradition of active non-governmental organizations (NGOs) that have enhanced the rights and well-being of a range of marginalized populations. In this tradition, a number of sex worker run NGOs across India were established against the backdrop of the HIV epidemic throughout the 1990s to further the health, human, and occupational rights of sex workers as well as to provide a forum that gives voice to sex workers. Although the Sonagachi Project is the most well known outside of India, a number of efforts throughout high prevalence states serve as examples of grass roots activism effecting change, a few of which are discussed above. Sex worker-run NGOS provide a venue in which sex workers set the agenda and engage in a number of activities including advocating for their legal rights and decriminalization of sex work, bringing attention to the extensive occurrence of police harassment, and leading educational seminars and workshops that raise awareness of sex worker empowerment among women involved in sex work.

Over the past decade, state and national conferences have provided forums for sex workers, policymakers, and law enforcement agencies to address sex workers rights. Such gatherings, which were held in Kerala and 2000 and 2003, raised public awareness and initiated a media debate on sexuality and morality (Jayasree 2004). These topics, which are taboo in India, are often the driving force of stigmatization and marginalization of sex workers and implicitly justify harassment and discrimination against sex workers. National efforts to modify ITPA and decriminalize sex work have been led by the Lawyer's Collective as well as the National Network of Sex Workers' Organizations.

Building on the successes of DMSC, Ashodaya Samithi (http://ashodaya. org/), a sex worker collective based in Mysore and Mandya districts, was initiated in 2004 through the Avahan Initiative. The organization, which was implemented by Karnataka Health Promotion Trust with funding from the Bill and Melinda Gates Foundation, reports 1800 active members located in Mysore and Mandya districts. Their stated objectives include: to "ensure, economic, social political and legal equality" for sex workers, to "engage in all forms of democratic activity alone or in collaboration with organizations and individuals with similar aims and uphold the rights and serve the need of sex workers", and to "strive for emancipation of sex workers from any form of exploitation, oppression, atrocities, and injustice". Programs run through Ashodaya Samithi include community mobilization and advocacy, STI services, health education, and literacy classes. The organization has further developed a learning site to share best practices in community mobilization among marginalized communities.

Gaps in Research and Practice

The sex worker community response to the Indian HIV epidemic is one of the most impressive in the world. The rise of HIV among Indian sex workers was met with a number of human rights, community-based organization that addressed a broad range of distal and proximal factors to reduce the burden of HIV among sex workers. Additionally, India provides an incredible example Government and private foundations, such as the Bill and Melinda Gates Foundation, have spent hundreds of millions of U.S. dollars to both document the nature of this complex epidemic and to respond through innovative and scaled up programs. Avahan programs are slated to be transitioned to the Indian government and community partners. The success of these transitions will greatly depend of the very nature of the transition, including how the community is involved in the process. Given the success of sex worker initiated efforts, their sustainability is key in turning the tide of the HVI epidemic among Indian sex workers.

Given the scope of the epidemic as well as the response over the past decades, India is likely one of the best examples of a country establishing extensive surveillance in a multipronged approach as well as funding numerous sustainable interventions. Generic ARTs are available in India, costing less than $1 USD per day. Access to these drugs could be improved, as even this modest cost is high for many Indians. Access to treatment could be incorporated into the extensive clinical and community infrastructure that has been established through the Indian Government, NGOs, and donors.

Although community mobilization efforts have helped to create an enabling environment for sex workers to access HIV prevention services in India, persisting stigma and discrimination as well as laws that indirectly criminalize sex work continue to increase female sex workers' risk for STIs and hinder their ability to access these services. There are currently no non-discrimination laws or regulations that specify protections for sex workers. Additionally, there are extensive gaps in research related to male and transgender sex workers.

Kenya

Introduction

Key Themes

- Though HIV prevalence in Kenya has been in decline in recent years since its peak in 2000, HIV prevalence among female sex workers remains extremely high at approximately 45%.
- The Kenyan Government has recognized the disproportionate burden of HIV among female sex workers and developed National Guidelines for HIV/STI Prevention among sex workers.
- Criminalization, as well as, stigma discrimination and violence are barriers to access to HIV prevention, treatment, and care services among Kenyan sex workers.

Kenya has a population of 39 million people and remains the largest economy in East Africa with a GDP of nearly 30 billion USD as compared to approximately 21 billion in Tanzania and 16 billion in Uganda. Kenya is at the upper end of low-income countries as defined by the World Bank with a GDP per Capita of 738 USD and a purchasing power parity that has been steady at $1,600 USD. The United Nations (UN) human development index of Kenya has been slowly increasing by 0.5% per year from 0.404–0.470 equating to a current rank of 128/169 countries and above the average of Sub-Saharan African countries (Beyrer 2011).

Historical Perspectives on and Trends of the HIV Epidemic and Response. The first case of HIV was estimated to have occurred in 1978 with the first AIDS case officially reported in 1984 (Kawewa 2005). The first and most clearly identified risk factor related to HIV infection at that time was sex work

(Kawewa 2005). By 1986, 286 cases had been observed with 38 AIDS-related deaths. The epidemic became generalized in the coming years and sentinel surveillance systems demonstrated prevalence of 5.1% by 1990, peaking at 13.4% in 2000 (Kimani, Kaul et al. 2008). As of 2007, Kenya had between 1.4 and 1.8 million reproductive age adults living with HIV of which approximately 68% were women and most of whom were living in rural areas (UNAIDS 2010). The disproportionate burden of HIV among women in Kenya has remained consistent throughout the history of the epidemic. Since 2000, there has been a decline in estimated HIV prevalence in the general population with current prevalence estimated at approximately 6% among adults which is slightly lower than the 7% which was observed in the Kenyan AIDS Indicator Survey in 2003.(Cheluget, Baltazar et al. 2006) (DHS). These declines are especially apparent in urban sites and have corresponded with reductions in higher risk sexual practices in the general population, the scale up of ART, and improved HIV surveillance (Unaids 2005; Unaids 2008). HIV Prevalence remains twice as high among females as it does among males with an estimated 8% of reproductive age women living with HIV as compared to 4% among men. In addition, there remains great geographic heterogeneity in the HIV epidemic in Kenya. Nyanza Province has the highest prevalence at 13.9% which is approximately twice the prevalence of the next highest province of approximately 7% in Nairobi and Western and less than one percent of adults living with HIV in Northeastern Province.

The national response to the HIV epidemic has focused on heterosexual partnerships and vertical transmission from mother to child though there has recently been increased attention to specific vulnerable populations including sex workers, injecting drug users, and men who have sex with men (NASCOP 2009). Kenya's HIV response is delivered under the 'Three-Ones' framework developed at International Conference on AIDS and STIs in Africa which encourages a single national AIDS coordinating authority, a single AIDS action framework to coordinate the work of partners, and a single national monitoring and evaluation system (NASCOP 2009). As part of this response, Kenya has adopted the third edition of the antiretroviral drug therapy treatment program that includes free treatment, though there is only 35% coverage among eligible HIV positive people in Kenya with a CD4 cutoff of 200 cells/ml (NASCOP 2009). As of December 2010, 430,000 people living with HIV were on treatment and 40,000 service providers have been supported to build additional capacity to continue scale up of treatment. While the most recent publicly available guidelines suggest a CD4 cutoff of 200 cells/ml, new guidelines adopting a cut off of 350 cells/ml are being adopted and operationalized. The strategy includes a focus on prevention-of-mother-to-child transmission (PMTCT) with counseling and testing in antenatal clinics in Kenya. Challenges remain in the implementation of this program as in 2006, only about 637,000 of the 1.5 million women in need of this program were appropriately tested. Approximately 60,000 women have tested positive for HIV infection, though less than 40% received appropriate treatment.

Nearly 98% of the entire HIV budget is derived from international donors including over 112 million USD already dispersed through the GF for HIV specifically in Kenya in addition to large scale investments as both a PEPFAR and Global Health Initiative focus country (Beyrer 2011). Specifically, the Government of Kenya contributed approximately 3.8 million USD in 2006/2007 out of a total of nearly 334 million USD total allocated to HIV (National Aids Control Council, World et al. 2009). More recently in 2009, the Kenyan National AIDS Council launched the third Kenya National AIDS Strategic Plan (KNASP III) (NASCOP 2009). The newest KNASP includes a significant component of prevention focused on most at risk populations given the increased understanding of the burden of HIV among these populations.

Scope, Typology, and Context of Sex Work

In Kenya specifically, according to the 2009 Kenyan Modes of Transmission (MoT) study, an estimated 14.1% of the national HIV infections to be among female sex workers and clients, ranging from 14.7% in Nairobi to 18.2% along the coastal region and 23.1% in Nyanza. While these estimates are based on mathematical models, they highlight that female sex work is a significant contributor to the HIV epidemic in Kenya.

Female sex workers commonly work at trucking stops along the trans-Africa highway and have been found to have HIV prevalence as high as 50% (Ferguson and Morris 2007; Morris, Morris et al. 2009). The MoT estimates that up to 6% of adult women report selling sex in Kenya; many of these women are also married and, while they use condoms with casual sexual partners, they are much less likely to use condoms with their regular male partners (National Aids Control Council, World et al. 2009). The populations of female sex workers are large with a recent capture-recapture population assessment approximating 1,350 sex workers in Kisumu alone (95% CI 1,261–1,443) (Vuylsteke, Vandenhoudt et al. 2010). Moreover, there are an estimated 8,000 female sex workers along the trans-Africa highway between Mombasa, Kenya and Kampala, Uganda, who report approximately 129 different sexual partners per year and approximately 634 annual sexual acts.

Map 3.5   Geographic Distribution of HIV Prevalence among Female Sex Workers in Kenya

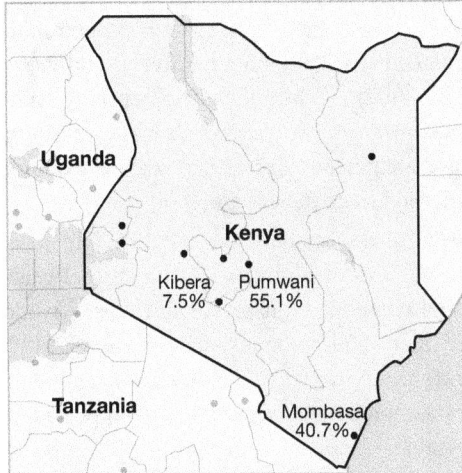

Source: Authors (developed from references HIV epidemiologic studies).

With these inputs, modeling exercises have estimated there to be an approximate 3200–4148 yearly HIV infections among sex workers along this highway which is significant in the context of the broader HIV epidemic in Kenya (Morris and Ferguson 2006). While not the focus of this assessment, drug use, including injection drug use, has also been increasingly recognized as an at-risk population in Kenya. To date, there has been a limited characterization of the role of drug use in increasing vulnerabilities to HIV and other sexually transmitted infections among sex workers in Kenya (Beckerleg, Telfer et al. 2005; Mathers, Degenhardt et al. 2008; Mathers, Degenhardt et al. 2010; Brodish, Singh et al. 2011).

Common Forms of Sex Work. There are three broad forms in which female sex workers in Kenya have been described in the literature including: self-defined sex workers working at established venues in urban centers; sex workers that sell sex on a part-time basis to supplement the household income; and those based along high volume transport corridors(Morison, Weiss et al. 2001; Hawken, Melis et al. 2002; McClelland, Hassan et al. 2006; Leclerc and Garenne 2008; Okal, Luchters et al. 2009; Singh, Brodish et al. 2011). HIV-related risks in terms of unprotected vaginal and anal intercourse and substance use are present among all three populations, though the interventions needed to address these risks need be individualized to each of these populations.

While the majority of studies presented throughout this case report have focused on full time female sex workers, there is an increasing amount of studies focused on part-time sex workers. A recent study by Hawken et al. explored part-time sex workers in a suburb of Mombasa (Hawken, Melis et al. 2002). These sex workers were described as part-time because their primary income is derived from other means including small businesses or more regular jobs. A convenience sample of 503 female sex workers reported an average of less than two partners per week, with an HIV prevalence of 30.6%. Condom use was low: 29% and 45% reporting never having used a condom with a client and non-paying partners, respectively. STIs were less common with 1.8% being infected with Gonorrhea, 4.2% with Chlamydia, and 2.0% with Syphilis (Hawken, Melis et al. 2002). While these women may have less sexual partners than full-time sex workers, trends towards less formal sex work may result in clients visiting a greater number of distinct sex workers which could also cause high transmission rates (Ghani and Aral 2005).

A geographical information systems assessment was completed to map patterns of sex work in the Northern Corridor highway that travels between Mombasa and Uganda, which demonstrated a high prevalence of sex work (Ferguson and Morris 2007). In 39 identified hot spots, an average of 2,400 trucks parked overnight where there were approximately 5,600 women in total. A further analysis of a convenience sample of sex workers (N=403) provided an estimate of 13.6 different clients and 54.2 sex acts in a month. One type of hot spot is related to places where mobility is delayed related to bureaucracy such as weigh bridges and border crossings. There are also hot spots that are exclusively directed to provide for the needs of travelers, such as the provision of fuel and food. Finally, there are certain truck stops that are integrated into urban centers including market centers (Morris and Ferguson 2006; Ferguson and Morris 2007). These truck stops are marked by at least one health care center at each of these facilities though the quality of and access to services is quite limited for sex workers and truckers. Access to HCT services are low and consequently there are low levels of HIV testing and knowledge with six percent of sex workers reporting a prior HIV test and 17% of truckers who were aware of their status. Moreover, there are a limited number of pharmacies available to provide appropriate antibiotics in response to sexually transmitted infections (Ferguson and Morris 2007). Further analyses of the context of sex work along this highway included an assessment of over 1,000 bars and lodgings (Morris, Morris et al. 2009). Only 26.8% of Kenyan sex workers reported 100% condom use, though these women reported higher rates of condom usage and access than Ugandan sex workers along the same highway.

Separate from populations of female sex workers, there have also been several epidemiological assessments of male sex workers. In fact, there is arguably more data characterizing self-identified male sex workers in Kenya than any other Sub-Saharan country (Geibel, van der Elst et al. 2007; Geibel, Luchters et al. 2008; Okal, Luchters et al. 2009). The majority of these studies have been completed in the context of studies evaluating men who have sex with men in Kenya, another identified vulnerable population in the country.

In an initial exploratory study of men who have sex with men, 14% reported sex work as their primary occupation (Sanders, Graham et al. 2007; Geibel, Luchters et al. 2008). In a sample of 285 men who have sex with men in Kenya, 74% reported selling sex for money or goods in the previous three months and 40% of these men reported buying sex during this same time frame(Sanders, Graham et al. 2006; Sanders, Graham et al. 2007). Only 17% of the sample reported not having bought or sold sex during the preceding 3 months. In a baseline behavioral study of 425 male sex workers sex, levels of HIV knowledge were very low, and alcohol was associated with lower levels of condom usage during sex work. A follow up study of 442 male sex workers completed after the provision of comprehensive preventive services. This study and intervention, to be discussed in greater detail, later in this chapter, demonstrated improvements across multiple domains of HIV risk status among male sex workers in Mombasa (Geibel, King'ola et al.). A population size estimation of male sex workers in Mombasa demonstrated a relatively large population of 739 men also in high need of basic preventive interventions. There is an emerging evidence of sex work among men who have sex with men in other settings such as Namibia, South Africa, Botswana, Lesotho, and Malawi though far more work is needed to characterize sex work among men who have sex with men in the African context (Smith, Tapsoba et al. 2009).

Legal and Policy Issues

There is limited peer-reviewed evidence evaluating structural risks affecting sex workers in Kenya. While sex work is common in Kenya, it is criminalized which ultimately limits the ability to characterize risk status among these populations as well as limits the possibility of providing comprehensive preventive services. In Kenya, the sale of sex is criminalized whereas the purchase of sex is not, exclusively targeting penalties at sex workers rather than clients.

A four country study completed by the African Sex Worker Alliance included Kenya assessed human rights violations and structural barriers to health care among female and male sex workers (Scorgie, Nakato et al. 2011). In this study, sexual violence was prevalent with common reports of police and related authorities being perpetrators of this violence. Gang rape by police was reported by both female and male SW and was also related to the need to commonly bribe the police. Police-perpetrated physical abuse was common as was humiliation during arrest including being forced to wear used condoms on their head or being publicly stripped. There are reports of a few female sex workers that have laid charges against the police in response to these abuses. However, these women report being bribed to drop these charges, or even abused, in response to the filing of these charges. Reports of arrest were common, but many reported being released before arriving at the station with by providing sexual favors or bribes and thus not formally charged. Detention was also reported with periods ranging from one week to as long as six months, and these reports were more common in eastern rather than southern African countries. The crime most commonly charged against female sex workers was related to loitering (Scorgie, Nakato et al. 2011). The study also demonstrated that health care access is limited and high prevalence of reported abusive or hostile interactions within health settings across the countries investigated, including Kenya. In response, female sex workers avoid health facilities where providers are known to be stigmatizing and tend to exclusively seek services at targeted and vertical services managed by community-based organizations (Scorgie, Nakato et al. 2011). While the results are not generalizable to the whole country of Kenya, they do indicate difficult contexts for HIV service provision and uptake for sex workers.

Epidemiology of and Risks Factors for HIV Among Sex Workers

Table 3.1 displays the recent prevalence trends of HIV among female sex workers in Kenya. The overall national prevalence of HIV among female sex workers in Kenya is approximately 45.1% (95% CI 43.4–46.8%), with ranges in prevalence from 3.4% to as high as 66.8%.

Table 3.1   Studies of HIV Prevalence among Female Sex Workers across Kenya, 2007–12

Year	Study design	Study location	Sample size	Number HIV positive	HIV prevalence	Reference
2011	Cohort	Mombasa	898	600	66.8%	McClelland, Richardson et al. 2011
2010	Cross-sectional	Mombasa	803	283	35.2%	Luchters, Vanden Broeck et al. 2010
2010	Cohort	Mombasa	148	5	3.4%	Tovanabutra, Sanders et al. 2010
2009	Cohort	Mombasa	176	55	31.3%	van der Elst, Okuku et al. 2009
2008	Cohort	Pumwani	2283	1279	56.0%	Kimani, Kaul et al. 2008
2008	Cross-sectional	Mombasa	991	317	32.0%	Chersich, Luchters et al. 2007
2008	Cohort	Kibera	466	35	7.5%	Hirbod, Kaul et al. 2008

(continued next page)

Table 3.1   *(continued)*

Year	Study design	Study location	Sample size	Number HIV positive	HIV prevalence	Reference
2008	Cohort	Pumwani	1090	580	53.2%	Lacap, Huntington et al. 2008
2007	Cross-sectional	Mombasa	689	249	36.1%	Chersich, Luchters et al. 2007
Total			7544	3403	45.1% (95% CI 43.4–46.8%)	

Source: Authors (developed from references HIV epidemiologic studies).
Note: CI = Confidence Interval.

In a prospective study of sex workers in Kenya, HSV-2 incidence of 23 cases per 100 person years was the highest observed for any population in the world (Chohan, Baeten et al. 2009). Genital ulcerative diseases, such as HSV-2, increased acquisition risks HIV by over 10 times with additional risk factors including recent entry into sex work, less frequent use of condoms, and working in a bar as compared to a night club (Chohan, Baeten et al. 2009).

Numerous harmful intravaginal practices have been reported among Kenyan sex workers including vaginal cleansing and the application of drying or astringent agents to the vagina preceding intercourse termed dry sex (Schwandt, Morris et al. 2006; Mehta, Moses et al. 2007; Low, Chersich et al. 2011). Such intravaginal practices can change natural vaginal flora including decreasing Lactobacillus colonization and cause enhanced epithelial damage during intercourse facilitating genital ulceration (Baeten, Hassan et al. 2009).

Figure 3.5   HIV Prevalence among Female Sex Workers in Kenya, 2007–12

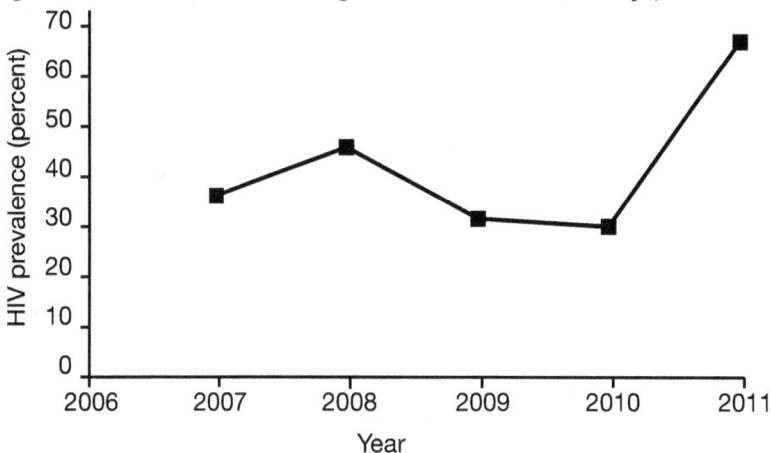

Source: Authors (developed from references HIV epidemiologic studies).

Among 147 participants randomly recruited from a prospective cohort of sex workers in Kenya, 36.1% reported having dry sex though most sex workers recognized that this was a higher risk sexual practice. Similar to anal intercourse, this sexual practice was nearly exclusively practiced during sex work rather than with spouse or committed partners. Among these women, dry sex was associated with lower rates of condom usage with both regular and causal clients (Schwandt, Morris et al. 2006). Vaginal cleansing is also extremely common. In a prospective study of 140 sex workers in Nairobi, 99% women reported vaginal cleansing in the previous 2 weeks for purposes of hygiene or to remove evidence of past coitus(Gallo, Sharma et al. 2010).

Anal intercourse has been established as a prevalent practice among female sex workers. Estimates of anal intercourse have ranged from 4.3% to over 40% of Kenyan sex workers with authors of the lower estimates interpreting that social desirability bias may cause underreporting of this sexual practice (Veldhuijzen, Ingabire et al. 2011). A study in Meru demonstrated that 40.8% (N=60/147) reported anal sex and that this was associated with reported symptoms of STI in previous year (OR 2.6, 95% CI 1.2–5.3) and higher risk sexual practices including lower levels of condom use (Schwandt, Morris et al. 2006). Notably, most sex workers charged higher rates for anal rather than vaginal intercourse and tended to nearly exclusively have anal intercourse (Schwandt, Morris et al. 2006). In Mombasa, anal intercourse was also recently reported by 4.3% (n=35/820) of a convenience sample of female sex workers with a HIV prevalence of 35.2% (95% CI 31.9–38.5). Reporting anal intercourse was also associated with higher numbers of partners (OR 2.2, 95% CI 1.1–4.3) and more inconsistent condom use (OR 2.1, 95% CI 1.1–4.2) (Veldhuijzen, Ingabire et al. 2011).

Knowledge of HIV serostatus and disease progression are associated with decreased high-risk sexual practices among sex workers in Kenya. The HIV-incidence in this group of women followed from 1993–2004 was 7.7%/100 person years (McClelland, Hassan et al. 2006). Reports of unprotected sex decreased from 27% in pre-seroconversion to 15% post-seroconversion (p<0.01) in these women. Overall there was a 31% decrease in reports of unprotected sex, an association that remained even in adjusted analyses (aOR 0.69, 95% CI 0.55–0.86) (McClelland, Hassan et al. 2006). Moreover with advanced HIV disease, as measured by lower CD4 counts, reported rates of unprotected sex continue to decrease in a dose-dependent manner (McClelland, Hassan et al. 2006).

Clients and Partners of Sex Workers. A recent study Ngugi et al compared 161 female sex workers in Kibera to 159 women in other occupations also living in Kibera (Ngugi, Benoit et al. 2011). Female sex workers reported a mean of over 5 partners in the last week as compared to a mean of less than 0.5 among women who are not sex workers. In this study, female sex workers reporting a romantic partner had less than 50% as many weekly sexual partners in both unadjusted and adjusted analyses. In addition, female sex workers were more likely to wear condoms with their sexual partners than were women who were not female sex workers.

Substance Use. Alcohol has also been established as being associated with high-risk sexual practices in multiple settings, including both high and low and middle income country settings. In the African context and Kenya specifically, the majority of data has been generated describing associations of alcohol use among adolescent populations and among sex workers. Investigators have employed different screening tools for alcohol abuse including the CAGE questionnaire (cite) and the Alcohol Use Disorders Identification Test (AUDIT) (Michel, Carrieri et al. 2010). Studies in Moshi, a rural district in the North of Tanzania, have also demonstrated increased risk of being HIV (aOR 3.1, 95% CI 1.1–8.9, P<0.05) or STI seropositive among sex workers (aOR 1.9, 95% CI 1.1–3.3, p<0.05) with alcohol use and further increased risk with alcohol abuse for both STI (aOR 3.6, 2.1–6.1, p<0.01) and HIV (aOR 4.0, 95% CI 1.6–10.2) (Norris, Kitali et al. 2009). These results corroborated earlier results from Tanzania demonstrating increased prevalence of high risk sexual practices associated with alcohol use and abuse (Mitsunaga and Larsen 2008). A study of 719 female sex workers in Kenya demonstrated 33.0% binge drinkers, 47% non-binge drinkers, and 22.4% lifetime abstainers from alcohol (Chersich, Luchters et al. 2007). When compared to non-binge drinkers, binge drinkers were more likely to report unprotected sex (aOR) 1.6, 95% CI 1.0–2.5) and sexual violence (a OR 1.9, 95% CI 1.3–2.7) and also carry higher burden of sexually transmitted infections. HIV prevalence was 39.9% in those who ever drank alcohol compared to 23.2% in abstainers (p<0.01). Other sexually transmitted infections were similarly higher among these women compared to alcohol abstainers (Chersich, Luchters et al. 2007).

HIV Prevention Interventions for Sex Workers

There are several ongoing HIV prevention, treatment, and care programs in place across Kenya with funding from both Global Fund grants as well as the United States Government through PEPFAR and USAID. Encouragingly, in September of 2010, the Kenyan National AIDS & STI Control Program (NASCOP) developed a set of National Guidelines for HIV/STI Programs for Sex Workers (NASCOP 2010). These guidelines were developed in response to the Kenya National HIV Strategic Plan (KNASP III) 2009–2013 identifying that female sex workers were a most at risk population and that there are barriers that limit their access to health and social services because some of their work is both criminalized and stigmatized in society (NASCOP 2009). These guidelines are progressive in that they are based in the following principles of respecting human rights, ensuring that interventions do no harm, and build capacity in the community of sex workers to facilitate participation and community ownership (NASCOP 2010).

The NASCOP HIV/STI Prevention Guidelines for Sex Workers in Kenya have biomedical, behavioral, and structural components. The biomedical components include HIV testing and counseling, STI screening and treatment, TB screening and referrals to treatment, and HIV care and treatment(NASCOP 2010). In addition, there is also a focus on reproductive health services including family planning, post-abortion services and cervical cancer screening. There are also urgent services including emergency contraception and post-exposure prophylaxis for HIV. Behavioral components including peer education and outreach, the distribution of condoms and condom-compatible lubricants, risk assessment with risk reduction counseling and skills building. Given the high levels of substance use among these women, there is a focus on the screening and treatment of drug and alcohol use. Structural components underpin this effort including services to mitigate sexual violence, psychosocial support, and family and social services. The services are intended to be implemented by peer educators, health workers, and other trained professionals.

Before the development of these national guidelines, the STD Control in Kenya Project was funded by the Canadian International Development Agency (CIDA)(Kimani, Kaul et al. 2008; Land, Luo et al. 2008; Oyugi, Vouriot et al. 2009). This project represented an implementation science project that refined and scaled-up the methodologies that had been developed for working with sex workers, and applied them at the community level. These methodologies included the mobilization of sex workers through trained peer leaders who were themselves identified and chosen by the sex workers themselves, the development of outreach strategies for working in the community, providing a comprehensive service that included both education messages and well as clinical care, and by bringing the sex workers together regularly in gatherings (locally called barazas), where they received feedback on the research studies, shared experiences, receive educational messages, and strengthened their own feelings of self-worth and esteem through group support (Ngugi, Wilson et al. 1996).

On a clinical level, the STD Control in Kenya Project was instrumental in establishing the guidelines for the syndromic treatment of STIs in Kenya, and establishing syndromic management as part of the national STI Control Programme (NASCOP) health policy. In 2005, the University of Manitoba and University of Nairobi group won a grant from PEPFAR, which allowed it not only to provide antiretroviral medication (ART) to its HIV-positive research population and their families, but also to expand the reach of its sex worker prevention activities. The two clinics in Majengo and Pumwani covered only a small portion of Nairobi, and were not close to some of the major "hot spots" in the city, so the group expanded to two existing City Council clinics in Baba Dogo and Korogocho slums, and also began intense mobilization activities within the Central Business District (CBD). However, by 2007 it was seen that only a quarter of those sex workers reached in the CBD ever found their way to the Majengo clinic, the remainder citing distance, disinterest in research participation, lack of bus fare, restricted opening hours and inconvenient location as reasons for not accessing the services available. What was needed was a clinic in the CBD specifically targeted to sex workers that could provide friendly, accessible and comprehensive STI/HIV care and services. The Sex Worker Outreach Programme Clinic, which quickly became known as the SWOP Clinic, opened its doors in August 2008. This is borne out by the numbers of clients who have come to the SWOP Clinic from all over Nairobi. By March 31, 2011, 20,717 clinical visits with sex workers had recorded by the SWOP Clinic alone, including 340 male sex workers, 6,515 had an HIV test for the first time (with about 28% testing positive), 825 had been initiated on ARTs and more than 3 million condoms had been distributed. Including the four other clinics also under the University of Manitoba / University of Nairobi PEPFAR program, 3,788 HIV-positive clients are on ART, with another 8,226 being followed, most of whom are sex workers.

The model of the SWOP services is focused on comprehensive service delivery including the a wide range of sexual and reproductive health services are offered, which represent what is generally considered to be a reasonable package of HIV prevention, care and treatment package for sex workers. This package includes information on safer sex practices, condom information, demonstration on use and provision, HIV testing and counseling, STI screening and treatment, risk reduction counseling services, ART and HIV basic care, family planning information and provision, TB screening and referral, Post-exposure prophylaxis (PEP) and emergency contraceptive provision, and Psychosocial support and referral.

Separate from this, Liverpool VCT (LVCT) has been providing services for sex workers in several regions of the country including Nairobi, Coastal Kenya, and Nyanza. LVCT has adopted a comprehensive package of services and focused providing these services in community setting as opposed to the centrally in clinics. These community settings have included moonlight settings or night events, and bars and night clubs with specific municipalities including Mlolongo, Thika, Huruma, Busia, Korogocho, and urban Nairobi.

While there are similarities in the package of services with the SWOP model, these services also include structural approaches such as information about gender based violence, as well as complementary services such as screening for tuberculosis. This program reached approximately 569 individual sex workers with high rates of observed HIV prevalence and STI prevalence. The benefits of these services were that there were limited barriers to service access including geographic or cost barriers. In addition, referrals were effective given that partnerships were developed with MOH facilities and private clinics in the area. There was a significant focus on creating an enabling environment for sex workers to facilitate open discussion of complicated health and rights issues including post-abortion trauma, substance use, and gender based violence.

The International Center for Reproductive Health in partnership with the Population Council also completed an evaluation of a multilevel intervention targeting male sex workers in Mombasa. Starting with the opening of a drop-in center for men who have sex with men in Mombasa, ICRH then trained 40 peer educators in HIV prevention in 2007—six of which were trained as HCT counselors (Geibel, King'ola et al.). These peer educators also received information about harm reduction in the context of alcohol and drugs. In addition, there was a significant effort to distribute condoms and water-based lubricants to sex workers. In total, over 100,000 condoms and 8,000 sachets of water-based lubricants were distributed. Given the significant uptake of lubricants, a further 20,000 sachets were ordered. The intervention also targeted the health sector with 20 service providers receiving sensitization training as well as clinical training on the specific needs of men who have sex with men including anal STIs. This study demonstrated significant increases in the knowledge and use of condoms and lubricants. In addition, there were significant increases in the uptake of HCT and the use of male sex worker-friendly clinical services. This study also demonstrated that in bivariate analyses, consistent condom use among male sex workers was significantly associated with exposure to peer educators, the use of men who have sex with men-friendly drop-in centers, and ever having been counseled or tested for HIV(Angala, Parkinson et al.; Horizons 2006).

Sex Worker Rights Organizations

There are several active service provision and advocacy entities for sex workers in Kenya including Liverpool Voluntary Counseling and Testing (Liverpool VCT), the International Centre for Reproductive Health (ICRH), the Bar Hostess Empowerment and Support Programme, African Sex Worker Alliance, and Sex Workers' Education and Advocacy Taskforce (SWEAT).

Gaps in Research and Practice

There is limited trend data available on the number of sex workers and patterns of sex work. Moreover, there is limited coverage data of HIV treatment and prevention programs among sex workers available in Kenya. Separately, the majority of peer-reviewed publications exploring risks of sex workers in Kenya have focused on the burden of disease including HIV prevalence and incidence along with individual-level risk factors or associations of infection. In reviewing the literature, there is a limited body of data characterizing higher order, structural, risk factors such as police-mediated violence and the relationship between these and HIV risk practices and burden of disease. In addition, while there is a relatively large body of data available characterizing HIV risk among male sex workers, there is only preliminary data on HIV prevention programs for these men. There is also no HIV prevalence data, known to the authors, characterizing the burden of HIV disease or effective HIV prevention strategies among transgender sex workers in the Kenyan context.

Nigeria

Introduction

Key Themes

• Female sex workers, both brothel-based and non-brothel based, have the highest prevalence of HIV of any sub-population within Nigeria.

• Men who serve in mobile occupations, such as truck drivers, police officers, and others are often the main client types for sex workers and are also vulnerable to HIV infection, warranting attention by HIV prevention programs.

• Criminalization of sex work, strong religious convictions, and inequitable gender norms within the general population, challenge sex workers' well-being and access to HIV prevention.

Since the identification of the first AIDS case in Federal Republic of Nigeria in 1986, the prevalence of HIV has noticeably increased from 1.8% in 1991 to its peak at 5.8% in 2001, the same year the government signed the Declaration of the Commitment on HIV and AIDS (National Agency for the Control of AIDS 2008). The current prevalence is now estimated at 3.6% (CI: 3.3–4.0%) (UNAIDS 2009). Accounting for approximately 9% of the global burden of HIV, Nigeria has the second highest number of people living with HIV worldwide (UNAIDS 2009).

The most populous country in Africa (total 2010 adult pop. 152 million), Nigeria is situated in West Africa and bordered by the Gulf of Guinea and by Cameroon, Niger, Chad, and Benin (Bureau of African Affairs 2011). Such a geographic orientation facilitates movement between countries (e.g., women may travel from Nigeria to Benin) and has implications for sex work and HIV prevention as sex workers are mobile and may migrate between countries and may face challenges in accessing HIV prevention and care services.

The expanse of this country is complemented by rich ethnic diversity, which is composed of over 250 ethnic groups, the majority which includes Hausa, Fulani, Yoruba, and Igbo. These four ethnic groups contribute four most common indigenous languages, in addition to the 500 other indigenous languages and to English, the official language in Nigeria (Bureau of African Affairs 2011; Central Intelligence Agency 2011). Fifty percent of the country is Muslim, whose presence is predominantly in the North, followed closely by Christian (40%) and indigenous religions (Steiner 2002; Bureau of African Affairs 2011; Central Intelligence Agency 2011). Religious and ethnic differences have led to underlying tensions and overt conflicts and have resulted in approximately 27,000 refugee and asylum seekers (UNHCR 2011) and an unknown number of internally displaced persons (Internal Displacement Monitoring Centre 2010).

During the start of the HIV epidemic, Nigeria was also experiencing a period of great social and political change. It was not until 1999 that a new democratic constitution was adopted following British rule that lasted until 1960 and then 16 years of military rule (National Agency for the Control of AIDS 2008; Central Intelligence Agency 2011). Within this context, and combined with endemic poverty, low levels of education, prevalence of other infectious diseases, Nigeria is in the throes of a complex epidemic. HIV is generalized among the adult population while high prevalence of infection is observed among vulnerable populations.

Historical Perspectives and Trends of the HIV Epidemic in Nigeria. Following the 2000 development of the Presidential Committee on AIDS and the National Action Committee on AIDS (NACA), which has now been transformed to the Agency for Control of AIDS), the HIV/AIDS Emergency Action Plan was developed with specific focus on prevention, care and support, and the creation of an enabling environment for community-based response. To enhance national efforts, Nigeria became a signing member of the Declaration of the Commitment on HIV and AIDS and the agreement to aim to achieve the consensus on a comprehensive framework to achieve the Millennium Development Goals of halting HIV epidemic by 2015. The national roadmap was developed in 2006 for scale-up for Universal Access to

HIV prevention, treatment, and care, that have since been incorporated and coordinated at the national, state, and local levels (National Agency for the Control of AIDS 2008). Additional steps towards addressing the vulnerability of women and girls have been taken by the National Women Coalition Against AIDS (NAWOCA), though, as of 2007, only four states had endorsed these efforts. Since this time, state chapters have been established with initiatives largely led by state governors and their wives, including in Cross River State (Ighodaro 2009), Lagos, Ekiti, Ondo, Ogun, Osun (2008), Anambra State (Anambra State Governor's Office 2011), Kaduna, Kano, Katsina, Kebbi, Zamfara, Sokoto, and Jigawa (2008).

Several policies, such as HIV/AIDS policies, National Workplace Policy on HIV and AIDS, and the National Reproductive Health policy have been adopted, while others, such as the National Gender Policy and the National Policy on Stigma and Discrimination for PLHIV have not yet been signed and ratified (National Agency for the Control of AIDS 2008). Since the review of the earlier National Strategic Framework (NSF), the new 2010–15 NSF has been revised to include the following policy domains: 1) Prevention of new infections and behavior change; 2) Treatment of HIV/AIDS and related health problems; 3) Care and support for people living with and affected by AIDS; 4) Institutional architecture and resourcing; 5) Advocacy, legal issues and human rights, and 6) Monitoring and evaluation (NACA 2010). Additionally, civil society organizations implement preventive interventions, including condom promotion and increased access to services, for vulnerable populations (National Agency for the Control of AIDS 2010).

The Federal Ministry of Health has made efforts to begin surveillance and track the HIV epidemic through clinic-based and population-based surveillance systems and, of four main survey systems, has developed the HIV/STI Integrated Biological and Behavioral Surveillance Survey (IBBSS) to focus on sexually transmitted infections and behaviors among vulnerable populations, including sex workers, men who have sex with men, injecting drug user, prison inmates, military servicemen, and transport workers (Federal Ministry of Health [Nigeria] 2008; National Agency for the Control of AIDS 2010; Federal Ministry of Health [Nigeria] 2011).

With the compilation of the first Integrated Biobehavioral Surveillance Survey (IBBSS) in 2007 and the 2009 Modes of Transmission Study (MOT), commissioned by the government, more attention turned to the increased vulnerability, risk, and prevalence of HIV among female sex workers as well as other at-risk populations, such as men who have sex with men, injecting drug users, prison inmates, military servicemen, and transport workers (National Agency for the Control of AIDS 2008; National Agency for the Control of AIDS 2010). Though these populations are estimated to comprise only one percent of the population, 40% of new infections are estimated to be associated with HIV risk behaviors among these groups and their sexual partners. Female sex workers bear the greatest burden of HIV infection among the groups with estimated prevalence ranging from 8.3 to 46% (National Agency for the Control of AIDS 2010) and HIV incidence was estimated between 11.97 to 12.36% among female sex workers in Nasarawa State in 2006 (Forbi, Entonu et al. 2011). Despite these findings and the feminization of the HIV epidemic, experts assert that little action was taken to prevent HIV transmission among women until those women who were not female sex workers started becoming infected (Garcia-Moreno 1996; Aniekwu 2002).

Figure 3.6   National Estimates of HIV Prevalence among Key Populations, 2010

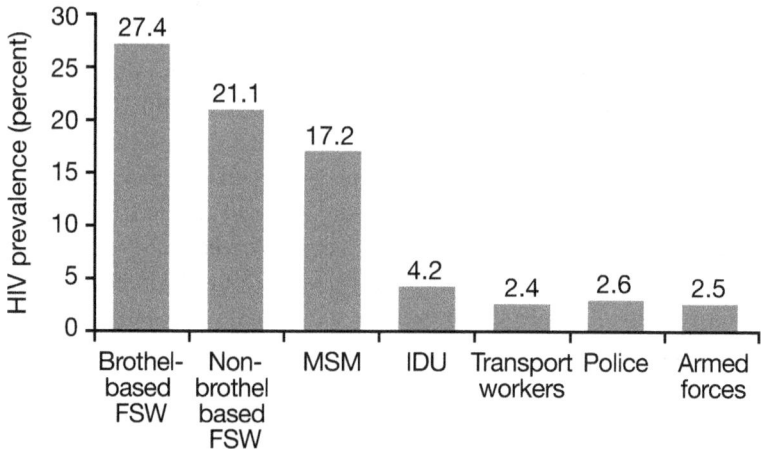

Source: Federal Ministry of Health (Nigeria) 2011.
Note: FSW = female sex worker; IDU = injecting drug user; MSM = men who have sex with men.

Scope, Typology, and Context of Sex Work

Sex work in Nigeria varies by geographic and social contexts, across the spectrum of formal or part-time sex work, and according to the level of acknowledgement and social acceptance of sex work. Differences in HIV prevalence and risk behaviors are observed between the different types of sex work as well as by geography.

Sex work in Nigeria is criminalized, less socially accepted and even condemned among more Islamic and Christian communities (Munoz, Adedimeji et al. 2010). In cities, sex-work may be brothel-based or organized within hotels and bars. This organization provides a situation that is easier to assess by HIV surveillance methods, as with the IBBSS, due to visibility of venues, peer networks, and self-identification as a sex worker whereas as in less formal situations, sex work may be conducted on the streets or in homes and thus more challenging for research and HIV surveillance (Munoz, Adedimeji et al. 2010; Oyefara 2007).

Common Forms of Sex Work. Brothels are typically characterized by an organizational structure led by the director, who owns the brothel, followed by a co-director and/or manager who assign the clients as well as runs the brothel, and a chairlady, who is a sex worker herself (Munoz, Adedimeji et al. 2010). An overview of brothel-based sex work in Lagos, the commercial capital of Nigeria, highlighted the presence of brothels across a variety of geographical and economic strata, ranging from lower economic slum areas to more affluent peri-urban areas. These venues may include hotels where sex workers take residence or brothels that house anywhere from four to 180 sex workers (Oyefara 2007). This environment varies geographically; for example, brothels in Ibadan have approximately 30 to 60 rooms for the sex workers, and women who cannot afford to rent a room on their own typically share with other women (Munoz, Adedimeji et al. 2010).

Map 3.6   Prevalence of HIV Infection among Brothel-Based Sex Workers by State in Nigeria, 2010

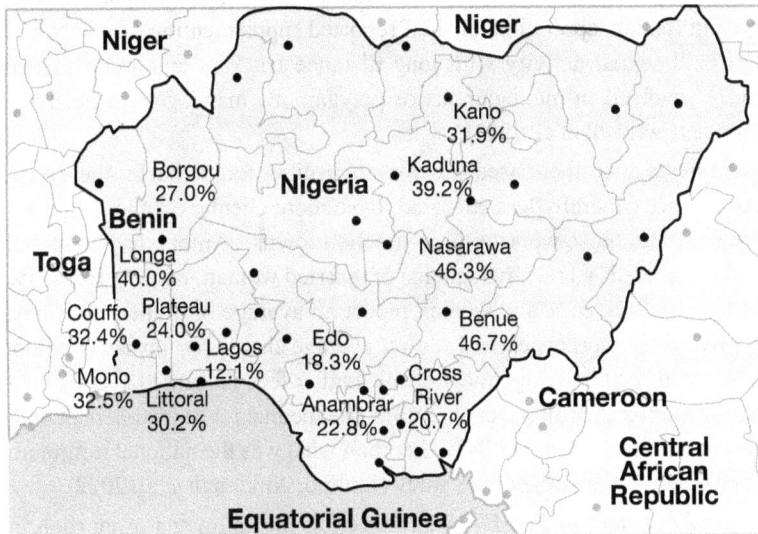

Source: Federal Ministry of Health (Nigeria) 2011

The population of brothel-based sex workers is a diverse one. In Enungu State, the majority (61.2%) of brothel-based sex workers interviewed for a survey of HIV knowledge and prevention practices reported working only in the sex work while smaller percentages supplemented their incomes with additional trades (15.7%) or were students (7.5%)(Onyeneho 2009). A similar study of brothel based sex workers in Lagos found that young women (20–24 years) represented 42.5% of the sex worker population (Oyefara 2007).

As observed across much of Africa, the history of road transport across Nigeria has led to the development of a social situation that allows for informal sex work to develop in relationship to this transport system. The Nigerian Transport Study was one of the first endeavors to study and describe the social factors and risk for HIV transmission in this context (Orubuloye, Caldwell et al. 1993). Along night truck stops, known as lorry parks, markets and 'junction' towns have developed to provide goods and services for long-haul truckers and truckers regularly stayed at the homes of local families; as a result truckers developed relationships with and financially supported local female hawkers (women who sell goods from portable trays balanced on their head or from temporary stalls in markets and often sell sex as well) and/or female residents of the guest houses of each town where they rest (Orubuloye, Caldwell et al. 1993). Brothels also exist in these towns, though a majority of transactional sex occurs in this informal setting. These women, however, may not necessarily identify as female sex workers. Among 467 female hawkers surveyed in Ibadan, approximately half reported supplementing their incomes through paid sexual activity with long distance truckers and some 14 and 13% were involved in monogamous or polygamous marriages, respectively (Orubuloye, Caldwell et al. 1993).

Assessments of brothel-based sex workers in cities found that brothel-based sex workers are generally less educated, have more clients, earn less, and are at more risk than those working in in junction towns. Among brothel-based sex workers, there is a lower percentage of married women, ranging from 11% (Onyeneho 2009) to 55% and women report an average of 4 clients per day. Brothel-based sex workers earned a lower average charge per sex act (Ladipo, Ankomah et al. 2002), though may receive higher fees for sexual acts without a condom (Munoz, Adedimeji et al. 2010). The income for sex workers in both settings, however, is substantially higher than what was the national minimum wage per month, at the time of the study (Ladipo, Ankomah et al. 2002).

Clients and Partners of Sex Workers. Overall, the estimated proportion in men reporting paying for sex has hovered around 10%, though has shown slight declines since 2005 (Carael, Slaymaker et al. 2006; Futures Group International 2010).

Early research demonstrated that a great proportion of sex work in Nigeria was associated with male clients' occupations that involve transportation and long durations spent away from home, such as trucking, oil production, and naval service; factors which are still fairly consistent today. This can encourage an establishment of relationships, either temporary or long-term, in transit or destination areas. Men in these occupations constitute a majority of the sex worker's clientele; for example, truckers may be the predominant clients in junction towns that are geographically distant from other areas of commerce. Seventy-eight percent of the male clients surveyed in the Nigerian Transport study were married, half of whom were involved in a polygamous marriage, spend approximately nine days away from home during trips, and have an average of 6.3 current partners with approximately 25 lifetime partners. Though all truckers were knowledgeable of HIV, only half had ever used a condom and 15% used them on a regular basis (Orubuloye, Caldwell et al. 1993).

A study of Naval personnel in Lagos found that 32.5% reported sexual contact with female sex workers and 19.9% within the last six months. These men reported an average of 5 lifetime partners and approximately 69.2% of the female sex workers' clients from the Navy were married. Low condom use was reported among Naval workers as well, 41% of whom did not use a condom at last sex with a female sex worker, and a majority reported being under the influence of alcohol at the time (Nwokoji and Ajuwon 2004). Low condom use may be an outcome of the high proportion of naval personnel who felt that they were not at their risk for HIV was low (68.8.%) and the perception that multiple partnerships is a tradition of naval officers, is common (Nwokoji and Ajuwon 2004). Through the course of qualitative research, investigators further found that naval personnel rejected condoms because of decreased sensation and pleasure, alcohol use, and the physical barrier between male and female partners (Nwokoji and Ajuwon 2004).

The 2010 IBBSS most recently reported lower figures of sex with sex workers in the last 12 months among these client groups, ranging from 5.0 to 8.9 among armed forces, transport workers and police, which may suggest a decline in high risk sex or a reporting bias. Nevertheless, the low proportions of these men who demonstrate accurate HIV knowledge (29.6 to 57.9%), suggests that interventions involving clients, particularly these occupational groups, are warranted (Federal Ministry of Health [Nigeria] 2011).

These findings highlight the cultural norms that influence sexual partnerships and potential risks. They further suggest that traditional concepts of sex work and risks for HIV associated with sex work, as utilized for HIV risk assessments and interventions, may under- or overestimate risk and miss some key populations, depending on the setting and surveillance methods employed.

Male Sex Workers. The population of male sex work has generally been assessed within the population of men who have sex with men. The prevalence of HIV among men who have sex with men is increasing in Nigeria with most recent estimates from the 2010 IBBSS suggesting a prevalence of 17.2% (Federal Ministry of Health [Nigeria] 2011). A cross-sectional study among men who have sex with men in Lagos and Kanos found that 24.4% and 36.0%, respectively, had sold sex to other men. These men also reported a range of 1–6 non-paying partners and a little less than 6.5% of the total sample of men who have sex with men had purchased sex from a female sex worker (Merrigan, Azeez et al. 2011). Among men who have sex with men in this study, approximately 34% (adjusted) in both towns reported consistent condom use when selling sex (Merrigan, Azeez et al. 2011). These figures are fairly consistent with national estimates, though condom use at last sex with a paying partner was estimated at 52.8% among men who have sex with men, according to national estimates. HIV testing, however, is more common among men who have sex with men than the general male population (34% compared to 15%, respectively) (Futures Group International 2010).

Legal and Policy Issues

The Penal Code, which governs the northern area of Nigeria, and the Criminal Code, which governs the south, both criminalize sex work in Nigeria (Onyeneho 2009). Though the existence of brothels is not rare in this country, criminal- ization of sex work forces sex workers underground and creates challenges for access to health and prevention services and also creates opportunity for violence against and exploitation of sex workers. As a result, brothels may be raided and women may experience a range of human rights abuses perpetrated by police and other officials including physical violence, harassment, being forced to provide sexual services, or blackmail (Munoz, Adedimeji et al. 2010). As a result, some brothels protect themselves by paying for protection from police or enforcement officers and, in some cases, officers may be involved in managing the brothel themselves (Munoz, Adedimeji et al. 2010). While the 2008 UNAIDS situation analysis indicated significant progress in the country as a whole with respect to response and scale-up of services, experts acknowledged the lack of access to services that remained among women and vulnerable populations, suggesting that criminalization of groups such as sex workers, men who have sex with men, and injecting drug users makes coverage of these populations particularly challenging (UNAIDS 2008).

Structural barriers facing sex workers are not only related to laws and policies but to religion as well. Sex workers in northern states may be further driven into hiding through the recent adoption of Muslim Sharia law that began in Zamfara State in the year 2000 and expanded to a total of 12 states in Northern Nigeria and which further bans sex work as well as homosexuality and pre-marital and extramarital sex (Pierce 2000; Onyeneho 2009). Punishments for these activities may range from flogging, amputation, stoning, to death for violation of the laws and have sentences for death by stoning have been reported for cases of extramarital sex and sodomy.(Steiner 2002; BBC News 2007)

Violence, Stigma and Discrimination.   In 2006, a report by Amnesty International documented the prevalence of rape against women and girls among the general population in Nigeria that is perpetrated by police and security forces while on and off duty. The stigma and blame that is often associated with rape and experience by victims has resulted in a lack of reporting which allows police to commit such violence without repercussion or justice. The report, in particular, highlighted the violence against sex workers, indicating that the criminalization of sex work creates an opportunity for police to raid streets frequented by sex workers, arresting and gang raping the women (Amnesty International 2006). Five years later, media continue to report on the culture of sexual violence against sex workers with impunity that exists within the police force that allows this trend to continue unchecked (see Box 3.1) (Salaudeen 2011).

Box 3.1   The Culture of Sexual Violence against Sex Workers
"Most often, the police will come to our brothel in the night, march us into their waiting van. They will take us to either Third Mainland Bridge or the Bar Beach. They will beat and rape us. They sleep with us without protection."
- Lagos Sex Worker
"Raping of sex workers is one of the fringe benefits attached to night patrol. We used to lobby for night patrol duties."
- Police Officer in the Ikeja Police Station
Source: Salaudeen 2011.

Violence perpetrated by clients is another one of many forms of violence that may be experienced by sex workers (Shannon and Csete 2010). Qualitative research was conducted among brothel-based, street working, and other informal sex workers in Abia State to specifically understand the experiences of violence and management/mitigation tactics of sex workers. Participants indicated fear of client violence—predominantly physical violence such as physical attack, murder, rape, torture, and ritual killings—in addition to sexually transmitted infections, as the greatest risks and potential for death of a sex worker. Women further reported being forced into unprotected sex or anal sex by clients, denied payment, or being paid with counterfeit money. With respect to condom use, women experienced clients who were uncooperative, sometimes violent, and even refused to use condoms when the woman suggested she may be infected with HIV and brutality may ensue if sex workers attempt to resist (Izugbara 2005).

Aside from clients, sex workers experience stigma and discrimination in the community and families as well. Women who are known or suspected to be involved in sex work may be viewed as sinful or indecent, called names, and further ostracized from the community or rejected by their families (Izugbara 2005). Opportunities for marriage may decline for known sex workers while risk of police arrest, detention and other forms of harassment may increase (Izugbara 2005).

A further challenge to addressing the HIV epidemic in the context of sex work is the general confusion of sex work with sexual exploitation and trafficking. In 2003, Nigeria was exposed as one of the major countries of origin for trafficked women and underage girls (Aborisade and Aderinto 2008) as well as a destination for trafficking victims from other African countries (UNODC 2009). These findings led to 2003 Trafficking in Persons (Prohibition) Law Enforcement and Administrative Act, the development of three specialized police forces led by the National Agency for the Prohibition of Traffic in Persons (NAPTIP) to enforce the law and identify and reintegrate victims (Aborisade and Aderinto 2008), and the 2006 development of the national action plan to combat trafficking (UNODC 2009). The development of the NAPTIP included a plan to rehabilitate and reintegrate trafficked victims and sex workers supported at the national and community levels. Though perhaps well intentioned from the perspective of those who are trafficked or seeking to provider services for trafficked women, a result of this program was the confounded perception that all sex work is associated with trafficking and meant that sex workers were enrolled into sexual trafficking rehabilitation programs with or without their consent or willingness. While positive results in the form of social rehabilitation may have been observed among women who were trafficked and willingly entered rehabilitation programs, others, predominantly female sex workers, were forced into rehabilitation programs or compulsory testing (Aborisade and Aderinto 2008). Non-consensual enrollment into rehabilitation programs are in violation of the human rights of those sex workers who were not trafficked and who did not agree to such enrollment.

Epidemiology and Risks Factors for HIV Among Sex Workers

In 1992, following a network and diffusion analysis of 488 men aged 15–50 in Ondo State, experts asserted that the slowly increasing HIV epidemic was different from what is observed in Sub-Saharan Africa. Based on this, it was assumed that the epidemic in Nigeria was not an epidemic with strong focus on sex work but likely related to the sexual diffusion within the population, despite the degree of sex work in Nigeria (Orubuloye, Caldwell et al. 1992). Since this time, however, the HIV epidemic has increased to a level that has brought Nigeria to the position of second highest number of people living with HIV worldwide and with very high HIV prevalence among sex workers in Nigeria (UNAIDS 2009).

Epidemiologic assessments report a range of prevalence of HIV among sex workers in Nigeria: peer reviewed publications report a range of 37 to 70% among sex workers (Munoz, Adedimeji et al. 2010; Forbi, Entonu et al. 2011) while national figures report an overall prevalence just less than 30% among female sex workers. These figures are in stark contrast to the 3.6% prevalence that is reported among the general population (2009). Figure 3.6 presents HIV prevalence trends, comparing national estimates of women screened during ANC visits (■) to the female sex work populations (▲ ▼) from 1991–2010. Recently, 900 female sex workers from 52 brothels in Nasarawa State were tested for HIV and incidence was estimated using the BED assay to prepare for a vaginal microbicide trial. Slightly lower than national estimates, the HIV prevalence was 37.2% among participants and, using two adjustment methods, the adjusted HIV incidence was estimated to be between 11.97% (95% CI: 8.51–15.43%) to 12.36% (8.18–16.34%) (Forbi, Entonu et al. 2011).

Based on IBBSS 2010, the highest prevalence of HIV was among female brothel-based sex workers (27.4%), closely followed by non-brothel-based sex workers (27.1%) (Federal Ministry of Health [Nigeria] 2011), figures that have dropped slightly since the IBBSS 2007 (Federal Ministry of Health [Nigeria] 2008). Among the nine surveyed states (Figure 3.7) , HIV prevalence was greatest among sex workers in Benue (46.7% among brothel-based and 27.5% among non-brothel based female sex workers) and Nasarawa (46.3% among brothel-based and 32.1% among non-brothel based female sex workers) (Federal Ministry of Health [Nigeria] 2011). In Kano, where HIV prevalence among injecting drug users is also high (4.9%), approximately 20% of the injecting drug user population reported sex with female sex workers (National Agency for the Control of AIDS 2010). Lowest prevalence estimates were observed in Lagos (12.1% among brothel-based and 13% among non-brothel based) (Federal Ministry of Health [Nigeria] 2011) where condom use with clients was reported above 98% among surveyed women (National Agency for the Control of AIDS 2010) as well as among non-brothel based sex workers in Cross River (8.3%) (Federal Ministry of Health [Nigeria] 2011).

Figure 3.7   HIV Prevalence among ANC Attendees and Female Sex Workers in Nigeria, 1991–2010

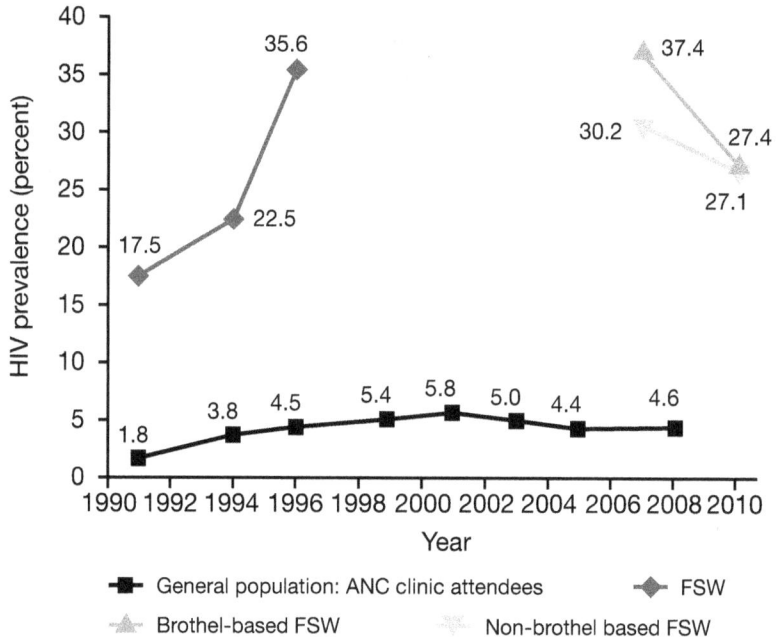

Source: National Agency for the Control of AIDS 2010.; IBBS, Federal Ministry of Health (Nigeria) 2008 and 2011.
Note: Surveillance data were not collected for female sex workers from 1999 to 2007; ANC = antenatal clinic; FSW = female sex worker.

Risk for HIV acquisition was only one of many perceived risks reported by younger sex workers who participated in qualitative interviews in Nigeria; these perceived risks also included violence, unwanted pregnancy, abortions, rape, STI, and being caught by police, though few had experienced any of these (Aderinto and Samuel 2008). Though HIV prevalence among the young population, in general has declined slightly over time (Futures Group

International 2010), the vulnerability of young female sex workers is as an important area of consideration for HIV programming.

Figure 3.8   Variations in HIV Prevalence by State and Type of Sex Work

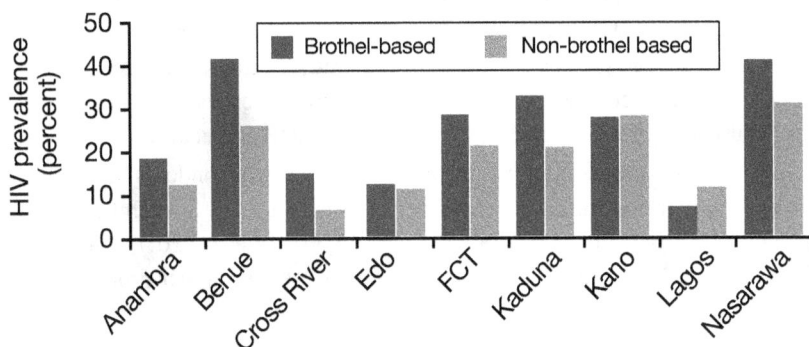

Source: Federal Ministry of Health (Nigeria) 2011.

The heightened risks for HIV among sex workers are also reflected in the overall reproductive health among sex workers in Nigeria. The most recent IBBSS reported that 15.7 and 24.4% of brothel-based sex workers and non-brothel based sex workers reported at least one STI symptom in the past 12 months (Federal Ministry of Health [Nigeria] 2011). These figures may approximate the findings of Oyefara and colleagues (2007) who demonstrated that approximately half of the sex workers surveyed reported having some type of STI during their time as a sex worker and 2.4% reported living with HIV. Unwanted pregnancy and induced abortions reported by this study also highlights other sexual health risks for sex workers, as 59.1% reported pregnancy during their course of sex work and 99.5% of these pregnancies underwent induced abortions, typically outside of modern hospitals (Oyefara 2007).

Condom Use.   Reported levels of condom use may be attributable to perceptions of HIV transmission risk and self-efficacy in addition to other environmental-structural factors which limit sex workers agency. Qualitative assessments from brothels in Ibadan, reported that women believed that only individuals who were unable to care for themselves would be infected with HIV and hence, did not consider themselves at risk (Munoz, Adedimeji et al. 2010). A large assessment of brothel-based sex workers found low numbers of women who know that a healthy looking person could be infected with HIV (24%) and only 39% knew that not using condoms could present risk for HIV transmission (Ladipo, Ankomah et al. 2002). Similarly, in the study conducted by Oyefara and colleagues, though all women had heard of HIV and knew of the male condom, 23.4% reported that condom use depended on the client's choice and 76.6% indicated that they would accept the client if he refused condoms (Oyefara 2007). While fewer women (3%) reported not using a condom at all, in a study conducted among brothel-based sex workers in Engugu State, 2006, women also reported that clients determined condom use, and some women reported practices such as douching with a salt solution if a condom was not used during intercourse (Onyeneho 2009). Across these studies, condom use decisions were often directed by the clients (Iyiani, Binns et al. 2011).

In Ajegunle, several factors, including low quality of condoms that resulted in breakage or painful sexual experiences, price, and low availability, served as additional barriers to condom use (Iyiani, Binns et al. 2011). Increased condom use self-efficacy translated to general use and higher proportions of sex workers in the cities reported consistent condom use compared to those in junction towns (58% compared to 43%) and 1/5 in junction towns had never used condoms (Ladipo, Ankomah et al. 2002). A later survey conducted among brothel-based sex workers in Enungu reported increased levels (96.2%) of condom use, though some 9.9% still reported prevention methods by washing after sex and 11.5% by prayers (Onyeneho 2009). Condom use may also vary by partner type, however, as IBBSS surveys indicated lower use during sexual relationships with boyfriends (38.1% in brothel based; 46.1% in non-brothel based) compared to casual paying partners (83.2% in brothel based and 84.8% in non brothel based)(Federal Ministry of Health [Nigeria] 2008). This difference in condoms use is also observed within marriages as cultural practices have placed men as the decision maker with respect to reproductive health and leave women without choice in when they will have sex or whether condoms can be used during sex (Iyiani, Binns et al. 2011).

Recent evidence from Nigeria also suggests the prevalence of violence and substance use and the influence this has on the use of condoms. Brothel-based sex workers in Ibadan reported that tactics used by clients ranged from subtle threats of taking business to another woman, use of alcohol and drugs for coercion, condom tampering and removal, to physical violence (Munoz, Adedimeji et al. 2010). Younger female sex workers were most often the recipients of these forms of violence (Munoz, Adedimeji et al. 2010). Further, brothel-based sex workers are expected to abide by an 'unwritten rule' to serve clients in any way necessary so as to keep their patronage; failure to do so would result in penalties or expulsion from the brothel (Munoz, Adedimeji et al. 2010). In other areas, however, such as Ajegunle, some female sex workers report that condom use is a part of the formal regulation of the hotel in which they work and one that they follow in order to maintain their employment (Iyiani, Binns et al. 2011).

HIV Testing. As of 2007, levels of HIV testing were also low; approximately half of women surveyed in Ibadan reported ever being tested (Munoz, Adedimeji et al. 2010). Women cited lack of confidentiality within existing testing services as a main deterrent from routine testing and even being seen within certain areas of the hospital lead to assumptions that a person was infected with HIV or another STI (Munoz, Adedimeji et al. 2010). Fear and stigma of HIV prevented women from being tested and the impact on one's ability to financially support themselves after diagnosis of HIV infection (Munoz, Adedimeji et al. 2010).

Pressures from within the brothel organizations further prevent women from testing for HIV: testing was not required of female sex workers; however, women who were tested were required to produce the results to confirm a negative status. Women who did not produce these results were judged to be hiding an infection and those with an infection were punished, ridiculed, or expelled from the brothel (Munoz, Adedimeji et al. 2010). As for many sex workers, HIV diagnosis not only has health implications and implications for their own earning potential but also serious economic consequences for those associated with sex workers living with HIV, such as their families and children.

Clients and Partners of Sex Workers. Little data exist that pertain to HIV male clients of female sex workers. One study, however, was identified by this report; conducted among 202 clients of brothel-based sex workers in Ibadan in 2004, 54% of the study population (n=202) screened positive for HIV. HIV serostatus did not vary by condom use, where approximately 84.7% had ever used a condom (Lawoyin 2004). The prevalence of HIV reported in this study is drastically higher than the national prevalence reported among the general male population (3.2% in 2007) (National Agency for the Control of AIDS 2010) and higher risk client populations such as transit workers and military personnel (approximately 2.5% in 2010) (Federal Ministry of Health [Nigeria] 2011). Specifically, the 2010 IBBSS preliminary findings reported a range of HIV prevalence among transport workers of 0.9% in Lagos to 8.0% in Benue, where prevalence among sex workers was also high (Federal Ministry of Health [Nigeria] 2011). Though the prevalence was slightly lower among police in Benue (2.6%), it was higher among armed forces (4.4%) and Nasarawa was equally affected (4.7% among police and 3.1% among armed forces) (Federal Ministry of Health [Nigeria] 2011).

Substance Use. Alcohol may be most commonly reported substance used by sex workers and clients: the IBSS highlighted the commonality of alcohol abuse among female sex workers, with over a quarter or more consuming alcohol daily; such figures which stand in stark contrast to other vulnerable populations, such as men who have sex with men, police, and transit workers which report less than 15% prevalence of daily consumption (Federal Ministry of Health [Nigeria] 2011). Interviewed sex workers suggested that alcohol was a necessary method to cope with having sex with such a number of men (Iyiani, Binns et al. 2011), while others suggested that substances boosted self-image and esteem and allowed them to deal with unhappiness (Izugbara 2005). With respect to client consumption of alcohol, women reported this often led to challenges for condom use when a client is intoxicated.

In addition to alcohol, injecting drug use has also become prevalent in Nigeria, particularly as heroin has become increasingly used across Africa (Dewing, Pluddenham et al. 2006). There is little data on the involvement of sex workers with injecting drug use. However, 31.4% of injecting drug users surveyed by the most recent IBBSS reported sex with a sex worker in the last 12 months (Federal Ministry of Health [Nigeria] 2011). Such a finding is relevant for HIV programming, given that the prevalence of HIV among injecting drug user is 4.2%, higher than among the general population (Federal Ministry of Health [Nigeria] 2011).

HIV Prevention Interventions Among Sex Workers

Nationally, the prevalence of exposure to HIV prevention in the last 12 months, particularly free condoms and education on safe sex practices, is approximately 80% for both brothel and non-brothel based sex workers. However, exposure to information about HIV is low and was reported only among 67.8% of brothel-based and 46.4% of non-brothel based sex workers (Federal Ministry of Health [Nigeria] 2011).

Formative research conducted in 2006 in Enungu State suggested that female sex workers supported the use of HIV knowledge building activities provided by the government (70.4%) and NGOs (52.65%), though fewer were supportive of peer education (26.7%), though researchers suggested this may be due to the fact that peer education was a new concept in this particular area at the time of the survey (Onyeneho 2009). Despite these suggestions for education and awareness building of HIV transmission and prevention, there are mixed reports on the success of such programs in Nigeria (Iyiani, Binns et al. 2011). A qualitative study to assess behavioral interventions suggested that women had sufficient knowledge of HIV prevention, particularly condom use, but other external social and economic factors prevented women from acting on their knowledge of HIV prevention methods (Iyiani, Binns et al. 2011).

Population Services International (PSI) studied the effects of condom advertising on consistent condom use and knowledge of HIV among 2,578 sex workers in Nigeria. Findings demonstrated that female sex workers who were exposed to "Gold Circle" or "Cool" condom brand advertisements (either heard or saw advertisements for one or both brands), were more likely to consistently use condoms than those who had not been exposed. While self-efficacy was the strongest predictor of consistent condom use, the findings encourage the use communication media to increase update and use of condoms, keeping in mind that exposure may have regional variations due to difference in access to media and timing in which advertisements air (Oladosu and Ladipo 2001).

The many qualitative findings that report general stigmatization and barriers to condom use suggest that implementation of HIV prevention activities must be evidenced based, coupled with rights affirming processes, and build on the agency of sex workers to lead prevention programs for themselves. One of the earliest intervention evaluations among sex workers, conducted in Cross River State and combining interventions which included peer-education, condom promotion, and STI testing and treatment, demonstrated the positive outcomes in condom use, STI treatment, and HIV awareness education that could be provided by peer educators and supported by chairladies who lead the sex work agencies. This project demonstrated impact on condom use by sex workers as well as HIV prevention knowledge and awareness among both sex workers and clients. Perhaps most importantly, the project involved sex workers, hotel managers, police, and the local Ministry of Health in the development and support of the intervention and resulted in trust and uptake by sex workers and their clients (Williams, Lamson et al. 1992).

Sex Worker Rights Organizations

Over the course of the epidemic, sex workers have organized to focus on increasing safety and decreasing stigma towards sex workers both for realizing their rights and increasing opportunities for HIV prevention. The Nigeria Vulnerable Women Association (NIVWA) for example, was formed by sex workers with both positive and negative HIV statuses to overcome stigma and discrimination and provide support for other women in the industry (Oyefara 2007). Motivated by the actions of sex workers in India, Nigerian sex workers have begun to emerge in number and have joined the international community of sex workers who march on the International Sex Workers Rights Day and International Day to End Violence Against Sex Workers. Organizations such as safe Haven International and other Nigerian NGOs have joined the African Sex Worker Alliance (ASWA) to continue to advocate for decriminalization of sex work (African Sex Worker Alliance 2010; Ehidiamen 2011).

Gaps in Research and Practice

Since the institution of the IBSS and subsequent findings of increased vulnerability of sex workers in Nigeria, HIV prevention, in the form of NGO supported activities and national strategies, have begun to include sex workers and other vulnerable populations. While social and epidemiologic data continue to emerge about these populations, little evaluation data exist on the implementation and impact of successful HIV prevention programs. These data are equally important for advocating for and ensuring effective and cost-efficient programs in low resourced and challenging settings.

Beyond high-risk client groups such as transit workers or uniformed men, there is also a dearth of data on HIV risk factors among clients of female sex workers and methods for prevention. Given the high proportion of married clients, this group may be particularly challenging to reach and information on successful interventions is necessary. An understanding of risks and prevention approaches for male sex workers is also lacking, yet the high prevalence of HIV suggests more knowledge of the population and successful intervention techniques are warranted.

Injecting drug use is also increasing as a risk factor for HIV in Nigeria. While the prevalence of HIV among injecting drug user is lower than that among female sex workers (4.2% compared to 34.0%) (Federal Ministry of Health [Nigeria] 2011), research and interventions should investigate prevention strategies for risk reduction among sex workers who may use drugs or who may be involved with clients who inject drugs.

The World Bank's assessment of policies related to HIV and female sex workers and clients highlighted that the high quality and high coverage of prevention programs in West Africa were mostly limited to male condoms and further suggested that the policies driving prevention and care for female sex workers is not well-developed (Lowndes 2008). While the risks for and prevalence of HIV among sex workers is undeniable and should continue be addressed, HIV prevention activities should be supported and programs should be implemented with caution to avoid unintentional restigmatization or 'blaming' of this population. Likewise, while advances have been made in HIV prevention, as a whole, effort should continue to focus on prevention, diminishing HIV related stigma, and further efforts should be taken to address stigma related blame for HIV transmission that is placed upon sex workers (Abdulraheem and Fawole 2009). These results highlight the continued need for implementation of HIV prevention programs within the broader context of community education and destigmatizion of sex work.

Thailand

Introduction

Key Themes

- Thailand is well-known for its comprehensive response to HIV including national mobilization, condom promotion, access to HIV/STI services, and early adoption of universal access to ARTs as national policy
- Sex worker rights organizations have been critical of the response to HIV in Thailand
- The context of sex work is changing in Thailand, with larger numbers of informal and street-based sex workers at high risk for HIV infection as are male and transgender sex workers

In the past two decades Thailand has been a global leader in the HIV response. The nation of 63 million people was one of the first in Asia to implement a national policy geared toward addressing the epidemic. It also was one of the first Asian countries to create a national HIV sentinel surveillance system and establish a national AIDS commission chaired by a top political leader (Beyrer, et al, 2011). Thailand, a middle-income country, was also the first nation in its region to lay out the critical goal of achieving universal access to antiretrovirals (Beyrer, et al, 2011).

As a result of its early prevention efforts, the country's HIV prevalence has generally been declining since 1996, but the nation's incidence continues to be greatest among key populations including non-establishment-based sex workers, men who have sex with men (men who have sex with men) and injecting drug users (IDU). Estimates from UNAIDS in 2009 suggest that there are currently about 530,000 people living with HIV in Thailand, or about 1.3% of the reproductive age population. Women aged 15 and up comprise 210,000 or almost half of estimated adult HIV infections in the country (UNAIDS, 2009).

A Modes of Transmission study conducted in 2006 utilized mathematical modeling methods developed by UNAIDS to estimate the proportion of new infections in Thailand in 2005 (Guows, 2006). This report estimated that female sex workers accounted for 3.9% of new infections in Thailand in 2005; their clients for 6.1%, and the regular partners of those clients for 8.4% of new infections. Overall, this component of the Thai epidemic was found to account for some 18% of new infections. In contrast, men who have sex with men accounted for some 21% of new infections, and general population reproductive aged adults for 43%. These modeled findings suggest that HIV remains a concern among sex workers and their clients, and that the industry overall accounts for approximately 1 in 5 new infections, a marked decline from the first decade of the epidemic, but still an important focus for HIV prevention interventions and programs (Commission on AIDS in Asia).

The systematic review and meta-analysis conducted for this report found an overall HIV prevalence of 11.9% (95% CI 8.4–15.5) among female sex workers in Thailand. The comparator HIV prevalence among all women of reproductive age (in 2011) was 1.15%. This yielded an odds of HIV infection (odds ratio, OR) of 11.6 (95% CI 8.3–16.2) for sex workers compared to all other women of reproductive age. Both HIV among sex workers and among women in the general in Thailand have declined in recent years, but female sex workers remain substantially more burdened by HIV infection.

Historical Perspectives on and Trends of the HIV Epidemic. The country's experience with the HIV epidemic spans three decades and include periods of vigorous intervention. The first recorded case of HIV in Thailand was reported in 1984. During the subsequent initial phases of the epidemic, from the mid- to late- 1980s, HIV spread was documented among men who have sex with men, female sex workers, and injecting drug users (Beyrer, 2011). The significant proportion of young Thai men having unprotected sex and high numbers of sex work related encounters led to a rapidly expanding epidemic among these men and to subsequent transmission to their female partners (Beyrer, 2011). By 1995, almost half of all new infections in the country were estimated to be transmitted from husbands to wives (43%). Sex workers and their clients accounted for most of the remaining new infections (35%) (Asian Epidemic Model, 2008). Just five years later, in 2000, transmission within male-female couples was estimated to be responsible for 56% of total new infections (Asian Epidemic Model, 2008).

The Thai epidemic was much more severe in the Northern Provinces, and particularly in the Upper North of the country. Among 21 year old military recruits from the upper north the HIV prevalence was 12.5% by 1991, the highest prevalence that had been reported among a male general population sample outside Africa (Nelson, et al, 1996). No HIV infections were found among female sex workers in surveys done by the Ministry of Health from 1985–1989, but the June 1989 sentinel survey done among women working in brothels in Chiang Mai, the largest city in the North, found 44% of these women to be HIV positive, an extremely rapid increase (Ungchusak, et al, 1989). Taken together, the these very high rates of new HIV infection among soldiers and female sex workers suggested that Thailand was undergoing the most explosive HIV epidemic that had ever been seen (Gray, et al. 1997). The rapidity of spread drove the Government into an escalated, and controversial, set of responses.

The Thai Government already had an extensive network of publicly funded sexually transmitted disease clinics, and these were quickly expanded. Widespread condom distribution and social marketing activities were undertaken, including the distribution of condoms to soldiers, and community education and outreach to the Thai people was undertaken on a national scale (Ainsworth, et al, 2003).

For female sex workers the programs were more controversial. The Ministry of Health launched its "100% Condom Campaign" and initially largely bypassed the organizations that were already working with sex workers prior to the HIV epidemic. The Thai campaign aimed at commercial sex venues with an effort to mandate condom use, but was seen by some stakeholders, including sex worker rights groups, as coercive and, in some cases, abusive, for people working in the sex industry.

The overall public health responses started to show impacts by the mid-1990s. Self-reported condom use rates among sex workers increased dramatically from about 50% to over 90%, and national STI clinic data showed that other sexual transmitted infections fell markedly over the same period (Ainsworth, et al, 2003). Even in the upper north, where rates had been the highest among young men and sex workers, prevalence peaked in 1995–1996 and steadily declined thereafter.

The epidemic among people who inject drugs, IDU, however, continued. And by 2005 it was evident that rapid spread was occurring among men who have sex with men (men who have sex with men) and Transgender populations. The Thai epidemic had become much more concentrated in these risk groups and this sub-epidemic continues in 2012 (van Griensven, 2010).

In 2011, the national HIV epidemic appears to have stabilized and overall HIV prevalence among the general population of reproductive aged adults 15–49 years old is currently 1.3% (UNAIDS, 2009). However, high HIV incidence continues to be reported among men who have sex with men and transgender persons in Bangkok, Phuket and Chiang Mai. However, with female sex workers and clients accounting for an estimated 1 in 5 new infections in Thailand in 2011, they remain an important population for HIV prevention, treatment, and care.

The Scope, Typology, and Context of Sex Work

The Thai sex industry is large and diverse. It includes female, male, and transgender sex workers, rural and urban contexts, and a wide range of venues, and economic levels. The majority of sex workers are women, and substantial proportions of these women are reportedly Burmese and ethnic minority peoples, especially in the Upper North. Many Hill Tribe people are not Thai citizens and they continue to work in the sex industry in large numbers. Sex workers are often a mobile population, in general, yet migration for sex work is criminalized in Thailand. While migrant sex workers may be the sole or primary provider for the family, the illegal migration places them at increased vulnerability and reduced access to HIV prevention compared to other sex workers who are Thai citizens (UNFPA 2010).

The Thai Ministry of Health has long characterized sex work by where sex is sold: it defines "direct" sex work as sex that is sold and occurs on the premises where women work, or "indirect," wherein sex services may be negotiated at work venues, but sex generally occurs off-premises. Direct venues include brothels and massage parlors. Indirect venues vary much more widely and include bars and clubs, Karaoke lounges, beer gardens, discos and others.

Map 3.7   Geographic Distribution of HIV Prevalence among Female Sex Workers in Thailand

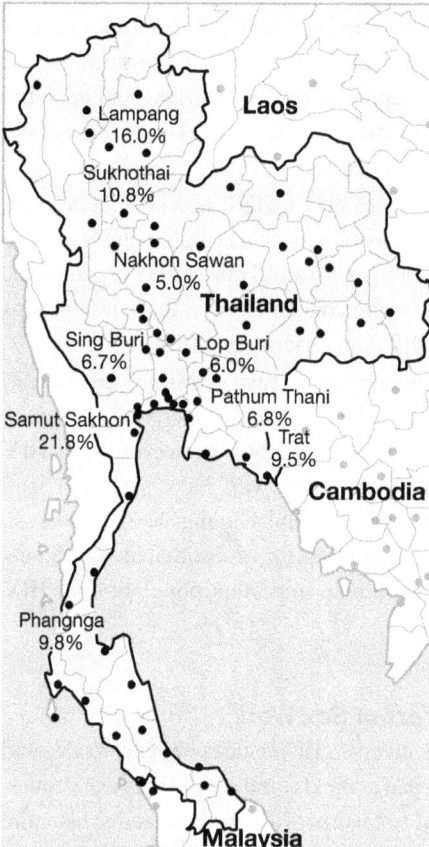

Source: UNGASS, 2010.

From the early periods of the epidemic and the subsequent national HIV sentinel surveillance it was clear that HIV rates were significantly higher among women classified by the Thai government as working in "direct" brothels. These differences have been attributed to greater numbers of clients, higher prevalence among lower-income brothel attending men, and reduced negotiating power among brothel-based sex workers.

HIV Among Female Sex Workers. Both direct and indirect sex workers, as defined by the Thai authorities, have had marked and steady declines in HIV prevalence since the 1990s (Figure 3.8). HIV prevalence among establishments based sex workers is now less than 3 percent in Thailand (UNGASS, 2010). However, street based sex workers, not included in these sentinel surveillance categories, have been found to have much higher HIV rates in specific studies (as do male and transgender street-based sex workers, who are also excluded from surveillance). These sex workers are of concern since they are less likely to access the social support system and HIV prevention services—especially if they are undocumented workers concerned about deportation.

Figure 3.9   HIV Prevalence among "Direct" and "Indirect" Female Sex Workers in Thailand, 1993–2009

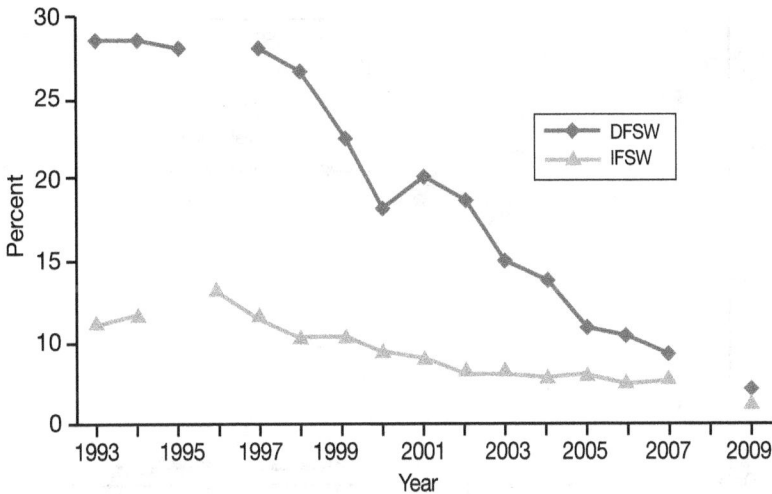

Source: Adapted from HIV and AIDS Data Hub for Asia-Pacific Evidence to Action: Thailand, 2011.
Note: DFSW = direct female sex worker; IFSW = indirect female sex worker.

One recent study out of the Bangkok Metropolitan Administration which looked at "street-based" sex workers in Bangkok found that this group had markedly higher HIV and syphilis prevalence than other sex workers—roughly 11 times greater than establishment based sex workers—underscoring the need to obtain more information and better access to this subpopulation in future information and intervention campaigns (Nhurod, et al, 2010).

Recent work from Shah et al, using respondent-driven sampling (RDS) found that approximately 20% of 540 street-based female sex workers were HIV positive (Shah, et al, 2011). Those findings are consistent with estimates from the Thai Ministry of Health which suggest that HIV prevalence stands between 18–30% among non-venue based sex workers (such as "street-based sex workers") (Akarasewi, 2010).

The HIV prevalence among pregnant women has also dropped, falling below 1% nationally and indicating there is no longer a generalized HIV epidemic in Thailand. The lowest prevalence of HIV among pregnant Thai women is in the youngest reported age bracket (women under age 20). These antenatal HIV prevalence data stand in contrast to those reported for women involved in sex work, particularly direct sex workers, in Thailand, though the gap is narrowing (Figure 3.9).

Figure 3.10   HIV Prevalence among Female Sex Workers and Pregnant Women in Thailand

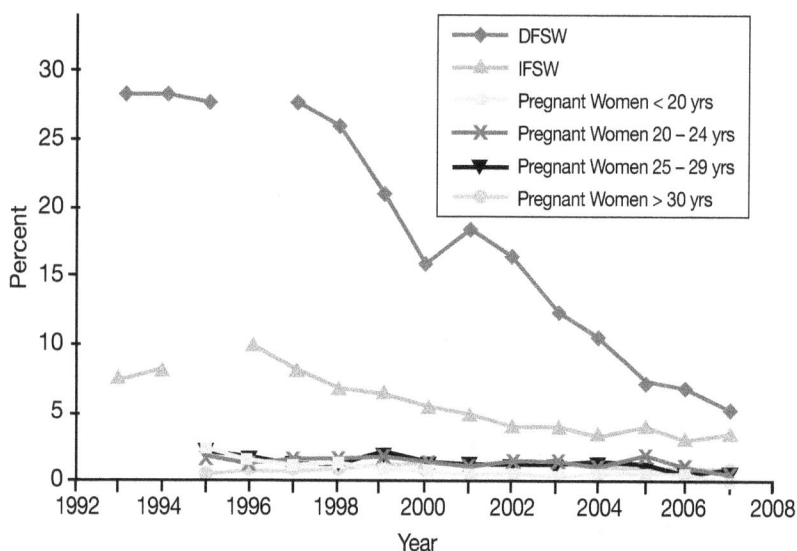

Source: Adapted from HIV and AIDS Data Hub for Asia-Pacific Evidence to Action: Thailand, 2011; Akarasewi, 2010, "Thailand: HIV Epidemiological Situation and Health Sector Response".
Note: DFSW = direct female sex worker; IFSW = indirect female sex worker.

The type and distribution of HIV among female sex workers is not consistent across Thailand. A 2007 RDS comparing HIV in Bangkok and Chiang Rai found that HIV rates were significantly higher in Bangkok. HIV prevalence was estimated at 19% in Bangkok and at 10% in Chiang Rai (Akarasewi, 2010). These differences may be due to differences in HIV infection seen among informal and street-based sex workers in the Bangkok sample. Meanwhile, other STI levels were lower and roughly equivalent (Akarasewi, 2010). Chlamydia prevalence hovered at 9% in both areas and gonorrhea was 2% in Chiang Rai and 1% in Bangkok (Akarasewi, 2010).

Substance Use. Though IDU populations continue to have high HIV rates, systematic tracking of injecting drug use or other substances such as alcohol among female sex workers has not been conducted. In general, use of such substances is associated with an increase in compromising behavior that could boost risk for HIV infection and STIs.

A government-sponsored crackdown on illegal drug use led by Prime Minister Thaksin Shinawatra in 2003 significantly hampered the country's ability to address HIV and protect the rights of those at risk. Human Rights Watch reports that mass arrests of individuals with a history of drug use and those targeted to help meet arrest quotas spawned a culture of fear among drug users that prevented them from accessing care (HRW, 2004). Those concerns about arrest, coupled with rampant discrimination against IDU, prevented drug users from accessing government-sponsored HIV treatment and from obtaining clean syringes. The massively overcrowded prisons and pre-treatment centers also gave rise to shared needle use during the crackdown and in its aftermath (Human Rights Watch, 2004).

There has been a limited amount of research exploring substance use among the clients of female sex workers. Shah et al.'s RDS work with female sex workers and their paying and non-paying partners in Bangkok found that most of the 178 clients of female sex workers and 79 non-paying partners in the study drank alcohol in the last month (60.6% and 70.1%, respectively). A few clients included in that survey (4.2%) also self-reported injection drug use and 8.3% of non-paying partners also reported injection drug use (Shah, 2011).

Clients and Male Partners of Sex Workers. Systematic data on the HIV status of male partners of female sex workers remains limited. HIV prevalence rates for military conscripts, a group that is often used as a proxy to represent the male clients for female sex workers, has fallen to approximately 0.5% (UNGASS, 2009). That figure represents a marked decrease since 1994 when prevalence numbers reached as high as 2.9% (Akarasewi, 2010). That same year prevalence of HIV among "direct" female sex workers reached 28.3% and was estimated to be at 7.6% among "indirect" female sex workers (Akarasewi, 2010). As previously discussed, HIV prevalence among military conscripts has typically been used as a stand-in for these rates since this group is known to engage with female sex workers in high numbers, but the prevalence may not be truly comparable or fully represent the male client population in Thailand. Shah et al.'s recent respondent driven sample study (RDS), however, present a more nuanced look at a 178-person sample of female sex worker's clients in Bangkok and their potential HIV risk factors. Among those clients, HIV infection was associated with men who engaged in sexual activity at a younger age (Shah, 2011).

Legal and Policy Issues

Sex work in Thailand continues to be illegal, but the nation's laws are geared toward penalizing sex business owners, managers, and customers. Against the backdrop of a larger national norm where there is tacit acceptance of sex work, however, it is not uncommon for police and local officials to receive bribes in exchange for allowing sex establishments to operate.

Under the relevant national law, amended in 1996, sex workers themselves are not technically subject to punishment (Rojanapithayakorn, 2006). However, in reality, the police in many localities do arrest and harass sex workers. Fear of arrest continues to shape sex workers daily lives. In qualitative interviews, sex workers reported that arrest, fines or being chased by police were of great concern (Ratinthorn, et al, 2009). To escape arrest, sex workers reported that they would be more prone to jump in the car of a prospective client without spending sufficient time to assess the client—potentially putting themselves in danger (Ratinthorn, et al, 2009). Female sex workers also reported that on days when sex work received publicity in the media or government officials spoke out about cracking down on drugs and Mafia-style crime, arrest rates among sex workers increased (Ratinthorn, et al, 2009).

Violence, Stigma, Discrimination. As in other settings, sex workers in Thailand suffer workplace harassment and physical and sexual violence in the context of sex work from a range of perpetrators. An estimated 14.6% of sex workers across four settings in Thailand reporting physical or sexual violence in the context of sex work in the past week (Decker et al., 2010). Reporting this violence is hindered by a general lack of responsiveness to the concerns of sex workers by police (Ratinthorn et al., 2009). Women working under the control of third parties can also suffer significant physical abuse, often perpetrated as a means of controlling women and ensuring their adherence to rules set forth by managers (Ratinthorn et al., 2009). Abuse from clients is often in the context of sexual and condom-related negotiation, with clients using physical force to obtain unprotected sex and forms of sex that have not been agreed to (Ratinthorn et al., 2009). Quantitative evidence has linked violence with condom failure and client condom refusal, as well as STI symptoms (Decker et al., 2010), indicative of the HIV implications of physical and sexual violence or rape. Severe forms of abuse, including kidnapping and gang rape, have also been reported among sex workers in Thailand (Ratinthorn et al., 2009). Other qualitative work speaks to an undercurrent of stigma and discrimination against sex workers. Evidence of sexual harassment and humiliation illustrate an environment that enables harassment and abuse against this population with little risk of punishment (Ratinthorn et al., 2009). Together, violence and other forms of harassment constitute significant threats to sex workers' ability to protect their health and human rights, and appear to confer significant risk for HIV. Given these risks, sex worker organizations have increased activities in the last decade and have demonstrated early successes in beginning to address violence and harassment of sex workers (see Sex Worker Organizations).

HIV Prevention Interventions for Sex Workers

In 2010, thirty years into the global AIDS epidemic, United Nations Secretary General Ban Ki-moon laid out a world-wide "Three Zero's" goal for HIV/AIDS: no new infections, no deaths, and no discrimination. Thailand has a vital role to play in fulfilling this goal, both for the welfare of its own nation and as a regional leader in fighting the epidemic. Thailand already has some of the infrastructure in place to attain these goals and has the opportunity to re-focus its programs on rights affirming and evidence-based approaches. New prevention approaches, including treatment as prevention and ART-based approaches should they prove safe and effective, could also help achieve the "Three Zeros."

It will be essential to revisit the fundamental aspects of that policy and consider ways to tailor that multi-faceted intervention to the needs of non-establishment "street-based" sex workers and other vulnerable communities. Sex workers need safe places to work and "street-based" sex work, as is indicated in the prevalence data, suggests that such non-establishment sex work does not afford needed protection for sex workers.

Sex worker led organizations have been instrumental in the HIV response in Thailand and have implemented many innovative approaches. EMPOWER's Can Do Bar is one such example. EMPOWER, a sex worker-led organization, founded a bar five years ago geared toward offering sex workers a venue with increased occupational health and safety. The "Can Do" bar is owned and operated by sex workers.

EMPOWER offers its employees (who run the bar): minimum wage or above (as defined by Thai Labor Law), a maximum working shift of 8 hours per night, vacation time sick leave, and safe sex education and access to free condoms and lubricant (Empower Foundation, 2012). Its employees are paid to manage the bar and any sex work they engage in after-business hours is considered private business.

There is no available data on the HIV prevalence among the Can Do staff as compared to sex workers in other settings, but anecdotally the group has heralded its success at offering sex workers safer working conditions to conduct their work versus other sites.

EMPOWER has been a vocal critic of the 100% condom program, arguing that the program was coercive in nature. The group states that sex work should be legalized and treated like any other type of work with consistent oversight and health and safety standards.

Planning future targeted interventions for sex workers will require the support of NGOs like EMPOWER as well as the ideological and financial backing of other private actors. Financing and education efforts from the private sector was a key factor that helped fuel the success of the brothel-based interventions in the early 1990s (Ainsworth, et al, 2003).

Specific coverage data for HIV prevention interventions among sex workers in Thailand is lacking. However reported coverage of voluntary counseling and testing for HIV among sex workers in the last six months was under 50%; condom use with clients appears to be slightly declining in recent years and HIV knowledge levels have stagnated at low levels (39%) indicating an important need for expanded HIV prevention and care services among sex workers in Thailand (UNGASS, 2010). Specific gaps in services include, for establishment and non-establishment-based sex workers, consistent funding to subsidize condoms (including access to female condoms), sexual health education and STI screening and management. Thailand will also need to ensure ARTs are widely available and remove structural obstacles to ART access particularly non-establishment based sex workers. Newer and less toxic regimes will also likely improve uptake and adherence.

Sex Worker Rights Organizations

Thailand has a robust network of sex worker NGOs and advocates that have pressed for legalization of sex work and improved health conditions for sex workers. Sex worker organisations like the Service Workers in Group (SWING) have provided funds to offset the cost of quality condoms for sex workers as part of an effort to minimize STIs for male and transgender sex workers in Bangkok and Pattaya (UNGASS, 2009). SWING and EMPOWER, have also pushed for sex workers to build up their own capacity to help themselves find and access health and social services including violence prevention services (UNGASS, 2009). In acknowledgement of the dedication and success of these organizations have both been recipients of several major human rights defenders awards, including the Red Ribbon, awarded to Empower, and Thailand's National Human Rights Commission Award and amfAR's men who have sex with men Initiative Award, awarded to SWING (amfAR 2009). Another leading NGO, Issarachon, has also worked for the past half-dozen years to deliver AIDS and sex education to street sex workers via mobile van services (UNGASS, 2009).

Sex worker organizations have also demonstrated capacity to address issues beyond HIV prevention, such as police-perpetrated violence and harassment. In 2005, SWING developed an internship program for incoming police cadets to work closely with SWING staff. Cadets are involved in SWING's condom use promotion activities for male sex workers in hotspot areas, teaching English and Thai lessons at SWING's drop-in center, and helping to lead games and energizers at workshops and outreach events. At the completion of the internship, the cadets are required to deliver a presentation on their experience to all 1,200 students in the police academy. The internship has proven to be widely successful and has developed into other HIV prevention curriculum for the academy and, among sex workers, fewer arrests and incidents of harassment have been reported (PACT, 2012).

Gaps in Research and Practice

Ramping up better policy and health conditions in this arena also hinges on gathering better data on changing sex work modalities in Thailand. Facilitating better access to care and providing targeted interventions for all sex workers will be key to this effort. Better access and engagement with the client population would also provide a clearer picture of the HIV risk for Thai sex workers.

Ensuring access to care and services for all sex workers, including non-Thai nationals, has been a substantial challenge for Thailand. ART treatment, now clearly shown to be both a treatment and preventive intervention, is essentially unavailable to migrants. This intervention should be prioritized for the next phase of the Thai response to HIV. Meanwhile, the fight against HIV will require substantial funding during the next phases of the response. Properly allocating resources during economically challenging times means thoroughly understanding the national epidemic and the groups most at-risk including a continued commitment to supporting sex workers through the application of interventions that are cost-effective and rights-based.

Ukraine

Introduction

Key Themes

* Ukraine continues to face a concentrated HIV epidemic with injection drug users, female sex workers, and men who have sex with men most affected.
* Ukraine is home to the highest HIV prevalence among female sex workers in a region facing a growing HIV burden; many cities have seen significant increases in HIV prevalence among female sex workers over the past five years.
* Heterosexual sex recently outpaced injection drug use as the primary HIV transmission mechanism, suggesting that Ukraine may be on the cusp of an expanding, and more generalized, epidemic, in which female sex workers are uniquely impacted.

Ukraine, the largest contiguous country on the European continent, is home to an estimated 45.4 million (State Statistics Committee of Ukraine 2011). Defined by the World Bank as a lower-middle-income economy, its gross national income per capita (GNI 2009; Atlas method) is $2,800 USD (The World Bank. 2009). The 2001 census indicates that the population is largely ethnic Ukrainian (77%), with Russians as the predominant minority group at 17% (State Statistics Committee of Ukraine 2011).

Historical Perspectives on and Trends of the HIV Epidemic. Ukraine has the highest adult HIV prevalence in all of Europe and Central Asia, and its epidemic is considered rapidly expanding (Kruglov, Kobyshcha et al. 2008). In 2007 the prevalence was 1.6% (1.2%–2.0%) (USAID. and Ministry of Health of Ukraine 2010) and decreased modestly to 1.2% in 2009, according to the Ukraine National Council on TB and HIV/AIDS (USAID. 2011). In 2009, 19,840 new cases were registered, (UNAIDS and Ministry of Health of Ukraine 2010) and an estimated 360,000 individuals aged 15 and over were living with HIV at the beginning of 2010 (UNAIDS and Ministry of Health of Ukraine 2010). The year 2009 witnessed the first decline in AIDS-related deaths in Ukraine, reflecting the success of antiretroviral therapy (ART) in this nation (UNAIDS and Ministry of Health of Ukraine 2010). Significant regional variation exists; the most affected southern and eastern regions are home to only a third of the total population, but contributed an estimated 70% of newly registered cases in 2007 (USAID. and Ministry of Health of Ukraine 2010). Urban settings are also disproportionately affected (USAID. and Ministry of Health of Ukraine 2010). Together with the Russian Federation, Ukraine accounts for nearly 90% of newly reported HIV infections in the region (USAID. and Ministry of Health of Ukraine 2011).

The first Ukrainian HIV case was reported in 1987. For several years, the epidemic initially seemed confined within a relatively small group of foreign students until an explosive epidemic emerged among injection drug users in 1995 (USAID. and Ministry of Health of Ukraine 2010). Injection drug use persisted as the primary transmission mechanism until it was overtaken by sexual transmission in 2008 (USAID. and Ministry of Health of Ukraine 2010). In 2009, an estimated 44% of new HIV infections were due to sexual transmission, with injection drug use responsible for 36% (UNAIDS and Ministry of Health of Ukraine 2010; USAID. and Ministry of Health of Ukraine 2010). As of 2009, the epidemic continues to be concentrated among most-at-risk populations including injection drug users (22.9%), men who have sex with men (8.6%), and female sex workers (13.2%) (USAID. and Ministry of Health of Ukraine 2011). Despite the high HIV prevalence among sex workers, Ukraine groups HIV cases among sex workers together with other sexual transmission cases for official registration purposes, rendering it difficult to know the extent of the proportion of HIV driven by sex work.(UNAIDS and Ministry of Health of Ukraine 2010).

The rising portion of new cases attributable to sexual transmission strongly suggests the possibility that HIV may begin to spread to and through the general population. Indicative of the rapid spread of HIV to the general population, HIV prevalence among pregnant women is now among the highest in Europe at 0.31% in 2006 (TAMPEP. and European Network for HIV/STI Prevention and Health Promotion Among Migrant Sex Workers. 2007). The high tuberculosis incidence (100 cases per 100,000 in 2008) further complicates Ukraine's HIV epidemic (USAID. and Ministry of Health of Ukraine 2011).

Ukraine's national response to HIV initiated in 1992 with the establishment of the National AIDS Committee however this committee was dissolved in 1998. In 1998, free HIV treatment was mandated, however the limited resources to carry out this mandate have effectively limited access to many in need. The 2005 establishment of the National Coordination Council on HIV/AIDS facilitated programming including opioid substitution therapy, HIV prevention, and harm reduction programming mandated for each oblast or district (USAID. and Ministry of Health of Ukraine 2010). The Ukrainian Institute for Social Research conducts regular behavioral surveillance with female sex workers, with support from the International HIV/AIDS Alliance in Ukraine, the Global Fund to Fight AIDS, Tuberculosis and Malaria, and the Futures Group International. In 2008, Ukraine committed upwards of 102 million USD$ towards the goal of HIV prevention and control (UNAIDS and Ministry of Health of Ukraine 2010).

Scope, Typologies, and Context of Sex Work

While estimates vary widely, 2010 estimates suggest that Ukraine is considered home to 65,000 to 93,000 female sex workers, with Donetsk, Odessa, and Kiev home to the largest populations.(International HIV/AIDS Alliance in Ukraine. 2010). Approximately 10% are immigrants, largely from Moldova and Russia (TAMPEP. and European Network for HIV/STI Prevention and Health Promotion Among Migrant Sex Workers. 2007). As in many other settings, Ukraine is home to a relative hierarchy of sex work which includes a top level of elite sex workers who are well paid and protected by security guards, personal doctors, and pimps. The middle category organizes in locations near hotels, bars and strip clubs as well as private residences. They often work with pimps or madams who take a portion of their salary in exchange for protection from police and clients. The lowest tier includes women working on the streets as well as those on highways, parking areas, train stations and bus stops; this group often includes drug and alcohol users as well as homeless women (TAMPEP. and European Network for HIV/STI Prevention and Health Promotion Among Migrant Sex Workers. 2007). Street-based sex work is considered the most common form of sex work at approximately 80% (TAMPEP. and European Network for HIV/STI Prevention and Health Promotion Among Migrant Sex Workers. 2007). The 2007 surveillance data suggests that the majority of female sex workers are ages 20–29 years, with a substantial portion of women aged 19 years and younger (18%).(Balakirye-va, Bondar et al. 2008). Most are unmarried and have completed secondary education (Balakiryeva, Bondar et al. 2008). Sex work is the sole source of income for an estimated 75% of female sex workers (Balakiryeva, Bondar et al. 2008). Almost half are supporting other individuals on their income, including parents, children and friends (Balakiryeva, Bondar et al. 2008).

Seasonal migration brings women from rural areas to the city to sell sex in the warmer months of the year (TAMPEP. and European Network for HIV/ STI Prevention and Health Promotion Among Migrant Sex Workers. 2007). An estimated 21% migrated in the past year to other cities or oblasts for sex work, and a small percentage (11%) travel to other countries for sex work, including Turkey, Russia, and Poland (Balakiryeva, Bondar et al. 2008). Kiev and Odessa have the highest portion of migrant sex workers at 82% and 62% respectively (Balakiryeva, Bondar et al. 2008); and likely includes both immigrants and migrants within the nation. Ukrainian women have been noted in the sex worker populations of neighboring nations, including Russia (Stachowiak, Sherman et al. 2005), where they can suffer substantial exploitation and human rights abuses with minimal recourse in the absence of official registration papers. The HIV implications of migration have not been explicitly examined in Ukraine but warrant consideration, because the need to preserve invisibility to police and other officials can render illegal migrants effectively invisible to social services and HIV prevention efforts.

Far less is known about male and transgender sex workers in Ukraine, however several situation analyses and surveillance related research efforts with men who have sex with men confirm the presence of these populations (Filipov 2005; Amjadeen L et al. 2005 [in Ukrainian]; TAMPEP. and European Network for HIV/STI Prevention and Health Promotion Among Migrant Sex Workers. 2007; Balakiryeva, Bondar et al. 2008; SWAN. 2009). Recent estimates suggest that 3,700 male sex workers exist in Ukraine (International HIV/AIDS Alliance in Ukraine. 2010); however no such estimates were provided for transgender sex workers. Surveillance data from 2008 on with men who have sex with men illustrates significant sexual risk in the context of paid sex; over one third reported condom non-use in this context with client condom refusal a primary reason for unprotected sex (Balakiryeva, Bondar et al. 2008). The stigma and discrimination against male and transgender sex workers within Ukraine and the region render these populations largely hidden, and comprehensive data are lacking.   Documentation of severe violence against male and transgender sex workers in Ukraine and elsewhere in the region recently emerged in the context of an investigation of violence against sex workers; the small group of male sex workers included described severe violence and exploitation at the hands of police (SWAN. 2009). Taken together, these reports illustrate the marginalized nature of male and transgender sex workers and the severe risks they face when identified. The need for further research to clarify the context of sex work and the HIV risk profiles for male and transgender sex workers is clear.

Legal and Policy Issues

The legality of sex work in Ukraine fluctuated significantly over the past decade.   Until 2001, sex work was considered an administrative offense, punishable by fine (TAMPEP. and European Network for HIV/STI Prevention and Health Promotion Among Migrant Sex Workers. 2007). From 2001 to 2005, it became a criminal offense, punishable by either a large fine or forced labor. Intensive advocacy and lobbying on the part of sex worker organizations and advocates ended this regulation in 2005. While sex work itself is once again considered an administrative offense, other aspects of sex work including pimping and brothel operations are criminal offenses punishable by imprisonment or fines. Despite these shifts in the severity of criminalization of sex work from administrative offense to criminal offense, and then reverting back, criminalization of sex workers continues with reports from the region indicating that police largely operate outside the law, with female sex workers subject to police abuse including extortion and arrest on false charges. Arrest on a range of charges can be invoked as a punishment for failing to submit to forced sex or pay bribes (SWAN. 2009). The legal climate has significant implications for the health and well-being of female sex workers. Policies that criminalize and stigmatize sex work are thought to create a context for, and effectively facilitate, the control and abuse of sex workers by agents of the state (SWAN. 2009).

Independent of the legal status of sex work, female sex workers in Ukraine face a myriad of forms of police exploitation. Severe police brutality has been documented; findings from a recent cross-national report which included 20 participants from Ukraine demonstrated that physical assault by police is almost ubiquitous; 85% of those surveyed reported past-year physical violence by police. Almost half (45%) reported sexual assault (SWAN. 2009). These encounters can also include kidnapping and gang rape. The practice of "subbotnik" continues, in which police demand sex without payment in exchange for freedom from arrest or allowing the pimp to continue operations. The HIV implications of such abuse were recently confirmed in neighboring Russia, where subbotnik was identified as a significant STI/HIV risk factor (Decker, Wirtz et al. 2012). In light of these abuses, female sex workers report significant barriers to obtaining legal justice, including being blamed by police for the violence perpetrated against them (SWAN. 2009). Confirming the findings from this relatively small sample, NGO workers describe this abuse as "absolutely typical" and "normal practice for law enforcement agents" (SWAN. 2009). Further corroborating these data are recent findings from female street youth in four Ukrainian cities, the majority of whom have been involved in sex work, illustrating that over half report experiences of forced sex and police harassment (Busza, Balakireva et al.).

Epidemiology of and Risks Factors for HIV Among Sex Workers
Ukraine leads the region in HIV prevalence among sex workers, estimated at 13.2% across 25 territories in 2008–2009 (USAID. and Ministry of Health of Ukraine 2011). Significant regional variation is noted. Recent 2008–2009 data illustrate Donetsk as the most affected setting with 39% infected; with prevalence estimates in Simferopol, Kyiv, and Mykolaiv all upwards of 20% (Map 3.8 [UNAIDS and Ministry of Health of Ukraine 2010]).

Map 3.8   HIV Prevalence among Ukrainian Female Sex Workers in 22 Cities, 2008–09

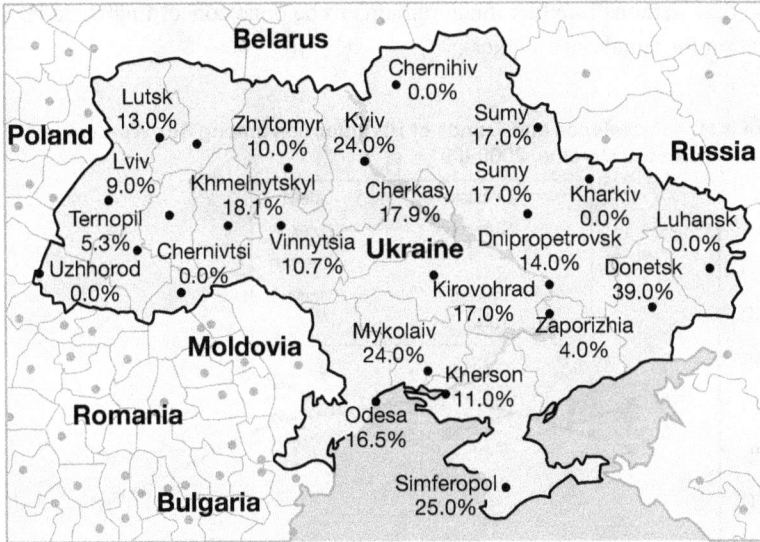

Source: UNAIDS and Ministry of Health of Ukraine 2010.

Many of these most affected cities have witnessed significant increases in HIV prevalence over the past five years, specifically Kyiv, Donetsk, and Simferopol (UNAIDS and Ministry of Health of Ukraine 2008; UNAIDS and Ministry of Health of Ukraine 2010). In other settings, such as Kherson, prevalence appears to have stabilized (Figure 3.10 [UNAIDS and Ministry of Health of Ukraine 2008; UNAIDS and Ministry of Health of Ukraine 2010]). In describing the reach of the outreach and HIV testing and counseling efforts, the International HIV/AIDS Alliance in Ukraine indicated that in 2009, over 20,000 sex workers received voluntary HIV testing and counseling; of whom 1,121 were infected (International HIV/AIDS Alliance in Ukraine. 2009).

HIV transmission knowledge is low among female sex workers but appears to be on the rise. The most recent behavioral surveillance data, collected in 2007 from 1,602 female sex workers across 12 oblasts, demonstrate that less than half of female sex workers (48%) have complete knowledge of HIV transmission mechanisms (i.e., could correctly answer five questions e.g., "can a healthy person have HIV?" and "Can a person get HIV through common use of a toilet, swimming pool or sauna with an HIV positive individual?")

(Balakiryeva, Bondar et al. 2008). Knowledge levels are higher among female sex workers over the age of 25 years relative to their younger counterparts. These data demonstrate that much remains to be done concerning basic HIV education for female sex workers.

Figure 3.11   Prevalence and Trends of HIV Infection among Sex Workers in High Risk Cities in Ukraine, 2006–09

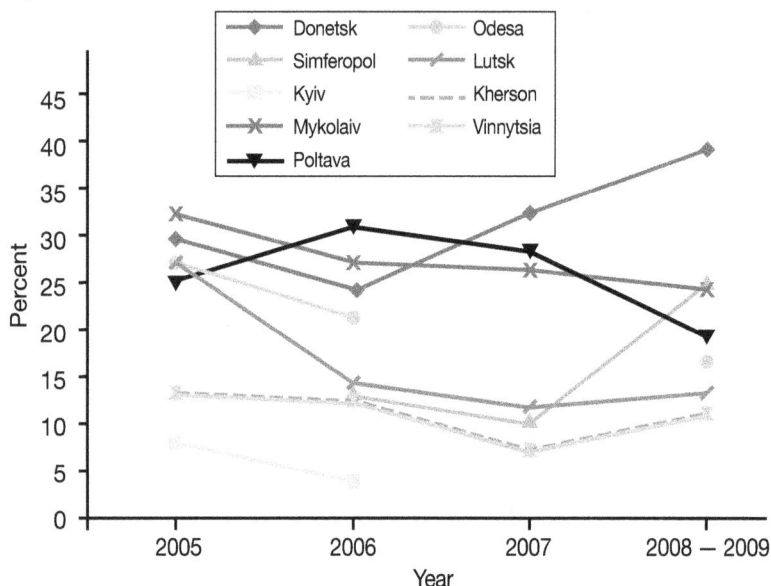

Source: UNAIDS and Ministry of Health of Ukraine 2008; UNAIDS and Ministry of Health of Ukraine 2010.

Behavioral surveillance data concerning condom use among female sex workers is mixed. Nationally, upwards of 80% of female sex workers report using a condom with their most recent client, (UNAIDS and Ministry of Health of Ukraine 2010) however estimates are significantly lower in some settings such as Vinnitsa (66%) (Kyrychenko and Polonets 2005). Consistent condom use is highest (66%) for vaginal sex, followed by oral sex (48%). While anal sex is common (about half report anal sex in the past year), only 28% report always using condoms for anal sex (Balakiryeva, Bondar et al. 2008), Client insistence on unprotected sex and receiving more money for unprotected sex are the dominant reasons for nonuse (Kyrychenko and Polonets 2005; Balakiryeva, Bondar et al. 2008), strongly suggesting the role of exogenous forces, including economic pressure, on female sex workers ability to successfully ensure condom use and thus HIV prevention. Together these data demonstrate significant risk for heterosexual HIV transmission among female sex workers in Ukraine, and bolster concerns for their role in an expanding heterosexual epidemic.

While HIV testing is largely considered accessible by female sex workers (88%) (Balakiryeva, Bondar et al. 2008), testing is far from universal. The 2007 surveillance data indicate that 46% of female sex workers had received HIV testing and obtained results; this prevalence is on the rise relative to prior years. More recent data further suggests strides in this domain with 58% of surveyed female sex workers indicating that they were tested in the past 12 months and are aware of their status (International HIV/AIDS Alliance in Ukraine. 2009; UNAIDS and Ministry of Health of Ukraine 2010). The success of the planned ART scale-up depends heavily on the ability of Ukraine to expand voluntary HIV testing among female sex workers as an essential step in linking those affected to available treatment.

Clients and Partners of Sex Workers. Relatively little is known about the clients of female sex workers in Ukraine, however a large, multi-site study conducted in 2009 suggested that 2.8% of clients were HIV positive, a higher prevalence than observed among the general population (International HIV/ AIDS Alliance in Ukraine. 2009).

Violence, Stigma, and Discrimination. To date, experiences of violence, stigma and discrimination against female sex workers in Ukraine have been primarily reported in the context of police. The severe nature of the assaults suggests both important human rights violations as well as substantial potential for HIV risk. The extensive police physical and sexual abuse of female sex workers clearly occurs in a broader context of discrimination with female sex workers also report other forms of humiliation at the hands of police as well as being forced to perform tasks such as washing cars or police stations (SWAN. 2009). These reports suggest that female sex workers may face stigma and discrimination in other settings, e.g., those related to health and other support services, however no formal investigation has begun. In addition to police violence, female sex workers in Ukraine appear to face severe physical and sexual violence from clients and pimps (SWAN. 2009), however little investigation has begun into the extent of this violence, nor its HIV risk implications, in the context of Ukraine. Globally, a growing body of evidence, including research conducted among female sex workers, illustrates the HIV risk associated with physical and sexual violence perpetrated by male partners and clients (Jewkes, Dunkle et al.; Ulibarri, Strathdee et al.; Sarkar, Bal et al. 2008). Additionally, violence by police against injection drug users in Ukraine has been found to prompt unsafe injection practices and limit access to exchange programs and drug treatment settings (Booth, Dvoryak et al. 2010); results from a recent modeling exercise indicated that reductions in police violence against injection drug users could have a significant impact on HIV reduction in settings where police brutality is most common (Strathdee, Hallett et al.). Taken together these data illustrate the need for further investigation of the scope of violence against female sex workers in Ukraine, including those involved in injection drug use, as well as its impact on HIV.

Substance Use. Injection drug use is a significant source of HIV risk to both male and female sex workers alike. The economic collapse of the early 1990s prompted significant increases in injection drug use in Ukraine and the broader former USSR region. Estimates from 2010 suggest an injection drug user population of 230,000–360,000 in Ukraine (International HIV/AIDS Alliance in Ukraine. 2010). As in most other nations, injection drug users are at heightened risk for HIV infection; data from 30 territories across Ukraine from 2008–2009 suggests that over one in five injection drug users are HIV infected (22.9%), with prevalence as high as 39% and 50% in some settings (USAID. and Ministry of Health of Ukraine 2011). Up to 16% of non-injecting sexual partners of injection drug users are HIV infected (International HIV/AIDS Alliance in Ukraine. 2009), highlighting the risk of sexual transmission from injection drug users to their non-injecting counterparts. Recent reports from Donetsk and Odessa suggest that over half of new HIV infections attributed to sexual transmission result from unprotected sex with injection drug user partners (TAMPEP. and European Network for HIV/STI Prevention and Health Promotion Among Migrant Sex Workers. 2007).

Concurrent injection drug use and sex work varies regionally, with over half of surveyed female sex workers reporting injection drug use in Cherkasy relative to 3% in Sumy (Balakiryeva, Bondar et al. 2008). Needle sharing and other risky practices have been documented among sex workers who inject in Vinnitsa (Kyrychenko and Polonets 2005). Substances are often used prior to sex work which may impair judgment and capacity to negotiate safe sex (Kyrychenko and Polonets 2005). Sexual risks are also heightened for female sex workers who also use injection drugs; this group is least likely to have used a condom at last sexual contact with a client (Balakiryeva, Bondar et al. 2008). Reflecting this confluence of risk, HIV prevalence is significantly higher among female sex workers who inject drugs (42.5% as compared 8.5% among non-injecting female sex workers) (UNAIDS and Ministry of Health of Ukraine 2010).

HIV Prevention Interventions for Sex Workers

The International HIV/AIDS Alliance Ukraine (Alliance-Ukraine) is the national leader, prevention implementer, and clearinghouse for HIV-related information, advocacy and research. A Global Fund recipient, Alliance-Ukraine supports ongoing behavior surveillance as well as in-depth research on sex workers and other vulnerable groups. Through the Alliance-Ukraine, over 25,000 sex workers received HIV prevention and social services, via 41 NGOs across 21 regions.

HIV intervention for female sex workers in Ukraine dates back to 1997, when a local NGO based in Odessa began training health professionals and law enforcement on the HIV and STD prevention needs for female sex workers. These efforts prompted female sex workers to initiate an HIV prevention project including a rapid assessment, behavioral survey, and prevention efforts including provision of counseling and condoms. By 2000, the project had reached over 2000 women. Peer intervention was the natural outgrowth of these efforts, with female sex workers sharing HIV prevention information, including that concerning violent clients (Nitzsche 2000). The Odessa-based efforts prompted other Ukrainian cities to take up HIV prevention for female sex workers. Across the nation now, HIV prevention interventions follow a similar format, primarily consisting of street outreach, peer training and education, cultivation of networks of trusted doctors, and drop-in centers.

Coverage and Access to HIV Prevention Services. Intervention coverage is difficult to estimate for marginalized, hidden populations such as female sex workers, and there is always concern that the most marginalized will also be hidden from both sentinel surveillance as well as programs themselves. The available behavioral surveillance data suggest that program coverage is on the rise. In 2004, only 34% of female sex workers had been reached by prevention programs, but more recent estimates suggest better coverage, with an estimated 69% of female sex workers reached (Balakiryeva, Bondar et al. 2008; UNAIDS and Ministry of Health of Ukraine 2010). A significant portion (39%) reported participation in peer education groups in 2007 (Balakiryeva, Bondar et al. 2008).

To date, far less is known about coverage for necessary ART treatment among HIV positive female sex workers. This dearth of knowledge may reflect the nature of Ukraine's epidemic, which until relatively recently was primary concentrated among injection drug users. Overall, Ukraine has set forth ambitious ART treatment goals (90% of those eligible by 2010). In practice, treatment coverage remains limited but increasing. In 2007, less than

10% of 91,000 eligible patients received treatment (UNAIDS and Ministry of Health of Ukraine 2008); by 2009, almost half of those eligible received this necessary care (UNAIDS and Ministry of Health of Ukraine 2010). No formal investigation has begun into ART coverage for female sex workers. Concerns have emerged that injection drug users may face unique barriers to accessing ART, including physician fears of noncompliance as well as police harassment and interference (Mimiaga, Safren et al.; Schleifer R. 2006; Bruce, Dvoryak et al. 2007). The overall climate of discrimination and harassment of female sex workers in Ukraine would suggest similar concerns for female sex workers, highlighting the need to investigate potential barriers to health services for HIV positive female sex workers.

Available Impact Evaluation Data. Available data indicate that HIV prevention intervention for female sex workers in Ukraine appear to be making an impact in the areas of greatest need; the 2007 surveillance data suggest that those exposed to prevention programs report higher levels of protected sex, and greater HIV knowledge (Balakiryeva, Bondar et al. 2008).

Sex Worker Rights Organizations

In 2006, following the successful advocacy to reverse the criminalization of prostitution and again consider it an administrative offense, Ukrainian sex worker organizations established a formal network with the help of the Ukrainian Harm Reduction Association (UHRA). A Sex Workers Rights Advocacy Network (SWAN) affiliate, the League Legalife works to mobilize the sex work community and prevent STI/HIV, TB and substance use among sex workers. These activities are intended to have a national impact; indeed, Legalife's 2009 meeting included representatives from five of Ukraine's regions. Their work also include advocacy and organizing around policy issues and those impacting the health and well-being of female sex workers, for example, as a component of their activities, League Legalife holds an annual press-conference in Kyiv on International Day against Violence towards Sex Workers, with support from Alliance- Ukraine to raise awareness about violence, and to call for legal reforms to better protect sex workers (International HIV/AIDS Alliance in Ukraine, 2009).

Gaps in Research and Practice

To date, Ukraine's HIV epidemic has been predominantly researched in the context of injection drug users, likely reflective of the rapid spread of HIV among injection drug users in the early stages of the epidemic. The rising prevalence of HIV among female sex workers coupled with the recent predominance of heterosexual transmission strongly suggests the need for further investigation among female sex workers as to their most relevant sources of HIV risk, as well as intervention coverage and access to ART. In light of the relatively low levels of HIV transmission knowledge among female sex workers, interventions would do well to increase basic knowledge and this important indicator should be closely monitored. In addition, the scope and extent of violence against female sex workers in Ukraine appears to be high. Interventions that can protect female sex workers from violent police and clients, and enable access to the criminal justice system to report such crimes are necessary. Finally, scaling up access to HIV testing services for sex workers is an urgent step in ensuring the success of the planned ART expansion.

From a research standpoint, the ongoing and recent behavioral surveillance data provide necessary insights into HIV risks for female sex workers in Ukraine. These efforts must be supported and expanded so as to continue monitoring HIV risk for female sex workers, and continue to clarify the coverage and impact of existing intervention efforts. To date, the behavioral surveillance has been largely designed to generate data for standard national HIV indicators. Little qualitative investigation has begun; mixed-methods research that blends qualitative methods with in-depth quantitative study would allow a better understanding of the context and nuances of HIV risk for female sex workers, as well as potential barriers to implementing HIV prevention in this setting. Such research is best done with a community-based participatory approach which supports the involvement of sex workers in all aspects of study design and interpretation of findings, so as to support a holistic understanding of the broader context of sex work.

Ukraine is home to the highest HIV prevalence among female sex workers in a region that faces a growing HIV burden. Increasingly across the nation and broader region, the primary transmission mechanism is heterosexual sex. Thus there exists an urgent need to better understand female sex workers and their HIV risk behavior, as well as the broader contexts such as police interference, discrimination, and related violence that may contribute to such risk.

Notes

1. Research and interventions with what in English might be referred to as "transgender women" in Brazil generally refers to travestis. Travesti is a complex social and cultural construct that has been the subject of important anthropological research (for more, see Silva 1993; Kulick 1998; Klein 1999; Parker 1999; Benedetti 2005). Yet the term tends to reference those who

perform femininity in their daily lives, have a penis, and adopt a gender identity as a "travesti". Given that research on transgender sex work overwhelming refers to this population, that the travesti activist organizations in Brazil prefer the term, and that the Brazilian National AIDS Program has most recently highlighted the specific vulnerabilities of this population by including an "Affirmative Plan for Travestis" as part of their National Plan to Confront AIDS and STDS among men who have sex with men, Gays, and Travestis, the term "travesti" will be used throughout the case study.

2. Relevant exchange rate—R$1.96 to US$1.00

References for Benin

Agbemavo, P. (2011). *Quarterly Newsletter of the U.S. Agency for International Development Mission in Benin.*

Agbemavo, P. (March 2011). "USAID Newsletter".

Ahoyo, A. B., Alary, M., Meda, H., Ndour, M., Batona, G., Bitera, R., et al. (2007). "Female sex workers in Benin, 2002. Behavioural survey and HIV and other STI screening." *Cahiers Sante* 17 (3), 143–151.

Cherabi, K., M. Greenall, et al. (2011). Synthèse de l'analyse de la situation épidémiologique et de la réponse nationale face au VIH/SIDA au Bénin. *CNLS Bénin Cadre Stratégique National de Lutte contre le VIH/SIDA/IST* 2006–2010

Guedeme, A., G. (2009). Ekanmian, et al. *Rapport de l'Etude sur les Modes de Transmission du VIH au Benin*, CNLS, UNAIDS.

Le Comité National de Lutte contre le Sida (CNLS) (2010). *Rapport De Situation National À L'intention De L'ungass* - Bénin.

Lowndes, C. M., M. Alary, et al. (2007). "Interventions among male clients of female sex workers in Benin, West Africa: an essential component of targeted HIV preventive interventions." *Sexually Transmitted Infections* 83 (7): 577–581.

Minani, I., M. Alary, et al. (2009). CO.36: Niveau élevé de comportements à risque pour le VIH rapporté en interview anonyme selon la technique de la cabine de vote (PBS) comparé aux résultats de l'interview face à face dans la population générale de Cotonou et ses environs. *2emes Journees Scientifiques Beninoises sur le VIH, le SIDA et les IST.* Contonou.

PNLS (2009). Enquete de Surveillance de Deuxieme Generation des IST/VIH/SIDA au Benin (ESDG 2008). *Tome 1: Travailleuses de sexe, Routiers et Clients des travaileuses.*

PSI Benin (2009). Evaluation de l'utilisation du condom chez les travailleuses de sexe de 15–29 ans des zones d'intervention des projets IMPACT et KfW au Bénin. *Deuxième Passage.* http://www.psi.org/benin.".

The Global Fund. "*Country portfolio - Benin.*" http://portfolio.theglobalfund.org/en/Grant/List/BEN.

U.S. Department of State. (2010, November 22, 2010). "*Background Note: Benin.*" Retrieved 10 July 2011. http://www.state.gov/r/pa/ei/bgn/6761.htm.

UNAIDS. "*2010 National Policy Composite Index Report - Benin.*" http://www.unaids.org/en/dataanalysis/monitoringcountryprogress/2010nationalcompositepolicyindexncpire-ports-countries/benin_2010_ncpi_fr.pdf.

UNAIDS *Global Report: UNAIDS Report on the global AIDS epidemic 2010.*

UNAIDS. (2009). "*Epidemiological Fact Sheet.*" Retrieved 10 July 2011. http://www.unaids.org/en/regionscountries/countries/benin/.

References for Brazil

Barbosa Jr., A., C. Szwarcwald, et al. (2009). "Trends in the AIDS epidemic in groups at highest risk in Brazil, 1980–2994." *Cadernos de Saúde Pública* 25(4): 727–737.

Bastos, F., D. Kerrigan, et al. (2001). "Treatment for HIV/AIDS in Brazil: strengths, challenges, and opportunities for operations research." *AIDScience* 1 (15). http://www.aidscience.com/Articles/aidscience012.asp.

Benedetti, M. (2005). *Toda Feita: O Corpo e o Genero das Travestis Rio de Janeiro*, Garamond Ltd.

Berkman, A., J. Garcia, et al. (2005). "A Critical Analysis of the Brazilian Response to HIV/AIDS: Lessons Learned for Controlling and Mitigating the Epidemic in Developing Countries." *American Journal of Public Health* 95 (7): 1162–1172.

Blanchette, T. and A.P. Silva. (2012). On bullshit and the trafficking of women: moral entrepreneurs and the invention of trafficking of persons in Brazil. Dialetical Anthropology. 36: 107-125. doi: 10.1007/s10624-012-9268-8

Brainard, L. and L. Martinez-Diaz, Eds. (2009). Brazil as an Economic Superpower?: Understanding Brazil's Changing Role in the Global Economy. Washington, DC: The Brookings Institute.

Consulta Nacional de DST/AIDS, Direitos Humanos e Prostituição. (2008). *Report and Recommendations*. Accessed on October 9, 2012 from: http://www.unfpa.org.br/Arquivos/consulta_nacional_dst_aids.pdf

Correa, S. and Olivar, Z. Forthcoming. *"The Politics of Prostitution in Brazil: Between "state neutrality" and "feminist troubles".* Paper commissioned to be published in a book being edited in India on the tensions between feminism and sex workers rights activism

Cortes, E., R. Detels, et al. (1989). "HIV-1, HIV-2, and HTLV-1 Infection in high-risk groups in Brazil." *New England Journal of Medicine* 320 (15).

Cortez, F., D. P. Boer, et al. (2010). "A psychosocial study of male-to-female transgendered and male hustler sex workers in Sao Paulo, Brazil." *Archives of Sexual Behavior.*

Damacena, G., C. Szwarcwald, et al. (2011). "Risk factors associated with HIV prevalence among female sex workers in 10 Brazilian cities." *Journal Acquired Immune Deficiency Syndrome* 57 (3): S144–S152.

Fonseca, M. G. and F. Bastos (2007). "Twenty-five years of the AIDS epidemic in Brazil: principal epidemiological findings, 1980–2005." *Cadernos de Saúde Pública* 23 (Sup 3): S333–S344.

Garcia, M. and Y. Lehman (2011). "Issues concerning the informality and outdoor sex work performed by travestis in Sao Paulo, Brazil." *Archives of Sexual Behavior.*

Grandi, J. L., S. Goihman, et al. (2000). "HIV infection, syphilis, and behavioral risks in brazilian male sex workers." *AIDS and Behavior* 4 (1): 129–135.

Grangeiro, A., L. Silva, et al. (2009). "Response to AIDS in Brazil: Contributions of social movements and sanitary reforms." *Revista Panamericana de Salud Publica/Pan American Journal of Public Health* 26 (1): 87–94.

Hinchberger, B. (2005). "Support for sex workers leaves Brazil without US cash." *The Lancet* 366: 883–884.

IBGE (2010). *2010 Census Instituto Brasileiro de Geografia e Estadistica*

Inciardi, J. A. (2000). *Sex, Drugs, and HIV/AIDS in Brazil*. Boulder: Westview Press.

Kerrigan, D., P. Telles, et al. (2008). "Community development and HIV/STI-related vulnerability among female sex workers in Rio de Janeiro, Brazil." *Health Education Research* 23 (1): 137–145.

Klein, C. (1999). "'The ghetto is over darling': Emerging gay communities and gender and sexual politics in contemporary Brazil." *Culture, Health & Sexuality* 1 (3): 239–260.

Larvie, P. (1999). Natural born targets: malehustlers and AIDS prevention in Brazil. men who sell sex: International perspectives on male prostitution and HIV/AIDS. *G. Herdt. ed.* New York: Oxford University Press.

Leite, G. (2010). *The impact of collaboration: sex workers and governments in Brazil. Human trafficking, HIV/AIDS, and the sex sector: Human rights for all.* Washington DC: American University and CHANGE: 59–68.

Lenz, F. (2008). *Daspu: Moda Sem Vergonha.* Rio de Janeiro, Objetivo.

Lenz, F. (2011). Decisão Historia: Prostitutas rejeitam financiamento para combate à Aids. *Beijo da Rua.* Rio de Janeiro, Davida.

Lenz, F. (2011). O Estado da Saúde e a "Doença" das Prostitutas: Uma Analise das Representações da Prostituição nos Discursos do SUS e do Terceiro Setor. *Comunicação em Saúde.* Rio de Janeiro, FIOCRUZ.

Lippman, S., M. Chinaglia, et al. (2012). "Findings from encontros: a multi-level STI/HIV intervention to increase condom use, reduce STI, and change the social environment among sex workers in Brazil." *Sexually Transmitted Diseases.* 39 (3):209–216.

Lippman, S., A. Donini, et al. (2010). "Social environmental factors are significantly associated with protective sexual behavior among sex workers: the Encontros intervention in Brazil." *American Journal of Public Health* 100 (Suppl 1): S216–223.

Longo, P. (1998). *The Pegacao Program: Information, prevention, and empowerment of young male sex workers in Rio de Janeiro. Global sex workers: Rights, resistance, and redefinition.* K. Kempado and J. Doezema. New York: Routledge.

Menezes, V., N. Brito, et al. (2010). *Resultados Consolidados: Coleta de Informacoes Sobre o Perfil do Publico Alvo. Projeto Transpondo Barreiras: Rede de Saude, Cidadania e Prevencao das DST/HIV.* Rio de Janeiro: Pact Brasil.

Ministry of Health. (2001). *Implementation and monitoring report - AIDS II - December 1998–May 2001.* World Bank Loan BIRD 4392/BR.

Ministry of Health. (2002). *Profissionais do Sexo:Documento Referencial para Acoes de Prevencao das DST e da aids.* P. N. d. DST/aids. Brasilia: Ministerio de Saude.

Ministry of Health. (2004). *Avaliação de Efetividade das Ações de Prevenção Dirigidas as Profissionais do Sexo, em Três Regiões Brasileiras Serie Estudos Pesquisas e Avaliação Brasilia,* National STD/AIDS Program.

Ministry of Health. (2010). *Gays e outros HSH sao mais escolarizados, tem maior poder aquisitivo e acessam mais o servico publico de saude do que os homens em geral.* Brasilia STD, AIDS and Viral Hepatitis Department, Brazilian Ministry of Health.

Ministry of Health. (2010). *Boltetim Epidemiologico AIDS DST.* Brasilia, Department of STDs, AIDS and Viral Hepatitis VII: Brazilian Ministry of Health.

Ministry of Health (2010b). UNGASS 2008–2009 *Country Progress Report Brasilia STD, AIDS, and Viral Hepatitis* Department - National STD and AIDS Commission.

Mitchell, G. (2011). *Organizational Challenges among male sex workers in Brazil's tourist zones. Policing pleasure: sex work, policy and the state in global perspective.* S. Dewey and P. Kelly ed. New York: New York University Press.

Mitchell, G. (2012). *Padrinhos gringos: turismo sexual, parentesco queer e famílias do futuro. Trânsitos Contemporâneos: turismo, migrações, gênero, sexo, afetos e dinheiro*. A. Piscitelli and G. Assis. Campinas, UNICAMP.

Munoz-Laboy, M., V. de Almeida, et al. (2004). "Promoting sexual health through action research among young male sex workers in Rio de Janeiro, Brazil." *Practicing Anthropology* 26 (2): 30–34.

Murray, L., S. Lippman, et al. (2010). "She's a professional like anybody else: Social identity among Brazilian Sex Workers." *Culture, Health & Sexuality* 12 (3).

Nunn, A. (2009). *The Politics and History of AIDS Treatment in Brazil*. New York: Springer.

Okie, S. (2006). "Fighting HIV-Lessons from Brazil." *New England Journal of Medicine* 354: 1977–1981.

Olivar, J. M. (2011). "Entre Nilce, a prostituta, e Isabel, a Princesa. Sobre redes, relacoes e arcabourcos libertarios" *Iluminuras* 12 (27).

Parker, R. (1992). *Male Prostitution, Bisexual behaviour and HIV transmission in urban Brazil. Sexual behaviour and networking: Anthropological and socio-cultural studies on the transmission of HIV*. T. Dyson. Belguim: International Union for the Scientific Study of Population: 109–122.

Parker, R. (2009). "Civil society, political mobilization, and the impact of HIV scale-up on health systems in Brazil." *Journal of Acquired Immune Deficiency Syndromes* 52 (1): S49–S51.

Parker, R. and K. Camargo Jr (2000). "Pobreza e HIV/AIDS: aspectos antropológicos e sociológicos." *Cadernos de Saúde Pública* 16 (Supp. 1): 89–102.

Parker, R. G. (1999). *Beneath the equator: cultures of desire, male homosexuality, and emerging gay communities in Brazil*. New York: Routledge.

Pelucio, L. (2009). *Abjeção e Desejo - uma etnografia travesti sobre o modelo preventivo de aids*. Sao Paulo: Editora Annablume.

Pimenta, M. C., S. Correa, et al. (2009). *Sexuality and Development: Brazilian National Response to HIV/AIDS amongst Sex Workers*. Study Report. Rio de Janeiro: ABIA.

Piscitelli, A. (2007). "Shifting Boundaries: Sex and Money in the North-East of Brazil." *Sexualities* 10 (4): 489–500.

Piscitelli, A. (2008). "Entre as 'mafias' e a 'ajuda': a construcao de conhecimento sobre trafico de pessoas." *Cadernos Pagu* 31: 29–64.

Prostitutas, R. B. d. (2009). *Human Rights and Female Prostitution* (Report). Rio de Janeiro: Rede Brasileira de Prostitutas

Rago, M. (1991). *Os Prazeres da Noite: Prostitucao e Codigos da Sexualidade feminina em Sao Paulo, 1890–1930*. Sao Paulo: Companhia das Letras.

Santos, A., V. Silva, et al. (2006). *Analise da Implementacao das Atividades de Prevencao ao HIV/AIDS Desenvolvidos pelo Programa Elos*. Sao Paulo: Pact Brasil.

Saude, M. d. (2002). *profissionais do sexo:documento referencial para acoes de prevencao das DST e da aids*. P. N. d. DST/aids. Brasilia: Ministerio de Saude.

Silva, A. P. and T. Blanchette (2005). "Nossa senhora da help: Sexo, turismo, e deslocamento transnacional em copacabana." *Cadernos Pagu* 25: 249–280.

Simões, S. (2010). Identidade e politica: a prostituição e o reconhecimento de um metier no Brasil. Revista de Antropologia Social dos Alunos do PPGAS-UFSCar. 2(1): 24-46

Simpson, K and G. Baby. (n/d). *E assim nasceu o movimento de travestis e transexuais*

Sutmoller, F., T. Penna, et al. (2002). "Human immunodeficiency virus incidence and risk behavior in the 'Project Rio': results of the first 5 years of the Rio de Janeiro open cohor of homosexual and bisexual men, 1994–8." *International Journal of Infectious Diseases* 6 (4): 259–265.

Szwarcwald, C., A. Barbosa, et al. (2008). "HIV testing during pregnancy: use of secondary data to esimate 2006 test coverage and prevalence in Brazil." *Brazil Journal of Infectous Disease* 12 (3): 167–172.

Szwarcwald, C., A. Barbosa Jr., et al. (2005). "Knowledge, practices, and behaviours related to HIV transmission among the Brazilian population in the 15– 54 years age group, 2004." *AIDS* 19 (suppl 4): S51–S58.

Szwarcwald, C., P. Souza Junior, et al. (2011). "Analysis of Data Collected by RDS Among Sex Workers in 10 Brazilian Cities, 2009: Estimation of the Prevalence of HIV, Variance, and Design Effect." *Journal of Acquired Immune Deficiency Syndromes* 57: S129–S135.

Toledo, L., C. Codeco, et al. (2011). "Putting Respondent-Driven Sampling on the Map: Insights from Rio de Janeiro, Brazil." *Journal of Aquired Immune Deficiency Syndrome* 57 (3).

Tun, W., M. Mello, et al. (2008). "Sexual risk behaviours and HIV seroprevalence among male sex workers who have sex with men and non-sex workers in Campinas, Brazil." *Sexually Transmitted Infections* 84: 455–457.

UNAIDS (2008). *Report on the global AIDS epidemic*. Geneva.

USAID. (2005). "*Acquisition & Assistance Policy Directive (AAPD) 05– 04.*" Retrieved October 13, 2008. http://www.usaid.gov/business/business_opportunities/cib/pdf/ aapd05_04.pdf.

Williams, E. (Forthcoming). *Ambiguous Entanglements: Sex, Race, and Tourism in Salvador, Brazil*. Champaign, IL: University of Illinois Press.

References for Dominican Republic

Barrington C, Latkin C, Sweat M, Moreno L, Ellen J, Kerrigan D. (2009) "Talking the talk, walking the walk: Social network norms, communication patterns, and condom use among the male partners of female sex workers in La Romana, Dominican Republic." *Social Science and Medicine*: vol. 68 (11), p. 2037–2044.

Brennan, D. *What's Love Got to Do With It? Transnational Desires and Sex Tourism in the Dominican Republic*. 2004. Duke University Press.

Cabezas, A. 2009. *Economies of Desire: Sex and Tourism in Cuba and the Dominican Republic*. Temple University Press: Philadelphia, PA.

Codigo Penal de la Republica Dominicana. 2007. Santo Domingo, República Dominicana.

COIN 2008. *Trabajo Sexual, Trata de Personas y VIH/SIDA*. Santo Domingo: COIN.

Consejo Presidencial del SIDA (COPRESIDA). 2009. *Iera Encuesta de Vigilancia de Comportamiento con Vinculacion Serologica en Poblaciones Vulnerables año 2008*. Santo Domingo, República Dominicana.

Centro de Estudios Sociales y Demográficos (CESDEM) y Macro International Inc. 2008. *Encuesta Demográfica y de Salud 2007*. Santo Domingo, República Dominicana: CESDEM y Macro International Inc.

Djomand G, Metch B, Zorrilla CD, Donastorg Y, Casapia M, Villafana T, Pape J, Figueroa P, Hansen M, Buchbinder S, Beyrer C; 903 Protocol Team (2008). "The HVTN protocol 903 vaccine preparedness study: lessons learned in preparation for HIV vaccine efficacy trials." *Journal of Acquired Immune Deficiency Syndrome* 1; 48 (1): 82–9.

Halperin DT, de Moya EA, Pérez-Then E, Pappas G, Garcia Calleja JM. (2009) "Understanding the HIV epidemic in the Dominican Republic: a prevention success story in the Caribbean. *Journal of Acquired Immune Deficiency Syndrome* 1; 51 Suppl 1: S52–9.

Kerrigan, D, Barrington, C, Moreno Montalvo, L. (2009). The State of HV/AIDS in the Dominican Republic: Guarded Optimism amidst Sustainability Concerns. *In. Public Health Aspects of HIV/AIDS in Low and Middle Income Countries.* Celentano, D and Beyrer, C ed. Springer: New York, New York.

Kerrigan D, Moreno L, Rosario S, Gomez B, Jerez H, Barrington C, Weiss E, Sweat M. (2006). "Environmental-structural interventions to reduce HIV/STI risk among female sex workers in the Dominican Republic." *American Journal of Public Health* 96 (1): 120–5. Epub 2005 Nov. 29.

Kerrigan, D, Moreno, L, Rosario, S, Gomez, B, Jerez, H, Weiss, E, van Dam, J, Roca, E, Barrington, C, and Sweat, M. (2004). *Combining Community Approaches and Government Policy to Prevent HIV Infection in the Dominican Republic.* Horizons/Population Council/ USAID. Washington. DC.

Kerrigan D, Ellen JM, Moreno L, Rosario S, Katz J, Celentano DD, Sweat M. (2003). "Environmental-structural factors significantly associated with consistent condom use among female sex workers in the Dominican Republic." *AIDS* 17 (3): 415–23.

Moreno, L. and Kerrigan, D. (2000). "The Evolution of HIV Prevention Strategies among Female Sex Workers in the Dominican Republic." *Research for Sex Work.* Volume 3: 8–10.

Murray L, Moreno, L, Rosario S, Ellen J, Sweat M, Kerrigan D. The role of relationship intimacy in consistent condom use among female sex workers and their regular paying partners in the Dominican Republic. *AIDS Behav.* 2007 May; 11 (3): 463–70. Epub 2006 Nov 10.

Movimiento de Mujeres Unidas (MODEMU) and Murray, L. (2001). *Laughing on the outside, crying on the inside.* MODEMU: Santo Domingo, Dominican Republic.

Padilla, M. (2007). *Caribbean Pleasure Industry: Tourism, Sexuality, and AIDS in the Dominican Republic.* Chicago: University of Chicago Press.

Padilla M. B, Guilamo-Ramos V, Bouris A, Reyes AM. (2010). HIV/AIDS and tourism in the Caribbean: an ecological systems perspective. *Am J Public Health* 100 (1): 70–7. Epub .

Padilla, M. B. (2010). The embodiment of tourism among bisexually-behaving Dominican male sex workers. *Arch Sex Behavior.* Oct;37 (5): 783–93.

Padilla, M. B, Castellanos, D., Guilamo-Ramos, V., Reyes, A. M., Sánchez Marte, L. E., M. A. Soriano (2008). Stigma, social inequality, and HIV risk disclosure among Dominican male sex workers. *Society Science Medicine.* 67 (3): 380–8. Epub 2008 Apr 12.

Padilla, M. B, Barrington, C, Matiz, A. (Forthcoming). Trajectories and Trans-Actions: Sexual Geographies of Transgender Sex Workers in the Eastern Dominican Republic.

Pantaleon, D. *Trabajadoras sexuales rechazan proyecto de zona rosa.* Listin Diario. Downloaded October 17, 2011. http://listindiario.com/la-republica/2011/6/23/193190/Rechazan-proyecto-sobre-zona-rosa.

Rojas P, Malow R, Ruffin B, Roth E, Rosenberg R. The HIV/AIDS Epidemic in the Dominican Republic: Key Contributing Factors. *J Int Assoc Physicians AIDS Care* (Chic). 2011 Mar. 2.

Sweat, M., Kerrigan, D., Moreno, L., Rosario, S., Gomez, B., Jerez, H., Weiss, E., Barrington, C. (2006). *Cost-effectiveness of environmental-structural communication interventions for HIV prevention in the female sex industry in the Dominican Republic. Journal Health Community* 11 Suppl 2: 123–42.

Tabet, S. R., de Moya, E. A., Holmes, K. K., Krone, M, R., de Quinones, M. R., de Lister, M. B., Garris, I., Thorman, M., Castellanos, C., Swenson, P. D., Dallabeta, G. A., Ryan, C. A. (1996). Sexual behaviors and risk factors for HIV infection among men who have sex with men in the Dominican Republic. *AIDS* 10 (2): 201–6.

Thanel, Barrington, C., Kerrigan, D. (2009). Santo Domingo, Dominican Republic.

UNAIDS. (2008). *Epidemiological Fact Sheet on HIV and AIDS*: Dominican Republic—2008 Update. Geneva.

UNAIDS. (2010a). Global Report. Fact Sheet: *The Caribbean*. Geneva.

UNAIDS. (2010b). *HIV Modes of Transmission Model: Analysis of the Distribution of new HIV infections in the Dominican Republic and Recommendations for Prevention*. Final Report. UNAIDS: Santo Domingo, Dominican Republic.

UNAIDS. (2010c). *Informe UNGASS 2010 República Dominicana*. Geneva.

UNFPA. (2010). Report Card: *HIV Prevention for Girls and Young Women*. Downloaded, August 10, 2011.

USAID. HIV/AIDS *Health Profile for the Dominican Republic*. Downloaded, August 10, 2011.

USAID. *HIV/AIDS Health Profile for the Caribbean*. Downloaded, January 22, 2012.

World Bank. (2011). World Bank Data Bank: *World Development Indicators & Global Development Finance*. Downloaded, August 10, 2011.

References for India

Basu, I., S. Jana, et al. (2004). "HIV prevention among sex workers in India." *Journal of Acquired Immune Deficiency Syndrome* 36 (3): 845–852.

Beattie, T. S., P. Bhattacharjee, et al. (2010). "Violence against female sex workers in Karnataka state, south India: impact on health, and reductions in violence following an intervention program." *BMC Public Health* 10: 476.

Blanchard, J. F., J. OíNeil, et al. (2005). "Understanding the social and cultural contexts of female sex workers in Karnataka, India: implications for prevention of HIV infection." *Journal of Infectious Diseases* 191 (Supplement 1): S139.

Brahmam, G. N., V. Kodavalla, et al. (2008). "Sexual practices, HIV and sexually transmitted infections among self-identified men who have sex with men in four high HIV prevalence states of India." *AIDS* 22 Suppl 5: S45–57.

Buzdugan, R., S. S. Halli, et al. (2009). "The female sex work typology in India in the context of HIV/AIDS." *Tropical Med International Health* 14 (6): 673–687.

Chakrabarty, I. (2004). Influence of rights-based approach in achieving success in HIV program and in improving the life of sex workers. Kolkata, India, *Durbar Mahila Samanwaya Committee Publication*.

Chandrasekaran, P., G. Dallabetta, et al. (2008). "Evaluation design for large-scale HIV prevention programmes: the case of Avahan, the India AIDS initiative." *AIDS* 22 Suppl 5: S1–15.

Chandrasekaran, P., G. Dallabetta, et al. (2006). "Containing HIV/AIDS in India: the unfinished agenda." *The Lancet Infectious Disease* 6 (8): 508–521.

Chatterjee, P. (2006). "AIDS in India: police powers and public health." *The Lancet* 367 (9513): 805–806.

Cornish, F. (2004). "Making context concrete: a dialogical approach to the society and health relation." *Journal of Health Psychology* 9 (2): 281.

Dandona, R., L. Dandona, et al. (2005). "High risk of HIV in non-brothel based female sex workers in India." *BMC Public Health* 5 (1): 87.

Dutta, M., D. Mandel, et al. (2002). Strategizing peer pressure in enhancing safer sex practices in brothel setting. *International Conference on AIDS*. abstract no. TuPeF5332.

Gangakhedkar, R. R., M. E. Bentley, et al. (1997). "Spread of HIV infection in married monogamous women in India." *JAMA: the journal of the American Medical Association* 278(23): 2090.

Ghose, T., D. Swendeman, et al. (2008). "Mobilizing collective identity to reduce HIV risk among sex workers in Sonagachi, India: The boundaries, consciousness, negotiation framework." *Social Science & Medicine* 67 (2): 311–320.

Go, V. F., A. K. Srikrishnan, et al. (2011). "High prevalence of forced sex among non-brothel based, wine shop centered sex workers in Chennai, India." *AIDS and Behavior* 15 (1): 163–171.

Halli, S. S., B. Ramesh, et al. (2006). "The role of collectives in STI and HIV/AIDS prevention among female sex workers in Karnataka, India." *AIDS Care* 18 (7): 739–749.

Hernandez, A. L., C. P. Lindan, et al. (2006). "Sexual behavior among men who have sex with women, men, and hijras in Mumbai, Indiaómultiple sexual risks." *AIDS and Behavior* 10: 5–6.

IIPS (2000). *National Family Health Survey* (NFHS-2), 1998–99. Mumbai, International Institute for Population Sciences and ORC Macro.

IIPS (2007). *National Family Health Survey* (NFHS-3), 2005–06: India: Volume 1. IIPS. Mumbai, International Institute for Population Sciences (IIPS) and *Macro International*.

IMF (2011). *World Economic Outlook Database-April 2011*, International Monetary Fund.

Jayasree, A. K. (2004). "Searching for justice for body and self in a coercive environment: sex work in Kerala, India." *Reproductive Health Matters* 12 (23): 58–67.

Jewkes, R. K., K. Dunkle, et al. (2010). "Intimate partner violence, relationship power inequity, and incidence of HIV infection in young women in South Africa: a cohort study." *The Lancet* 376 (9734): 41–48.

NACO. (2007). "*HIV/AIDS: Facts and Figures.*" Retrieved Jan 30, 2007. http://www.nacoonline.org.

NACO (2010). *UNGASS Country Progress Report 2010*. Reporting Period: 2008–2009. New Delhi, National AIDS Control Organization, Ministry of Health and Family Welfare: Government of India.

NARI (2007). *National Interim Summary Report-India*. Integrated Behavioral and Biological Assessment Round 1, Indian Council of Medical Research and Family Health International.

National AIDS Control Organization (2008). *HIV sentinel surveillance and HIV estimation in India 2007: A Technical Brief.*

National Network of Sex Workers and L.C.H.A. Unite (2011). *Sex Workers Meet Law Makers.* New Dehli.

Ramesh, B. M., S. Moses, et al. (2008). "Determinants of HIV prevalence among female sex workers in four south Indian states: analysis of cross-sectional surveys in twenty-three districts." *AIDS* 22 Suppl 5: S35–44.

Rao, A., K. Thomas, et al. (2009). "HIV/AIDS epidemic in India and predicting the impact of the national response: mathematical modeling and analysis." *Mathematical Biosciences and Engineering* 6 (4): 779–813.

Reed, E., J. Gupta, et al. (2010). "The context of economic insecurity and its relation to violence and risk factors for HIV among female sex workers in Andhra Pradesh, India." *Public Health Report* 125 Suppl 4: 81–89.

Sangram (2002). "Rehabilitation: against their will? Of veshyas, vamps, whores and women: Challenging preconceived notions of prostitution and sex work." *VAMP* 1 (2).

Sangram (2002). "Turning a blind eye. Of veshyas, vamps, whores and women: Challenging preconceived notions of prostitution and sex work." *VAMP* 1 (3).

Sarkar, K., B. Bal, et al. (2008). "Sex-trafficking, violence, negotiating skill, and HIV infection in brothel-based sex workers of eastern India, adjoining Nepal, Bhutan, and Bangladesh." *Journal of Health Population Nutrition* 26 (2): 223–231.

Setia, M. S., C. Lindan, et al. (2006). "Men who have sex with men and transgenders in Mumbai, India: An emerging risk group for STIs and HIV." *Indian Journal of Dermatology, Venereology, and Leprology* 72 (6): 425.

Shahmanesh, M., F. Cowan, et al. (2009). "The burden and determinants of HIV and sexually transmitted infections in a population-based sample of female sex workers in Goa, India." *Sexually Transmitted Infections* 85 (1): 50–59.

Shahmanesh, M., S. Wayal, et al. (2009). "Suicidal behavior among female sex workers in Goa, India: the silent epidemic." *American Journal of Public Health* 99 (7): 1239–1246.

Shinde, S., M. S. Setia, et al. (2009). "Male sex workers: Are we ignoring a risk group in Mumbai, India?" *Indian Journal of Dermatology, Venereology, and Leprology* 75 (1): 41.

Silverman, J. G., M. R. Decker, et al. (2008). "Intimate partner violence and HIV infection among married Indian women." *JAMA: the Journal of the American Medical Association* 300 (6): 703.

Simoes, E., P. Babu, et al. (1987). "Evidence for HTLV-III infection in prostitutes in Tamil Nadu (India)." *Indian Journal of Medical Research* 85: 335–338.

Steinbrook, R. (2007). "HIV in India—a complex epidemic." New England Journal of Medicine 356 (11): 1089–1093.

Surtees, R. (2003). "Brothel raids in Indonesia—ideal solution or further violation?" *Research for Sex Work* 6: 5–7.

Swain, S. N., N. Saggurti, et al. (2011). "Experience of violence and adverse reproductive health outcomes, HIV risks among mobile female sex workers in India." *BMC Public Health* 11: 357.

UNAIDS (2005). *"AIDS Epidemic Update 2005."* www.unaids.org/en/media/unaids/.../irc.../ epi_update2005_en.pdf

UNAIDS. (2008). *"Global Report on HIV/AIDS."* Retrieved Jan 30, 2009. http://www.unaids. org/en/KnowledgeCentre/HIVData/EpiUpdate/EpiUpdArchive/2007/default.asp.

UNICEF. (2011). *"Information by Country."* Retrieved June 20, 2011. www.unicef.org/ infobycountry/

Verma, R., A. Shekhar, et al. (2010). "Scale-up and coverage of Avahan: a large-scale HIV-prevention programme among female sex workers and men who have sex with men in four Indian states." *Sexually Transmitted Infections* 86 Suppl 1: i76–82.

Verma, R. K., N. Saggurti, et al. (2010). "Alcohol and sexual risk behavior among migrant female sex workers and male workers in districts with high in-migration from four high HIV prevalence states in India." *AIDS and Behavior* 14 Suppl 1: S31–39.

Weiss, H. A., V. Patel, et al. (2008). "Spousal sexual violence and poverty are risk factors for sexually transmitted infections in women: a longitudinal study of women in Goa, India." *Sexually Transmitted Infections* 84 (2): 133.

Xu, J., K. Brown, et al. (2011). "Factors associated with HIV testing history and HIV-test result follow-up among female sex workers in two cities in Yunnan, China." *Sexually Transmitted Diseases* 38 (2): 89–95.

References for Kenya

Angala, P., A. Parkinson, et al. Men who have sex with men (MSM) as presented in VCT data in Kenya. Abstract no. MOPE0581. AIDS 2006 - XVI International AIDS Conference, 2006.

Baeten, J. M., W. M. Hassan, et al. (2009). "Prospective study of correlates of vaginal Lactobacillus colonisation among high-risk HIV-1 seronegative women." *Sexually Transmitted Infections* 85 (5): 348–353.

Beckerleg, S., M. Telfer, et al. (2005). "The rise of injecting drug use in East Africa: a case study from Kenya." *Harm Reduction Journal* 2: 12.

Beyrer, C., Wirtz, A., Walker, D., Johns, B., Sifakis, F., Baral, S. (2011). *The Global HIV Epidemics among Men Who Have Sex with Men: Epidemiology, Prevention, Access to Care and Human Rights.* Washington, DC: World Bank.

Brodish, P., K. Singh, et al. (2011). "Evidence of high-risk sexual behaviors among injection drug users in the Kenya PLACE study." *Drug and Alcohol Dependence* 119 (1–2): 138–141.

Cheluget, B., G. Baltazar, et al. (2006). "Evidence for population level declines in adult HIV prevalence in Kenya." *Sexually Transmitted Infections* 82 Suppl 1: i21–26.

Chersich, M. F., S. M. F. Luchters, et al. (2007). "Heavy episodic drinking among Kenyan female sex workers is associated with unsafe sex, sexual violence and sexually transmitted infections." *International Journal of STD & AIDS* 18 (11): 764–769.

Chohan, V., J. M. Baeten, et al. (2009). "A prospective study of risk factors for herpes simplex virus type 2 acquisition among high-risk HIV-1 seronegative women in Kenya." *Sexually Transmitted Infections* 85 (7): 489–492.

Ferguson, A. G. and C. N. Morris (2007). "Mapping transactional sex on the Northern Corridor highway in Kenya." *Health Place* 13(2): 504–519.

Gallo, M. F., A. Sharma, et al. (2010). "Intravaginal practices among female sex workers in Kibera, Kenya." *Sexually Transmitted Infections* 86 (4): 318–322.

Geibel, S., N. King'ola, et al. *Impact of Male Sex Worker Peer Education on Condom Use in Mombasa, Kenya.* 5ᵗʰ IAS Conference on HIV Pathogenesis, Treatment and Prevention, Cape Town, South Africa.

Geibel, S., S. Luchters, et al. (2008). "Factors associated with self-reported unprotected anal sex among male sex workers in Mombasa, Kenya." *Sexually Transmitted Diseases.* 35 (8): 746–752.

Geibel, S., E. M. van der Elst, et al. (2007). "'Are you on the market?': a capture-recapture enumeration of men who sell sex to men in and around Mombasa, Kenya." *AIDS.* London, England 21 (10): 1349–1354.

Ghani, A. C. and S. O. Aral (2005). "Patterns of sex worker-client contacts and their implications for the persistence of sexually transmitted infections." *The Journal of Infectious Diseases* 191 Suppl 1: S34–41.

Hawken, M. P., R. D. Melis, et al. (2002). "Part time female sex workers in a suburban community in Kenya: a vulnerable hidden population." *Sexually Transmitted Infections* 78 (4): 271–273.

Hirbod, T., R. Kaul, et al. (2008). "HIV-neutralizing immunoglobulin A and HIV-specific proliferation are independently associated with reduced HIV acquisition in Kenyan sex workers." *AIDS* 22 (6): 727–735.

Horizons, P. (2006). *Understanding the HIV/STI Prevention Needs of Men Who Have Sex with Men in Kenya.* Nairobi: Population Council.

Kawewa, J. (2005). *Situational Analysis on HIV/AIDS in Kenya.* UNESCO. Nairobi: University of Nairobi.

Kimani, J., R. Kaul, et al. (2008). "Reduced rates of HIV acquisition during unprotected sex by Kenyan female sex workers predating population declines in HIV prevalence." *AIDS* 22 (1): 131–137.

Lacap, P. A., J. D. Huntington, et al. (2008). "Associations of human leukocyte antigen DRB with resistance or susceptibility to HIV-1 infection in the Pumwani Sex Worker Cohort." *AIDS* 22 (9): 1029–1038.

Land, A. M., M. Luo, et al. (2008). "High prevalence of genetically similar HIV-1 recombinants among infected sex workers in Nairobi, Kenya." *AIDS Research and Human Retroviruses* 24 (11): 1455–1460.

Leclerc, P. M. and M. Garenne (2008). "Commercial sex and HIV transmission in mature epidemics: a study of five African countries." *International Journal of STD & AIDS* 19 (10): 660–664.

Low, N., M. F. Chersich, et al. (2011). "Intravaginal practices, bacterial vaginosis, and HIV infection in women: individual participant data meta-analysis." *PLoS Medicine* 8 (2): e1000416.

Luchters, S. M., D. Vanden Broeck, et al. (2010). "Association of HIV infection with distribution and viral load of HPV types in Kenya: a survey with 820 female sex workers." *BMC Infectious Diseases* 10: 18.

Mathers, B. M., L. Degenhardt, et al. (2010). "HIV prevention, treatment, and care services for people who inject drugs: a systematic review of global, regional, and national coverage." *The Lancet* 375 (9719): 1014–1028.

Mathers, B. M., L. Degenhardt, et al. (2008). "Global epidemiology of injecting drug use and HIV among people who inject drugs: a systematic review." *The Lancet* 372 (9651): 1733–1745.

McClelland, R. S., W. M. Hassan, et al. (2006). "HIV-1 acquisition and disease progression are associated with decreased high-risk sexual behaviour among Kenyan female sex workers." *AIDS*. London, England 20 (15): 1969–1973.

McClelland, R. S., B. A. Richardson, et al. (2011). "Association between participant self-report and biological outcomes used to measure sexual risk behavior in human immunodeficiency virus-1-seropositive female sex workers in Mombasa, Kenya." *Sexually Transmitted Diseases* 38 (5): 429–433.

Mehta, S. D., S. Moses, et al. (2007). "Identification of novel risks for nonulcerative sexually transmitted infections among young men in Kisumu, Kenya." *Sexually Transmitted Diseases*. 34 (11): 892–899.

Michel, L., M. P. Carrieri, et al. (2010). "Harmful alcohol consumption and patterns of substance use in HIV-infected patients receiving antiretrovirals (ANRS-EN12-VESPA Study): Relevance for clinical management and intervention." *AIDS Care - Psychological and Socio-Medical Aspects of AIDS/HIV* 22 (9): 1136–1145.

Mitsunaga, T. and U. Larsen (2008). "Prevalence of and risk factors associated with alcohol abuse in Moshi, northern Tanzania." *Journal of Biosocial Science* 40 (3): 379–399.

Morison, L., H. A. Weiss, et al. (2001). "Commercial sex and the spread of HIV in four cities in sub-Saharan Africa." *AIDS* (London, England) 15 Suppl 4: S61–S69.

Morris, C. N. and A. G. Ferguson (2006). "Estimation of the sexual transmission of HIV in Kenya and Uganda on the trans-Africa highway: the continuing role for prevention in high risk groups." *Sexually Transmitted Infections* 82 (5): 368–371.

Morris, C. N., S. R. Morris, et al. (2009). "Sexual behavior of female sex workers and access to condoms in Kenya and uganda on the trans-Africa highway." *AIDS and Behavior* 13 (5): 860–865.

NASCOP (2009). Kenya National AIDS Strategic Plan 2010–2013 - *Delivering on Universal Access to Services*. Nairobi: Office of the President.

NASCOP (2010). *National Guidelines for HIV/STI Programs for Sex Workers*. Nairobi: MOPHS.

National Aids Control Council: Office of the President, Kenya., World Bank, et al. (2009). Kenya HIV *Prevention response and Modes of Transmission Analysis*. Nairobi, NACC.

Ngugi, E., C. Benoit, et al. (2011). "Partners and clients of female sex workers in an informal urban settlement in Nairobi: Kenya." *Culture, Health & Sexuality*.

Ngugi, E. N., D. Wilson, et al. (1996). "Focused peer-mediated educational programs among female sex workers to reduce sexually transmitted disease and human immunodeficiency virus transmission in Kenya and Zimbabwe." *The Journal of Infectious Diseases* 174 Suppl 2: S240–247.

Norris, A. H., A. J. Kitali, et al. (2009). "Alcohol and transactional sex: how risky is the mix?" *Social Science & Medicine* 69 (8): 1167–1176.

Okal, J., S. Luchters, et al. (2009). "Social context, sexual risk perceptions and stigma: HIV vulnerability among male sex workers in Mombasa, Kenya." *Culture Health & Sexuality*: 1.

Oyugi, J. O., F. C. M. Vouriot, et al. (2009). "A common CD4 gene variant is associated with an increased risk of HIV-1 infection in kenyan female commercial sex workers." *Journal of Infectious Diseases* 199 (9): 1327–1334.

Sanders, E. J., S. Graham, et al. (2006). *Establishing a high risk HIV-negative cohort in Kilifi, Kenya*. Amsterdam, AIDS Vaccine 2006 Conference.

Sanders, E. J., S. M. Graham, et al. (2007). "HIV-1 infection in high risk men who have sex with men in Mombasa, Kenya." *AIDS*. London, England 21 (18): 2513–2520.

Schwandt, M., C. Morris, et al. (2006). "Anal and dry sex in commercial sex work, and relation to risk for sexually transmitted infections and HIV in Meru, Kenya." *Sexually Transmitted Infections* 82 (5): 392–396.

Scorgie, F., D. Nakato, et al. (2011). "I expect to be abused and I have fear": *Sex workers' experiences of human rights violations and barriers to accessing healthcare in four African countries*. A. S. W. Alliance. Johannesburg.

Singh, K., P. Brodish, et al. (2011). "A Venue-Based Approach to Reaching MSM, IDUs and the General Population with VCT: A Three Study Site in Kenya." *AIDS and Behavior*.

Smith, A. D., P. Tapsoba, et al. (2009). "Men who have sex with men and HIV/AIDS in sub-Saharan Africa." *The Lancet* 374 (9687): 416–422.

Tovanabutra, S., E. J. Sanders, et al. (2010). "Evaluation of HIV type 1 strains in men having sex with men and in female sex workers in Mombasa, Kenya." *AIDS Research and Human Retroviruses* 26 (2): 123–131.

UNAIDS (2005). *Update on the Global HIV/AIDS Pandemic*. Geneva.

UNAIDS (2008). *2008 Report on the global AIDS epidemic*. Geneva.

UNAIDS (2010). *Report on the global AIDS epidemic 2010*. Geneva.

van der Elst, E. M., H. S. Okuku, et al. (2009). "Is audio computer-assisted self-interview (ACASI) useful in risk behaviour assessment of female and male sex workers, Mombasa, Kenya?" *PloS One* 4 (5): e5340.

Veldhuijzen, N. J., C. Ingabire, et al. (2011). "Anal intercourse among female sex workers in East Africa is associated with other high-risk behaviours for HIV." *Sexual Health* 8 (2): 251–254.

Vuylsteke, B., H. Vandenhoudt, et al. (2010). "Capture recapture for estimating the size of the female sex worker population in three cities in Cote d'Ivoire and in Kisumu, western Kenya." *Tropical Medicine & International Health* 15 (12): 1537–1543.

References for Nigeria

(4 Nov 2008). "*First Lady launches North West chapter of NAWOCA.*" Retrieved 5 Jan, 2012. http://www.nigeriafirst.org/printer_8464.shtml.

(2008). NAWOCA South West Zone Launched. *Action: A Quarterly Bulletin of the Lagos State AIDS Control Agency.* Lagos State AIDS Control Agency: Governor's Office. 2:4.

Abdulraheem, I. S. and O. I. Fawole (2009). "Young People's Sexual Risk Behaviors in Nigeria." *Journal of Adolescent Research* 24 (4): 505–527.

Aborisade, R. A. and A. A. Aderinto (2008). "Adjustment Patterns and Obstacles Against Social Rehabilitation of Sex Workers in Nigeria." *African Sociological Review/Revue Africaine de Sociologie* 12 (2): 128–143.

Aderinto, A. and E. Samuel (2008). "Adolescents at risk: A qualitative study of adolescent sex workers in Ibadan." *South African Review of Sociology* 39 (1): 38–50.

Adeyi, O. (2006). AIDS in Nigeria; A Nation on the Threshold, HARTard University Press, *HARTard Series on Population and International Health.*

African Sex Worker Alliance (2010) "*Female Sex Workers in Nigeria Call for Recognition and Respect of their Rights.*" http://africansexworkeralliance.org/content/female-sex-workers-nigeria-call-recognition-and-respect-their-rights

Amnesty International (2006). *Nigeria: Rape - the Silent Weapon.* London.

Anambra State Governor's Office. (2011). "*The profile of the landmark achievements of Her Excellency: Mrs. Margaret Peter-Obi, the First Lady of Anambra State.*" Retrieved 5 Jan, 2012. http://www.anambrastate.gov.ng/first-lady.html.

Aniekwu, N. I. (2002). "Gender and human rights dimensions of HIV/AIDS in Nigeria." *African journal of reproductive health* 6 (3): 30–37.

BBC News (2007). *Gay Nigerians face Sharia death.* London. http://news.bbc.co.uk/2/Hi/6940061.stm

Bureau of African Affairs. (2011, 20 Oct 2011). "*Background note: Nigeria.*" Retrieved 5 Jan, 2012. http://www.state.gov/r/pa/ei/bgn/2836.htm.

Carael, M., E. Slaymaker, et al. (2006). "Clients of sex workers in different regions of the world: hard to count." *Sexually Transmitted Infections* 82 Suppl 3: iii26–33.

Central Intelligence Agency. (2011). "*World Fact Book: Nigeria.*" Retrieved 27 Aug, 2011. https://www.cia.gov/library/publications/the-world-factbook/geos/ni.html.

Dewing, S., A. Pluddenham, et al. (2006). "Review of injection drug use in six African countries: Egypt, Kenya, Mauritius, Nigeria, South Africa and Tanzania." *Drugs: Education, Prevention and policy*, 13 (2): 121–137.

Ehidiamen, J. (2011) "Sex Workers Advocate for Decriminalization of Their Profession in Nigeria." *Global Press Institute.*

Federal Ministry of Health (Nigeria) (2008). *HIV/STI Integrated Biological and Behavioral Surveillance Survey* (IBBSS): 2007.

Federal Ministry of Health (Nigeria) (2011). *Nigeria: 2nd Round Integrated Biological and Behavioural Surveillance Survey* (2010): Key Findings.

Forbi, J. C., P. E. Entonu, et al. (2011). "Estimates of human immunodeficiency virus incidence among female sex workers in north central Nigeria: implications for HIV clinical trials." *Transactions of the Royal Society of Tropical Medicine and Hygiene* 105 (11): 655–660.

Futures Group International (2010). Strategic Review of the Sexual Transmision Prevention Program in Nigeria: Data Analysis and Triangulation for Evaluation (DATE) Project. *Final Technical Report.* Washington, DC. USAID.

Garcia-Moreno, C. (1996). *Presentation on women's health and development*. Report of the second meeting of interested parties. http://www.bioline.org.br/request?rh02032

Global Health Observatory. (2009). "Nigeria: Statistics." Retrieved 09 Nov, 2011, from http://www.who.int/countries/nga/en/.

Ighodaro, J. (2009). Imoke Commends Nawoca's Efforts on HIV/Aids. *Vanguard*.

Internal Displacement Monitoring Centre (2010). *Nigeria: Simmering tensions cause new displacement in the "middle belt"*, Norweigen Refugee Committee.

Iyiani, C., T. Binns, et al. (2011). "Talking past each other: Towards HIV/AIDS prevention in Nigeria." *International Social Work* 54 (2): 258–271.

Izugbara, C. O. (2005). "'Ashawo suppose shine her eyes': Female sex workers and sex work risks in Nigeria." *Health, Risk, & Society* 7 (2): 141–159.

Ladipo, O., Z. Ankomah, et al. (2002). *A comparative analysis of brothel-based commercial sex work in cities and junction-towns in Nigeria*. XIV International AIDS Conference. S. f. F. Health. Barcelona, Spain 235–239.

Lawoyin, T. (2004). *Characteristics of Male partners of brothel-based sex workers in Ibadan, Nigeria: Implications for intervention and program development* (abstract no. ThPeE8201). International Conference on AIDS. Bangkok 15.

Lowndes, C. M. (2008). *West Africa: HIV/AIDS Epidemiology and Response Synthesis: Implications for prevention*. The Global HIV/AIDS Program, The World Bank,. Global AIDS Monitoring and Evaluation Team. Washington, DC.

Merrigan, M., A. Azeez, et al. (2011). "HIV prevalence and risk behaviours among men having sex with men in Nigeria." *Sexually Transmitted Infections* 87 (1): 65–70.

Munoz, J., A. Adedimeji, et al. (2010). "'They bring AIDS to us and say we give it to them': Sociostructural context of female sex workers' vulnerability to HIV infection in Ibadan Nigeria." *Sahara-J: Journal of Social Aspects of HIV/AIDS/Journal de Aspects Sociaux du VIH/SIDA* 7 (2): 52–61.

National Agency for the Control of AIDS (2008). *Nigeria UNGASS Report, 2007*. UNAIDS. Geneva.

National Agency for the Control of AIDS (2010). *Nigeria UNGASS Country Progess Report*, Reporting Period: January 2008 – December 2009. Geneva.

Nwokoji, U. A. and A. J. Ajuwon (2004). "Knowledge of AIDS and HIV risk-related sexual behavior among Nigerian naval personnel." *BMC Public Health* 4: 24.

Oladosu, M. and O. Ladipo (2001). *Consistent condom use among sex workers in Nigeria*. PSI Research Division, Working Paper No. 39, Population Services International.

Onyeneho, N. G. (2009). "HIV/AIDS risk factors and economic empowerment needs of female sex workers in Enugu Urban, Nigeria." *Tanzania Journal of Health Research* 11 (3): 126–135.

Orubuloye, I. O., J. C. Caldwell, et al. (1991). "Sexual networking in the Ekiti district of Nigeria." *Studies in Family Planning* 22 (2): 61–73.

Orubuloye, I. O., J. C. Caldwell, et al. (1992). "Diffusion and focus in sexual networking: identifying partners and partners' partners." *Studies in family planning* 23 (6 Pt 1): 343–351.

Orubuloye, I. O., P. Caldwell, et al. (1993). "The Role of High-Risk Occupations In the Spread of AIDS: Truck Drivers and Itinerant Market Women in Nigeria." *International Family Planning Perspectives* 19: 43–48, 71.

Oyefara, J. L. (2007). "Food insecurity, HIV/AIDS pandemic and sexual behaviour of female commercial sex workers in Lagos metropolis, Nigeria." *Sahara-J* 4 (2): 626–635.

Panchaud, C., V. Wong, et al. (2002). "Issues in measuring HIV prevalence: The case of Nigeria." *African Journal of Reproductive Health* 6 (3): 11–29.

Pierce, J. (2000). *Analysis: Sharia takes hold.* BBC News. London, BBC News Online.

Quinn, T. C. and J. Overbaugh (2005). "HIV/AIDS in women: An expanding epidemic." *Science* 308 (5728): 1582–1583.

Salaudeen, L. (2011). Nigerians raise concern over incidence of police brutality. *The Nation.* Matori, Mushin, Vintage Press Limited.

Shannon, K. and J. Csete (2010). "Violence, condom negotiation, and HIV/STI risk among sex workers." *JAMA* 304 (5): 573–574.

Steiner, S. (2002). *Sharia Law.* Guardian. London.

UNAIDS (2008). *Nigeria: Country Situation.* Geneva: 1–3.

UNAIDS. (2009). *"UNAIDS: Epidemiological Fact Sheet, Nigeria."* Country Reports, from http://92.52.112.217/downloadpdf.htm?country_id=AFRNGA&lng_code=en&pdfoption=e-pi.

UNHCR. (2011). *"2011 Regional Operation Profile- West Africa: Nigeria."* Retrieved 23 Aug, 2011. http://www.unhcr.org/pages/49e484f76.html.

UNODC (2009). *The Global Report on Trafficking in Persons: West and Central Africa.* UNODC. Geneva 105–106.

USAID (2010). *USAID/Nigeria: Draft Program Description.* Washington, DC.

Williams, E., N. Lamson, et al. (1992). "Implementation of an AIDS prevention program among prostitutes in the Cross River State of Nigeria." *AIDS* 6 (2): 229–230.

References for Thailand

Ainsworth, M., Beyrer, C., Soucat, A. 2003. AIDS and Public Policy: The Lessons and Challenges of 'Success' in Thailand. *Health Policy.* 64: 1 13–37.

Akarasewi, Pasakorn. "(Brief) *Overview of the HIV Epidemic and the National HIV/AIDS surveillance.*" Powerpoint. Thailand Ministry of Public Health, 2010.

amfAR. *Director of Thai Sex Workers' Group Honored as Human Rights Champion. 2009.* Available at http://www.amfar.org/content.aspx?id=7413

Beyrer, C., Wirtz, A., Walker, D., Johns, B., Sifakis, F., and Baral, S. 2011. *"The Global HIV Epidemics among Men Who Have Sex with Men."* World Bank.

Chandeying, V. 2005. "Epidemiology of HIV and sexually transmitted infections in Thailand." *Sexual Health* (1) 209–216.

Decker, M.R., McCauley, H.L., Phuengsamran, D., Janyam, S., Silverman, J.G. 2011. "Sex Trafficking, Sexual Risk, Sexually Transmitted Infection and Reproductive Health Among Female Sex Workers in Thailand." *Journal of Epidemiology and Community Health,* 65 (4), 334–339.

Ditton, M., Lehane, L. "Towards Realizing the Health-Related Millenium Development Goals for Migrants from Burma in Thailand." 2009. *Journal of Empirical Research on Human Research Ethics.* 1556–2646: 37–48.

Empower Foundation website. Accessed 1 Aug. 2011. http://www.empowerfoundation.org/barcando_en.html.

Gray JA, Gregory J, Dore, Y L, Supawitkul S, Effler P, and John M. Kaldor. (1997) HIV-1 infection among female commercial sex workersin rural Thailand. *AIDS,* 11:89–94.

Guadamuz, T., W. Wimonsate, A. Varangrat, P. Phanuphak, R. Jommaroeng, P.A. Mock, J.W. Tappero, F. van Griensven. 2011. "Correlates of Forced Sex Among Populations of Men Who Have Sex with Men in Thailand." *Archive Sexual Behavior.* 40: 259–266.

Hayashi, K., Wood, E., Suwannawong, P., Kaplan, K., Qi, J., Kerr, T. (2011). "Methamphet-amine Injection and Syringe Sharing Among a Community-Recruited Sample of Injection Drug Users in Bangkok, Thailand." *Drug and Alcohol Dependence.* 115 (1–2): 145–9. Epub 2010. Dec. 3.

"*HIV and AIDS Data Hub for Asia-Pacific Evidence to Action: Thailand.*" 2011. http://www.aidsdatahub.org/en/country-profiles/thailand

Leiter, K., I. Tamm., C. Beyrer., V. Iacopino., et al. (2004). "*No Status: Migration, Trafficking and Exploitation of Women in Thailand: Health and HIV/AIDS Risk for Burmese and Hill Tribe Women and Girls.*". Physicians for Human Rights.

Liamputtong, P., Haritavorn, N., Kiatying-Angsulee, N. (2009). "HIV and AIDS, Stigma and AIDS Support Groups: Perspectives from Women Living with HIV and AIDS in Central Thailand." *Social Science and Medicine,* (69), 862–868.

Nhurod, P.,Bollen, L, Smutraprapoot, P., Suksripanich, O., Siangphoe, U., Lolekha, R., Manomaipiboon, P., Nandavisai, C., Anekvorapong, R., Supawitkul, S., Subhachaturas, W., Akarasewi, P., Foxx, K., 2010. "Access to HIV Testing for Sex Workers in Bangkok, Thailand: a High Prevalence of HIV Among Street-based Sex Workers." *Southeast Asian Journal of Tropical Medicine and Public Health.* Jan; 41 (1), 153–62.

PACT. *Turning an enemy into an ally: SWING's police cadet internships on HIV prevention among sex workers.* 2012. http://www.pactworld.org/cs/reach_news_and_media_swing_story

Ratinthorn, A., Meleis, A., Sindhu, S. 2009. "Trapped in Circle of Threats: Violence Against Sex Workers in Thailand." *Health Care for Women International,* 30:3, 249–269.

Rojanapithayakorn, Wiwat. 2006. "The 100% Condom Use Programme in Asia." *Reproductive Health Matters.* 14 (28), 41–52.

Scambler, Graham, Paoli, F. 2008. "Health Work, Female Sex Workers and HIV/AIDS: Global and Local Dimensions of Stigma and Deviance as Barriers to Effective Interventions." *Social Science and Medicine.* (66), 1848–1862.

Shah, N.S., R. W. Shiraishi, W. Subhachaturas, A. Anand, S. J. Whitehead, S. Tanpradech, C. Manopaiboon, K. M. Sabin, K. K. Fox, A. Y. Kim. 2011. "Bridging Populations—Sexual Risk Behaviors and HIV Prevalence in Clients and Partners of Female Sex Workers, Bangkok, Thailand 2007." *Journal of Urban Health: Bulletin of the New York Academy of Medicine,* Vol. 88, No. 3.

Schwartlander, B., J, Stover, T. Hallett, R. Atun, C.Avila, E.Gouws, M. Bartos, P.D. Ghys, M. Opuni, D.Barr, R. Alsallaq, L. Bollinger, M. de Freitas, G. rey Garnett, C. Holmes, K. Legins, Y. Pillay, A.E. Stanciole, C. McClure, G. Hirnschall, M.Laga, N. Padian. "Towards an Improved Investment Approach for an Effective Response to HIV/AIDS." 2011. *The Lancet;* 377: 2031–41.

Thailand Burma Border Consortium. *Thailand Burma Border Annual Report.* 2011.

"*Thailand: HIV Epidemiological Situation and Health Sector Response.*" (Powerpoint). Ministry of Public Health, Thailand. http://www.searo.who.int/LinkFiles/Facts_and_Figures_HIV_Thailand.pdf

"Thailand: Not Enough Graves: The War on Drugs, HIV/AIDS, and Violations of Human Rights." June 2004, *Human Rights Watch.* Vol. 16, No. 8.

"The Asian Epidemic Model (AEM) Projections for HIV/AIDS in Thailand: 2005–2025." 2009. *The Analysis and Advocacy Project and The Thai Working Group on HIV/AIDS Projections.*

"*The National Plan for Strategic and Integrated HIV and AIDS Prevention and Alleviation 2007–2011.*" November 2007. National Committee for HIV and AIDS Prevention and Alleviation.

Tieu, H., Phanuphak, N., Ananworanich, J., Vatanparast, R., Jadwattanakul, T., Pharachetsakul, N., Mingkwanrungrueng, P., Buajoom, R., Teeratakupisarn, S., Teeratukupisarn, N., Methajittiphun, P., Hammer, S., Chiasson, M., Phanuphak, P., 2010. "Acceptability of Male Circumcision for the Prevention of HIV Among High-Risk Heterosexual Men in Thailand." *Sexually Transmitted Diseases.* 37 (6), 353–355.

UNAIDS. 2009. *Thailand, Epidemiological Fact Sheets on HIV/AIDS and Sexually Transmitted Infections.*

UNFPA. *Building partnerships on HIV and sex work: Report and recommendations from the first Asia and the Pacific Regional Consultation on HIV and Sex Work.* 2010. Available at: http://asiapacific.unfpa.org/webdav/site/asiapacific/shared/Publications/2011/Building%20 Partnerships%20on%20HIV%20and%20Sex%20Work%202.pdf

UNGASS (United Nations General Assembly Special Session on HIV/AIDS) *Country Progress Report Thailand: Reporting Period January 2008-December 2009.* National AIDS Prevention and Alleviation Committee.

Ungchusak K, Sriprapandh S, Pinichpongse S, Kunasol S, Thanprasertsuk S.(1989) "First national sentinel surveillance seroprevalence survey of HIV-1 infection in Thailand." 1989. *Thai AIDS Journal,* I, 57–74.

van Griensven, F., J.W. de Lind van Wingaarden. "A Review of the Epidemiology of HIV Infection and Prevention Responses Among men who have sex with men in Asia." 2010. *AIDS,* 24 (suppl 3): S30–S40

References for Ukraine

Amjadeen L et al. (2005 [in Ukrainian]). *Report on the survey "Monitoring behaviours of MSM as a component of second-generation surveillance".* Kiev: International HIV/AIDS Alliance in Ukraine.

Balakiryeva, O., T. Bondar, et al. (2008). Report on the survey *"Monitoring behaviours of men having sex with men as a component of second generation surveillance".* Kiev: International HIV/AIDS Alliance in Ukraine.

Balakiryeva, O. N., T. V. Bondar, et al. (2008). Report on the survey *"Monitoring behaviours of men having sex with men as a component of second generation surveillance".* Kiev: International HIV/AIDS Alliance in Ukraine.

Booth, R. E., S. Dvoryak, et al. (2010). *Police brutality is independently associated with sharing injection equipment among injection drug users in Odessa, Ukraine.* XVI Conference of the International AIDS Society. Vienna, Austria.

Bruce, R. D., S. Dvoryak, et al. (2007). "HIV treatment access and scale-up for delivery of opiate substitution therapy with buprenorphine for IDUs in Ukraine—programme description and policy implications." *International Journal of Drug Policy* 18 (4): 326–328.

Busza, J. R., O. M. Balakireva, et al. "Street-based adolescents at high risk of HIV in Ukraine." *Journal of Epidemiol Community Health.*

Decker, M. R., Wirtz, A. L., Baral, S. D., Peryshkin, A, Mogilnyi, V., Weber, R. A, Stachowiak, J., Go, V., Beyrer, C., Injection drug use, sexual risk, violence and STI/HIV among Moscow female sex workers. Sexually Transmitted Infections. 2012 Jun;88(4):278-83. Epub 2012 Jan 27.

Filipov, D. (2005). "The research of risky behaviour in the context of HIV among MSM in Kiev." *The HIV/AIDS News* 3(5 [in Russian]).

International HIV/AIDS Alliance in Ukraine. (2009). *Annual Report, 2009.* Kiev.

International HIV/AIDS Alliance in Ukraine. (2010). *Estimation of the size of populations most-at-risk for HIV infection in Ukraine in 2009*. Kiev.

Jewkes, R. K., K. Dunkle, et al. "Intimate partner violence, relationship power inequity, and incidence of HIV infection in young women in South Africa: a cohort study." *The Lancet* 376 (9734): 41–48.

Kruglov, Y. V., Y. V. Kobyshcha, et al. (2008). "The most severe HIV epidemic in Europe: Ukraine's national HIV prevalence estimates for 2007." *Sexually Transmitted Infections* 84 (Suppl 1): i37–i41.

Kyrychenko, P. and V. Polonets (2005). "High HIV risk profile among female commercial sex workers in Vinnitsa, Ukraine." *Sexually Transmitted Infections* 81 (2): 187–188.

Mimiaga, M. J., S. A. Safren, et al. "'We fear the police, and the police fear us': structural and individual barriers and facilitators to HIV medication adherence among injection drug users in Kiev, Ukraine." *AIDS Care* 22(11): 1305–1313.

Nitzsche, A. S. (2000). *HIV/STD prevention among FSWs in Ukraine*. International conference on AIDS.

Sarkar, K., B. Bal, et al. (2008). "Sex-trafficking, violence, negotiating skill, and HIV infection in brothel-based sex workers of eastern India, adjoining Nepal, Bhutan, and Bangladesh." *J Health, Population & Nutrition* 26 (2): 223–231.

Schleifer R. (2006). *Rhetoric and risk: human rights abuses impeding Ukraine's fight against HIV/AIDS*. New York: Human Rights Watch.

Stachowiak, J. A., S. Sherman, et al. (2005). "Health risks and power among female sex workers in Moscow." *SEICUS Report*. 33 (2): 18–25.

State Statistics Committee of Ukraine. (2011). *"Population Census of Ukraine (1926 – 2001)."* English language. Retrieved 31 May 2011. http://ukrcensus.gov.ua/

Strathdee, S. A., T. B. Hallett, et al. "HIV and risk environment for injecting drug users: The past, present, and future." *The Lancet* 376 (9737): 268–284.

SWAN. (2009). *Arrest the Violence: Human rights abuses in Central and Eastern Europe and Central Asia*. http://www.harm-reduction.org/library/1673-arrest-the-violence-human-rights-violations-against-sex-workers-in-11-countries-in-central-and-eastern-europe-and-central-asia-report-by-swan.html

TAMPEP. and European Network for HIV/STI Prevention and Health Promotion Among Migrant Sex Workers. (2007). *National Report on HIV and Sex Work*. Kiev.

The World Bank. (2009). *"World development Indicators database"* (7 October, 2009) http://web.worldbank.org/WBSITE/EXTERNAL/DATASTATISTICS. Retrieved 18 July 2011

Ulibarri, M. D., S. A. Strathdee, et al. "Injection drug use as a mediator between client-perpetrated abuse and HIV status among female sex workers in two Mexico-US border cities." *AIDS Behavior* 15 (1): 179–185.

UNAIDS and Ministry of Health of Ukraine (2008). *Ukraine: National report on monitoring progress toward the UNGASS Declaration of Commitment on HIV/AIDS*. Reporting period: January 2006–December 2007. Kiev.

UNAIDS and Ministry of Health of Ukraine (2010). *Ukraine: National report on monitoring progress toward the UNGASS Declaration of Commitment on HIV/AIDS*. Reporting period: January 2008–December 2009. Kiev.

USAID. (2011). *"Ukraine."* Retrieved July 18, 2011. http://www.usaid.gov/our_work/global_health/aids/Countries/eande/ukraine.html.

USAID. and Ministry of Health of Ukraine (2010). *Ukraine: HIV/AIDS Health Profile*. Kiev.

USAID. and Ministry of Health of Ukraine (2011). *Europe and Eurasia Region: HIV/AIDS Health Profile*. Kiev.

CHAPTER 4

HIV Prevention Interventions for Sex Workers: Modeling the Impacts

Key Themes

- Expanding a community empowerment-based, comprehensive HIV prevention intervention among female sex workers in Brazil, Kenya, Thailand and Ukraine in the period 2011–2016 could avert up to 10,800 or between 8 –12% of new HIV infections among sex workers. The intervention demonstrates secondary benefits and could avert up to 20,700 or between 1–4% of new HIV infections among all adults within five years.

- Impact of community empowerment among sex workers is greatest in countries where the prevalence and incidence of HIV is high among female sex workers, their clients and adults generally.

- Combined expansion of ART and the community empowerment intervention may avert 16 to 40% of new infections among female sex workers across these epidemics, using a model of equal access to HIV testing and treatment services.

- An expansion of ART for all adult risk groups is expected to significantly reduce transmission of HIV. The empowerment intervention could help enable ART expansion among sex workers through a community-based outreach and mobilization approach.

The objectives of the mathematical modeling analysis presented here are to provide information and evidence on the possible impacts of scaling up HIV prevention interventions for sex workers. Analyses have been conducted with the objective of determining the impact of various combinations and coverage levels of key interventions in countries with different HIV epidemic scenarios.

The efforts are intended to assist policy makers and program planners in making decisions about resource allocation in the context of constrained funding environments across population groups and varied epidemic contexts. It will also enable researchers to focus the next generation of intervention research, including research around the scale-up and roll-out of novel interventions such as community empowerment-based, comprehensive HIV prevention which is developed and owned by the sex worker community in a given context and epidemic setting.

Interventions Overview and Descriptions

A range of HIV prevention interventions have been developed over the past two decades in response to the need for improved HIV prevention among sex workers. These interventions span biomedical, behavioral and structural approaches to HIV prevention and care among sex workers. The demonstrated efficacy of many of these interventions suggests significant promise in reducing the global epidemics of HIV among sex workers if carried out to scale.

Many of the leading interventions developed to prevent HIV infection among sex workers have been tested in the context of concentrated epidemics, thus, the impact of their widespread implementation across epidemic scenarios has not been well characterized. It is currently unclear if and how proven approaches to preventing HIV among sex workers can be adapted to generalized HIV epidemic settings and if adapted what their impact on curbing HIV incidence might be. In order to respond to such questions, we conducted mathematical modeling exercises on distinct and combined approaches to HIV prevention among sex workers described herein.

HIV prevention interventions are often categorized into three general areas: 1) Biomedical interventions that may include STI screening and management and increased access to ART; 2) Behavioral interventions including strategies such as peer education, condom distribution and social marketing, and HIV counseling and testing; and 3) Structural interventions focused on addressing social and economic inequalities through community and economic empowerment and the promotion of a supportive legal and policy environment for sex worker's rights. Ultimately, a comprehensive and combination approach to HIV prevention is understood by the sex worker community (NSWP 2011) and the field of HIV prevention (UNAIDS 2009) as optimal in reducing HIV infection and is in turn what we modeled in relation to sex workers.

We started however by examining the evidence for separate components of what might be a combination or comprehensive approach to HIV prevention among sex workers. Our initial, broad literature reviews conducted on HIV prevention among sex workers suggested that STI screening and management, peer education, and community empowerment-based approaches may be the most common forms of HIV prevention interventions among female sex workers in lower and middle income country settings. Additionally, given the emphasis on prevention, treatment and care and recent evidence regarding the importance of access to ART as prevention, we also examined the independent and combined impact of access to ART among sex workers.

While government-sponsored, policy-level approaches such as the Thai 100% condom program have received significant attention in the peer reviewed literature regarding HIV prevention among sex workers and their clients, such approaches were excluded from the combination HIV prevention package modeled here given concerns by the sex worker community regarding the lack of a human rights-based approach associated with such programs in the past (NSWP 2011).

To review, evaluate, and synthesize data on HIV prevention, treatment, and care interventions targeted to sex workers in LMIC, we built on existing reviews, utilizing intervention effect size data from recent systematic reviews sponsored by the World Health Organization (WHO). These reviews included those of community empowerment, STI screening and management, and periodic presumptive treatment (PPT) for STIs (WHO, UNFPA et al. 2012). A systematic review of HIV peer education, which included but was not limited to sex workers, was also identified (Medley, Kennedy et al. 2009).

After examining the findings from the community empowerment systematic review conducted we found that all included studies had an HIV peer education component, in addition to community development and mobilization strategies, and in turn the use of a separate review on HIV peer education in conjunction with these other components among sex workers was considered duplicative (WHO, UNFPA et al. 2012). Additionally, non-empowerment oriented, HIV peer education among sex workers did not demonstrate a significant positive impact on consistent condom use with clients in the systematic review identified (Medley, Kennedy et al. 2009).

Standalone STI screening and management as well as PPT interventions were not found to be effective in reducing HIV based on the WHO systematic reviews conducted (WHO, UNFPA et al. 2012). It should also be noted that NSWP members rejected the implementation of PPT with the exception of limited emergency circumstances given concerns that an over-emphasis on STI treatment in the absence of other critical social, behavioral and structural interventions could be created by the widespread adoption of such an approach (NSWP 2011).

While initially promising, recent negative randomized controlled trial findings on the impact of PreP and vaginal microbicides on HIV outcomes for women in addition to NSWP rejection of the implementation of these interventions at the current time led the team not to include these HIV prevention interventions in mathematical modeling and costing analyses. Data on the effects of early initiation of ART on HIV incidence among serodiscordant couples was drawn from a recent peer-reviewed publication from the multi-center, HPTN 052 trial (Eshleman, Hudelson et al. 2011). In turn, the two major areas of intervention modeled here independently and in combination are: "community empowerment-based, comprehensive HIV prevention" and "Early initiation of ART".

Community-Empowerment-based, Comprehensive HIV Prevention

The concept of community empowerment-based, comprehensive HIV prevention is understood here as a collective process through which structural constraints to health, human rights, and well-being are jointly addressed by sex workers to create new possibilities for social and behavioral change and access to health services to reduce their risk for acquiring HIV. The search upon which we relied for effect size data for community empowerment-based, comprehensive HIV prevention involved interventions emphasized the role of the sex worker community in organizing and mobilizing around sex worker priorities and needs. In such a community empowerment-based approach to HIV prevention among sex workers one often sees an initial focus placed on the creation of a safe space for and stimulating a sense of social cohesion among sex workers (Kerrigan, Moreno et al. 2006; Kerrigan, Telles et al. 2008), that can then later be built upon to advocate for increased collective power and control in society and to challenge power structures that deny sex workers access to social and materials resources including but not limited to HIV and health-related services (Lippman, Donini et al. 2010; Lippman, Chinaglia et al. 2012).

The systematic review of sex worker, community empowerment HIV prevention interventions was conducted by searching electronic databases such as PubMed, PsycINFO, Sociological Abstracts, CINAHL (Cumulative Index to Nursing and Allied Health Literature), and EMBASE from January, 1990-October, 2010, reviewing secondary references, and contacting experts to identify articles. Peer-reviewed studies were included in the analysis if they evaluated a community empowerment intervention among sex workers in a low- or middle-income country and if they provided pre-post or multi-arm measures of one of three key outcomes: HIV infection, STI infection, and condom use. The following terms were entered into all computer databases: ("sex work*" OR prostitut*) AND (empower* OR power OR mobiliz* OR mobilis* OR "community development" OR "community led" OR "community-led" OR collective OR solidarity OR "social cohesion" OR "social capital" OR "social vulnerability" OR "social inclusion" OR "social exclusion" OR "social environment" OR participat* OR rights OR environmental OR structural OR peer) AND (HIV OR AIDS OR STI OR STD OR "condom use").

Of the over 6,600 initial citations screened, 10 peer-reviewed studies met the criteria for inclusion in the full analysis. See the flow chart below detailing the sex worker, HIV prevention and community empowerment systematic review search and screening process.

Figure 4.1   Disposition of Citations During the Systematic Review Search and Screening Process for Community Empowerment and HIV Prevention Interventions among Sex Workers in Low to Middle Income Countries

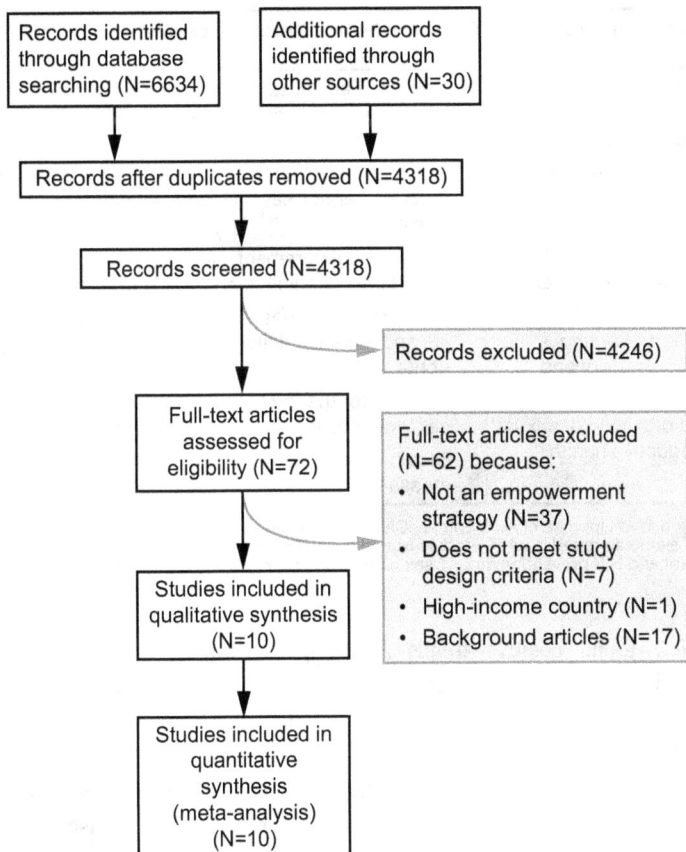

Source: Authors.

We found that all 10 studies which met the inclusion criteria included not only a community empowerment approach focused on the organizing and mobilization of sex workers, but also included some minimum form of the three most common HIV prevention elements conducted among sex workers, including: 1) peer education or education between sex workers describing HIV transmission and risk factors and the importance of safer sexual behaviors including condom use; 2) condom distribution and/or condom social marketing; and 3) the promotion of or greater access to sex worker friendly clinical services for the screening and treatment of STIs. Table 4.1 offers illustrative examples of the key components of the community empowerment based comprehensive HIV prevention interventions documented, signaling those elements with an asterisk which were common to all 10 studies included in the analysis.

Table 4.1   Select Examples of Community Empowerment-based Comprehensive HIV Prevention

Individual and Interpersonal Levels:	Community and Structural Levels:
• Peer education and outreach promoting HIV prevention and collective action[a]	• Collective activities and events to encourage stigma reduction and promote social integration[a]
• Provision of free condoms through clinics, outreach, public events[a]	• Practical skills building workshops on topics such as literacy, savings, and violence prevention[a]
• Enhanced access to STI/HIV prevention, testing and treatment[a]	• Forging of government, NGO and community-based partnerships to support sex workers[a]
• Counseling reinforcing protective behaviors and destigmatization	• Mobilization to engage sex workers in public life and increase dialogue on sex workers' rights
• Increased provision of sexual and reproductive health services	• Support for the formation of an association of sex workers, led and run by sex workers
	• Distribution of materials and local media messages destigmatizing sex workers

Sources: Adapted from Lippman et al.; Lippman, Chinaglia et al. 2012.
a. Intervention elements found in all 10 studies from the WHO systematic review on community empowerment and HIV prevention among sex workers in lower-middle income countries

This review found positive trends regarding the impact of community empowerment interventions among female sex workers on HIV-related outcomes, including HIV infection, STI infection, and condom use. Two observational studies measured the impact of community empowerment on HIV infection itself. The combined effect size was significantly protective (OR: 0.84, 95% CI: 0.709, 0.988). For condom use, one randomized controlled trial demonstrated a significant improvement in consistent condom use with all clients (Beta: 0.3447;

p=0.002), as did six additional observational studies documenting changes in the same outcome.

For our purposes, we meta-analyzed, using a random effects model, the seven studies from the review which measured changes in consistent condom use among female sex workers and all clients. Results of this meta-analysis showed a 51% reduction in the percent of inconsistent condom use among female sex workers exposed to community empowerment-based, comprehensive HIV prevention services (RR 1.77; 95% CI 1.41–2.203) as compared to those non-exposed to services.

Early Initiation of ART

Effect size data on early initiation of ART comes from the HPTN 052 trial, a multi-center phase III, randomized controlled trial which studied HIV transmission dynamics among serodiscordant couples. At baseline, HIV-infected index participants had not yet started ART and had a CD4 cell count of 350–550 cells/mm^3. Their sexual partners were HIV uninfected at baseline. Enrolled couples were randomized to initiate ART in the index at the time of enrollment or to initiate ART in the index when CD4 counts dropped below 250 cells/mm^3 or an AIDS-defining illness occurred. From April 2005 through May 2010, 1,763 couples with an HIV-infected partner were enrolled at 13 sites in Africa, Asia, and North and South America. Initial study findings demonstrated a 96% reduction in HIV transmission among partners where the index initiated ART early. Subsequent linked analyses showed an 88.6% percent reduction in HIV transmission among participating serodiscordant couples (Eshleman, Hudelson et al. 2011).

Methods

We have used mathematical models reflecting the HIV epidemic in four of the selected case study countries, Kenya, Thailand, Brazil, and Ukraine, to study the impact and cost-effectiveness of HIV prevention interventions for sex workers. These models depict the current HIV epidemic in these countries and are further utilized to estimate the number of new HIV infections among sex workers and the adult population with and without one of the effective interventions, and delivered at different levels of coverage and independently or in combination. We have sought to include both regional diversity as well as diversity in epidemic scenarios, including both concentrated and generalized epidemics as well as those with significant injection drug use. The impact of the identified interventions on the number of HIV infections among the general population is also explored. Such an assessment can drive the proper allocation of HIV prevention resources.

Model Description: The Goals Model

Using the updated Spectrum 2011 suite (v. 4.14 Beta 16), developed by Futures Institute, the research team applied the Goals projection model to selected case countries to predict how HIV incidence and prevalence will change among female sex workers as well as in the general adult population in lower and middle income countries when an intervention to prevent HIV transmission among sex workers is brought to scale. The projections are based on combined rollouts of biomedical, behavioral, and structural preventive interventions. The Goals model, often used by countries to estimate national prevalence of HIV infection and future incidence projections, was applied here to investigate the impacts of interventions for female sex workers on the sex work population as well as on the adult population.

The Goals model is a deterministic model, integrated within the Spectrum suite of models/tools as a 'module,' that uses data in several key areas to project HIV prevalence and incidence: demography; sexual behavior; and HIV and sexually transmitted infection (STI) rates. These inputs are specific to the selected country and defined risk groups; Goals uses population level demographic and epidemic projections from other Spectrum modules, such as the AIDS Impact Model (AIM) and DemProj (population).

The population risk groups within Goals are divided into: low, medium and high risk heterosexuals, injecting drug users and men who have sex with men. Specifically, the Goals model allows for comprehensive analysis of HIV epidemic and the impact of interventions targeted to the sex worker population; within Goals sex workers pertain to the category 'High Risk Female Heterosexual' and male clients of female sex workers pertain to 'High Risk Male Heterosexual'. The estimated duration of time within a given risk group can be specified according to research findings and, for sex workers, when this duration has been met, they are re-allocated to the 'Medium Risk Female Heterosexual' category. Though the report will not focus on other risk groups such as men who have sex with men, transgender, people who inject drugs, the inclusion of these groups in the modeling efforts will allow research-ers ensure that the variety of behaviors and differential risk observed in each modeled country is properly assessed. Risk group parameters are obtained and incorporated into the model through additional research, communication with country or risk group experts. Goals then estimates the number of new HIV infections occurring in the adult population and sub-population risk groups based on behavioral data and the intervention effectiveness and coverage.

Within Goals, behavioral parameters, such as numbers of partners, condom use, etc. are edited according to research or surveillance data that are available. Baseline intervention coverage levels are estimated based on country level reporting or expert input, presented as percentages. Goals then projects the number of new infections according to changes in interventions which effect changes to behaviors, and thus risk for HIV transmission. Change in coverage of an intervention is mapped to a change in the behavior of those risk groups reached by the intervention, ultimately changing risk behavior and the number of new infections. Depending on intervention effect, the risk group reached, and associated behaviors, some interventions therefore have wider impact than others. Further description of the Goals model assumptions internal validity and model mechanisms is available in Modeling Annex 4.A and online at http://futuresgroup.com/resources/software_models/goals_model.

Model Parameterization

Data inputs for selected countries are derived from the most recent and highest quality data available from population studies, UNGASS or UNAIDS country reports, other surveillance reports, and country expert opinion, when data were unavailable. Data were inputted for sex worker, sex work client, men who have sex with men, male and female people who inject drugs, and heterosexual risk populations. The initial model fitting and calibration stage of this work fit the Goals HIV epidemic projections to the most recent official national projections. Adult and risk group epidemic curves were developed and then calibrated against UNAIDS projections for adult prevalence. Surveillance estimates or pooled estimates from epidemiologic research studies, when surveillance was unavailable, were used to calibrate the Goals models against historical HIV epidemics among sex work populations. Sex work populations are heterogeneous populations in most countries and, as this report's case studies attest, sex workers demonstrate an array of behaviors and HIV prevalence proportions that vary across geography and contexts. Thus, a limitation to the Goals model is the need to assess sex workers as a single population with a specified behavior and risk. To meet this need, we conducted pooled analyses when faced with multiple and varied estimates, and readers should thus take this into consideration when reviewing the results.

Following parameterization, the models were cross-validated to analyze incidence and prevalence graphs against historical trends for further model adjustments and calibration, as necessary. For Thailand, Kenya, and Brazil models, the study baseline projections were calibrated against 2011 (unpublished) national projections. The 2011 UNAIDS AIM projection was unavailable for calibration at the time of this analysis, thus the UNGASS

2010 country report for Ukraine was referenced for calibration of the Ukraine model.

Model Fitting, Brazil

Data collected from national surveilancence and published studies on the HIV epidemics in Brazil to populate input parameters (see Brazil Case Study). Figure 4.2 depicts the fitted Goals model to the median UNAIDS estimations for the prevalence of HIV infection among the adult population; the model was fit to within the 95% confidence intervals around the projected UNAIDS estimates (Malta, Magnanini et al. 2010; UNAIDS 2010). The model was also fit against prevalence estimates for the female sex work (Malta, Magnanini et al. 2010; comparison not shown), before further modeling scenarios were run.

Figure 4.2   Brazil Model: Comparison of Goals Adult HIV Prevalence Estimates to UNAIDS Estimates

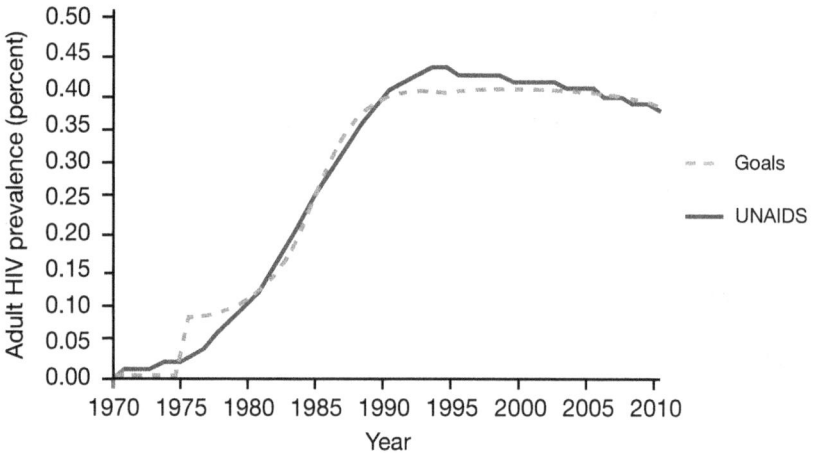

Source: Authors.

Model Fitting, Kenya

Behavioral and epidemiological data obtained through the case study review of published studies and surveillance reports were used to population the parameters for the Goals model (see Kenya Case Study).

The MoT was referenced for missing inputs and to serve as a check while country experts were contacted for any missing data. Figure 4.3 depicts the fitted Goals model to the median UNAIDS estimations for the prevalence of HIV infection among the adult population, fit to within 95% confidence intervals around the projected UNAIDS estimates. The Goals estimates of HIV prevalence among female sex workers was also compared against published studies to assess model fit (not displayed) (Chersich, Luchters et al. 2007; Hirbod, Kaul et al. 2008; Lacap, Huntington et al. 2008; van der Elst, Okuku et al. 2009; Luchters, Vanden Broeck et al. 2010; Tovanabutra, Sanders et al. 2010; McClelland, Richardson et al. 2011).

Figure 4.3   Kenya Model: Comparison of Goals Adult HIV Prevalence Estimates to UNAIDS Estimates

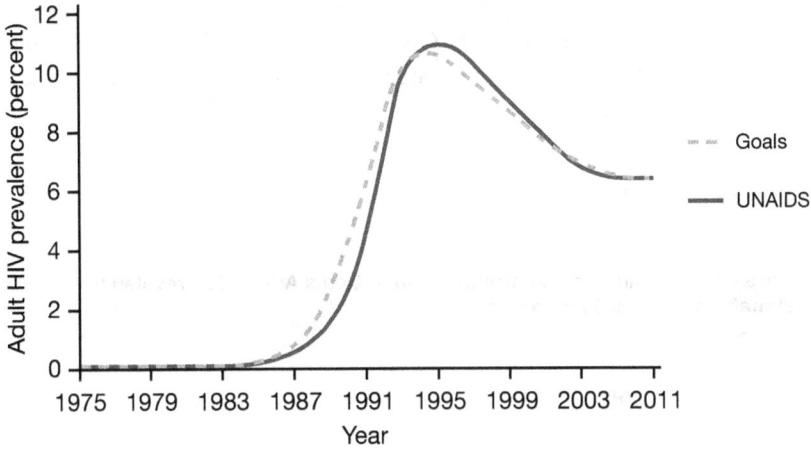

Source: Authors.

Model Fitting, Thailand

Figure 4.4   Thailand Model: Comparison of Goals Adult HIV Prevalence Estimates to UNAIDS Estimates

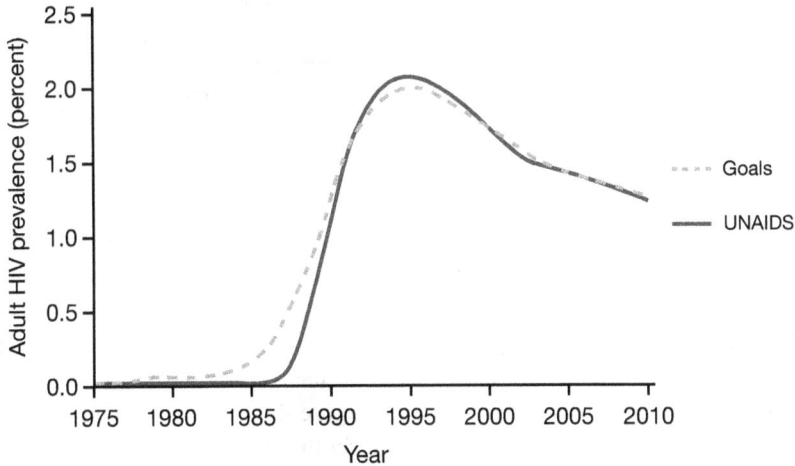

Source: Authors.

Behavioral and epidemiological data obtained through the case study review of published studies and surveillance reports were used to populate the parameters for the Goals model (see Thailand Case Study). The Thai Modes of Transmission study was referenced for missing inputs and to serve as a check on model assumptions. Country experts were contacted for any missing data. Figure 4.4 depicts the fitted Goals model to the median UNAIDS estimations for the prevalence of HIV infection among the adult population; when fitting the models we tried to stay within 95% confidence intervals around the projected UNAIDS estimates. The Goals estimates of HIV prevalence among female sex workers was also compared against published studies to assess model fit (not displayed).

Model Fitting, Ukraine

Figure 4.5   Ukraine Model: Comparison of Goals Adult HIV Prevalence Estimates to UNAIDS Estimates

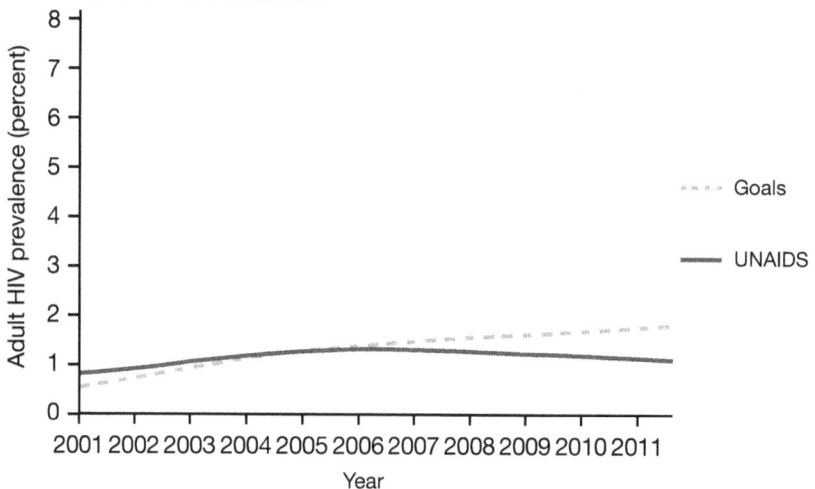

Source: Authors.

The case study review of published studies and AIDS Alliance surveillance reports provided behavioral and epidemiological data which were used to populate the parameters for the Goals model (see Ukraine Case Study). AIDS Allaince Ukraine conducts epidemiological and behavioral surveilance among risk groups in Ukraine and these published data were used to populate the model (AIDS Alliance Ukraine 2011). Figure 4.5 depicts the fitted Goals model to the median UNAIDS estimations for the prevalence of HIV infection among the adult population; when fitting the models we tried to stay within 95% confidence intervals around the projected UNAIDS estimates (UNAIDS and Ministry of Health of Ukraine 2008). The Goals estimates of HIV prevalence among female sex workers was also compared against published studies to assess model fit (not displayed).

Model Scenarios and Analysis Plan

Mathematical modeling scenarios for the select countries are focused on two key interventions: community empowerment of sex workers and scale-up of antiretrovirals (ART) for the adult population who are infected with HIV, according to national estimates and initiation criteria. Behavioral intervention impacts are taken into consideration in the Goals model through the impact matrix. This study focuses on the reduction in condom non-use associated with an intervention for sex workers. Another behavioral impact typically utilized to assess prevention of sexual transmission, is the reduction in number of sexual partners (or clients, in the case of sex workers); however, given the occupational perspective of sex work and that reduction in number of partners or clients would contradict an empowerment approach for sex workers, recognizing sex work as an occupation; this study did not investigate such a reduction in clients or partners and focused, instead, on reduction in condom non-use.

Table 4.2   Goals Model Impact Values for Key Interventions among Female Sex Workers

Parameter	Intervention impact (goals inputs)	Source
Impact of community empowerment-based, comprehensive HIV prevention on condom non-use with all clients	-51.0%	Intervention review
Reduction in transmission on ART	0.13	(Eshleman, Hudelson et al. 2011)
CD4 count at ART initiation[a]	<350 cells/mm^3	(WHO 2010)

Source: Authors.
a. Separate analyses were conducted for Thailand with ART initiation beginning at CD4 <200 cells/mm^3. These methods and results are described in Modeling Annex 4.A.

The systematic review of HIV interventions for sex workers provided the updates necessary for value for the impact of an intervention for sex workers, to be included in the impact matrix. The impact value for the reduction in condom non-use related to community empowerment was drawn from the recent systematic review, commissioned by the WHO. Data from relevant publications were further meta-analyzed all studies related to consistent condom use with all clients across study designs, which ultimately calculated a risk ratio in condom use of 1.77 (95% CI: 1.44, 2.203). This value was recalculated using the formula for relative decrease in non-use: D=(RR-1) x (1-cl)/cl in which cl was the pooled condom use at baseline of the intervention. This calculation estimated a value of -51.0% reduction in condom non-use associated with the intervention.

Given the importance of recent findings from the HPTN 052 study, we also modeled the impact of earlier initiation of treatment, according to the recent change in standards (WHO 2010). These models utilized an initiation of ART at a CD4 count of 350 cells/mm^3 and the demonstrated effectiveness value of 88.6% reduction in risk associated with ARTs at this initiation (Eshleman, Hudelson et al. 2011). For this study, we used a slightly conservative estimate of 87% (0.13 reduction in transmission when on ART). Recent updates to the Spectrum suite include provision of ART according to manually variable CD4 criteria. Specifically for Thailand, this option was used to create two models, estimating impacts at initiation of CD4<350 cells/mm^3, as the most recent international standard,(WHO 2010) as well as initiation at CD4<200 cells/mm^3, as this new initiation criterion has not yet been implemented in-country. Modeling projections for Thailand at CD4<200 cells/mm^3 are included in Modeling Annex 4.C.

Modeling projections followed to analyze and depict impacts on incidence and prevalence among the adult and female sex work populations using several scenarios of varying coverage and intervention combinations. Within Goals, behavioral interventions may be applied and brought to scale among specified risk groups, though ART coverage is applied to the adult population. To focus on the community-empowerment-based, comprehensive HIV prevention scenarios and investigate the impact of this intervention, we held ART coverage among adults constant from the 2011 estimated coverage levels forward through 2016. For the various Empowerment scenarios, we then incrementally expanded coverage, through changes occurring in 2012 through 2016. Likewise, the coverage of the community-empowerment-based, comprehensive HIV prevention was held constant from 2011 forward through 2016 for the first ART scenario, to allow for investigation of the impact among female sex workers when ART is scaled up among the general adult population. For all following ART scenarios, we then incrementally expanded coverage, through changes occurring in 2012 through 2016. Modeling scenarios are presented in the description of results for each of the four case study countries.

For all scenarios, ART coverage and scale-up was based on each country's national estimates, either in percent coverage or absolute numbers that may be covered by ART. Unlike behavioral interventions in Goals, ART can be scaled-up only among the overall adult populations, according to CD4 criterion, and cannot be specifically brought to scale among specified risk groups, such as sex workers. The final ART scenario combines the scale-up of the Community-empowerment-based, comprehensive HIV prevention to what is assumed to be the maximum, feasible coverage reached by 2016 and combined with the national scale-up of ART. Projections depict new infections observed among female sex workers, HIV prevalence among the female sex work population, as well as the new infections among the adult population according to the modeling scenarios.

Uncertainty Analysis

The final step in the modeling process includes uncertainty analyses around the scenarios generated for each country, focusing on the historical fit and future projection. The Spectrum software now has an Uncertainty tool built into the Goals module. Uncertainty estimates around future projections are then created using the historical estimates and impact matrix. Using triangular distribution of the variation around the intervention impact, based on the 95% confidence intervals of the intervention risk ratio, in addition to variation of the historical fit, we ran 500 iterations to generate outcomes. Outcomes are depicted as 1) the 95% plausibility range of adult infections averted when the community-empowerment-based, comprehensive HIV prevention is brought to scale among sex workers, without expansion of ART among adults; and 2) the 95% plausibility range of adult infections averted that are attributed to the scale up of the community-empowerment-based, comprehensive HIV prevention among sex workers, in the presence of expanding of ART coverage among adults.

Results of Modeling Analyses

Figures 4.6 to 4.30 present the modeling analyses grouped per modeled country, Brazil, Kenya, Thailand, and Ukraine. Values corresponding to these figures are displayed in Tables B1 to B.15, which display the number of new HIV infections and HIV prevalence (%) among female sex workers and adult populations. These tables are provided in Annex 4.B which follows this chapter. Table 4.11 and 4.12 present that summary results across the four modeled countries. Within the results presented for each country, we present first the modeling results of the expansion of the community empowerment-based, comprehensive HIV prevention among sex workers. The projections associated with the expansion of ART among the general population are depicted after the empowerment projections in each country. These projections also include one scenario with the combined expansion of ART among the adult population and empowerment among sex workers. Intervention scenarios are compared against that Status Quo, which represents maintained coverage levels of ART and empowerment from 2011 through 2016. Results are presented as new infections among the female sex work population, HIV prevalence among the female sex work population, and number of new HIV infections among the adult population (male and female combined).

Brazil: Community-empowerment-based, comprehensive HIV prevention among female sex workers

Table 4.3 displays the scenarios used to model the scale-up of the community empowerment-based, comprehensive HIV prevention among sex workers in Brazil.

Table 4.3   Community Empowerment-based, Comprehensive HIV Prevention Modeling Scenarios

Scenario		Coverage by 2016
Status quo	Baseline coverage of community empowerment-based, comprehensive HIV prevention held constant among female sex workers (2011–16)	10.0%
	ART held constant among total population (2011–16)	45%
Scenario 1:	Interpolated scale-up of community empowerment-based, comprehensive HIV prevention coverage from 2011 to additional 30% by 2016	40.0%
	ART held constant among total population (2011–16)	45%
Scenario 2:	Interpolated scale-up of community empowerment-based, comprehensive HIV prevention coverage from 2011 to additional 60% by 2016	70.0%
	ART held constant among total population (2011–16)	45%
Scenario 3:	Interpolated scale-up of community empowerment-based, comprehensive HIV prevention coverage from 2011 to reach 100% by 2016	100.0%
	ART held constant among total population (2011–16)	45%

Source: Authors.
Note: ART = antiretroviral therapy.

Figure 4.6 (Table 4.B.1) presents the number of new HIV infections and trends of these infections among female sex workers in Brazil when the community empowerment-based, comprehensive HIV prevention is brought to scale from a baseline coverage level of 10% to reach 40, 70, and 100% by 2016. A total of 2,717 new infections are averted between 2012 and 2016 among female sex workers when the intervention reaches a maximum, 100% coverage, compared to the status quo—a cumulative 15.1% reduction. Reaching a 70% coverage by 2016, a figure that is perhaps more feasible in this time period, more than 1,800 new infections may be averted (10.2% reduction in new infections) between 2012 and 2016 when compared to status quo.

Figure 4.7 (Table 4.B.2) displays the prevalence of HIV infection among female sex workers. The HIV epidemic among female sex workers, as well as the adult population is declining; a trend that is evident during the Status Quo scenario. Bringing the community empowerment-based, comprehensive HIV prevention to scale, however, begins to effect a decrease in prevalence. This decrease is relatively minor, due to the prevalence, which is relatively low, compared to what may be observed among female sex workers in other countries. When viewing these results, it is important to recognize that HIV prevalence typically does not decline in the short term; however, infections averted now will lead to a prevalence drop later.

Figure 4.6   Modeling Scale-up of the Community Empowerment-based, Comprehensive HIV Prevention in Brazil: Trends in Number of New HIV Infections among Female Sex Workers

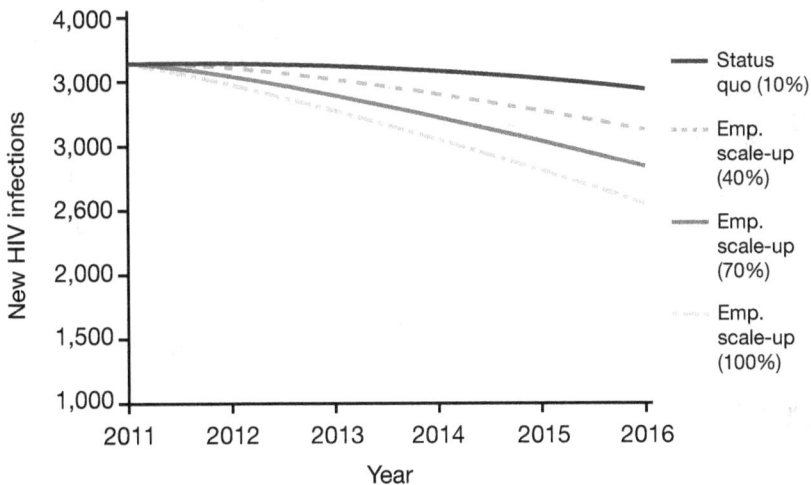

Source: Authors.
Note: Emp. = empowerment.

Figure 4.7   Modeling Scale-up of the Community Empowerment-based, Comprehensive HIV Prevention in Brazil: Trends in Prevalence (%) of HIV Infection among Female Sex Workers

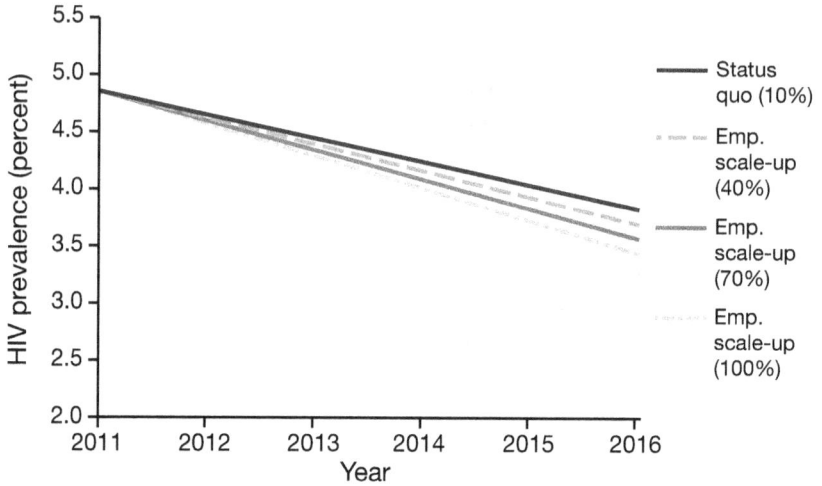

Source: Authors.
Note: Emp. = empowerment.

Figure 4.8   Modeling Scale-up of the Community Empowerment-based, Comprehensive HIV Prevention in Brazil: Annual Number of New HIV Infections among the Adult Population

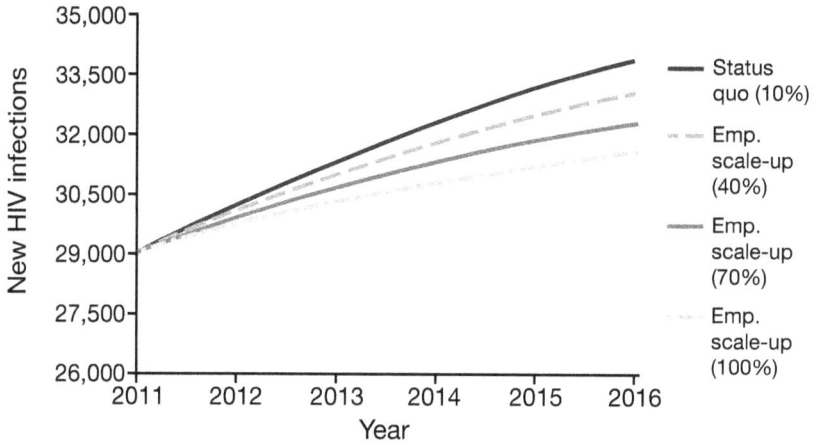

Source: Authors.
Note: Emp. = empowerment

Figure 4.8 (Table 4.B.3) depicts the number of new infections among the adult population when the community empowerment-based, comprehensive HIV prevention is increased to 40, 70, and 100% among the female sex work population. When ART coverage does not increase among the adult population, the number of new infections in Brazil will increase (Status quo). With coverage of the community empowerment-based, comprehensive HIV prevention that reaches 70% among sex workers, however, a total of 4,700 new infections among the adult population may be averted between 2012 and 2016 (a 2.9% reduction). Even greater impact is observed when coverage reaches 100% and more than 7,000 new infections may be averted during this time period.

Brazil: Population-wide ART scale-up and combination with the community empowerment-based, comprehensive HIV prevention for female sex workers

Table 4.4 displays the scenarios used to model the scale-up of ART among adults and the combination of ART and the community empowerment-based, comprehensive HIV prevention for female sex workers in Brazil.

Table 4.4   ART[a] Modeling Scenarios

Scenario		Brazil
Status quo	ART held constant among total population (2011–16)	45%
	Baseline coverage of community empowerment-based, comprehensive HIV prevention held constant among female sex workers	10.0%
Scenario 1:	Scale-up in coverage of ART by 2016 according to country estimations	270,000
	Baseline coverage of community empowerment-based, comprehensive HIV prevention held constant among female sex workers	10.0%
Scenario 2:	Scale-up in coverage of ART by 2016 according to country estimations	270,000
	Interpolated scale-up of community empowerment-based, comprehensive HIV prevention coverage from 2011 of additional 60% by 2016	70.0%

Source: Authors.
Note: ART = antiretroviral therapy.
a. Baseline ART and scale-up among adults based on county UNAIDS projections estimate, absolute numbers.

Figure 4.9 (Table 4.B.4) present the number of new HIV infections and trends of these infections among female sex workers in Brazil when ART is expanded among eligible adults, according to national estimates, by 2016.

An additional scenario depicts the impact when the expansion of ART is combined with expanded coverage of the community empowerment-based, comprehensive HIV prevention, reaching 70% by 2016. These scenarios are compared against that Status Quo, which represents maintained coverage levels of ART and empowerment from 2011 through 2016. A total of 6,000 new infections among sex workers are averted between 2012 and 2016 among female sex workers as ART expands among the adult population, without additional sex worker HIV prevention intervention scale-up. This represents a 33% reduction in new infections among female sex workers. With the addition of the community empowerment-based, comprehensive HIV prevention to ART expansion, a total of 7,123 new infections are averted, resulting in a 40% reduction in new infections between 2012 and 2016. In the presence of ART expansion, the community empowerment-based, comprehensive HIV prevention may avert more than 1,100 infections among sex workers.

Figure 4.9   Expansion of ART among Adult Population and Combination with Community Empowerment-based, Comprehensive HIV Prevention: Trends in New HIV Infections among Female Sex Workers in Brazil

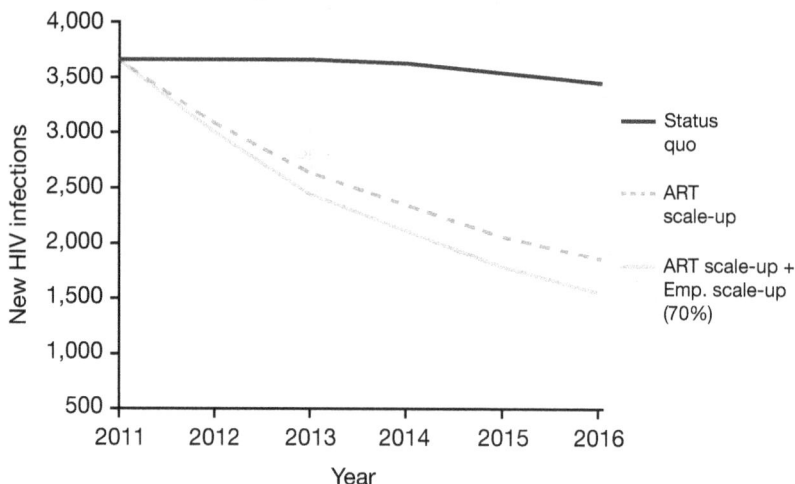

Source: Authors.
Note: Emp. = empowerment; ART = antiretroviral therapy.

Figure 4.10 (Table 4.B.5) displays the prevalence of HIV infection among female sex workers. The HIV epidemic among female sex workers, as well as the adult population is declining; a trend that is evident during the Status Quo scenario. Expanding ART initiates a further decline in the prevalence, which is enhanced with the addition of the community empowerment-based, comprehensive HIV prevention. It is important to keep in mind that HIV prevalence does not change rapidly in the short-term, but comes about through long term changes in new infection. Additionally, considering that ART saves lives, the proportion of people living with HIV will actually begin to increase as ART improves longevity of the population living with HIV.

Figure 4.11 (Table 4.B.6) present the number and trends of new HIV infections among the adult population in Brazil, between 2011 to 2016, when ART is expanded among eligible adults, according to national estimates. An additional scenario depicts the impact when the expansion of ART is combined with expanded coverage of the community empowerment-based, comprehensive HIV prevention from 10% to 70% coverage of the female sex worker population by 2016. Among adults, almost 55,000 new infections may be averted between 2011 and 2016 when ART expands alone. This represents a 34% reduction in new infections among the adult population, between 2012–2016. With the additional scale-up of the community empowerment-based, comprehensive HIV prevention, approximately 57,700 new infections are averted, resulting in a 36% reduction in new infections between 2012 and 2016. In the presence of ART expansion, the community empowerment-based, comprehensive HIV prevention averts an additional 2,800 infections among adults.

Figure 4.10   ART Expansion among the Adult Population and Combination with Community Empowerment for Sex Workers in Brazil: Prevalence of HIV (%) among Female Sex Workers, 2011–16

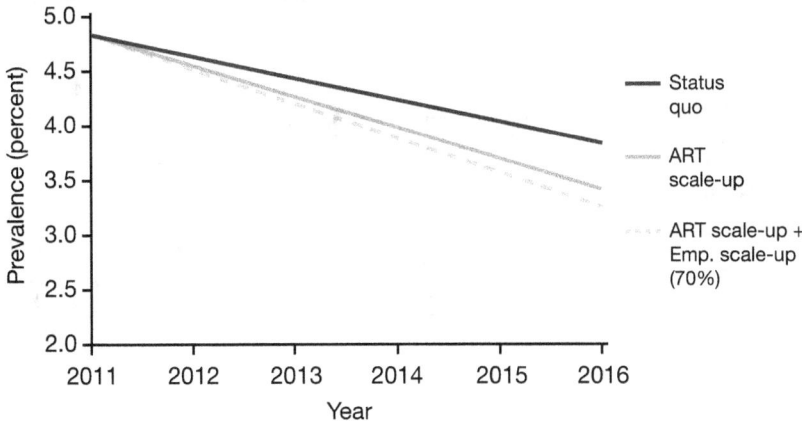

Source: Authors.
Note: Emp. = empowerment; ART = antiretroviral therapy.

Figure 4.11   ART Expansion among the Adult Population and Combination with Community Empowerment for Sex Workers in Brazil: Number of New Infections among the Adult Population

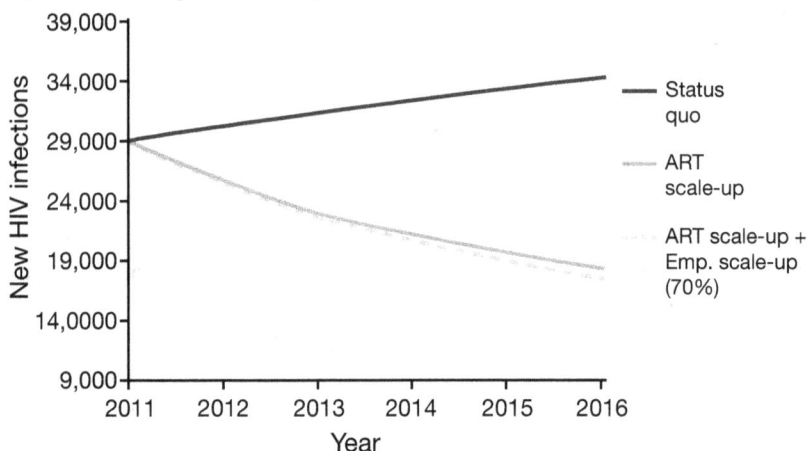

Source: Authors.
Note: Emp. = empowerment; ART = antiretroviral therapy.

Kenya: Community empowerment-based, comprehensive HIV prevention among female sex workers

Table 4.5 displays the scenarios used to model the scale-up of the community empowerment-based, comprehensive HIV prevention among female sex workers in Kenya.

Table 4.5   Community Empowerment-based, Comprehensive HIV Prevention Modeling Scenarios

Scenario	Coverage reached by 2016	
Status quo	Baseline coverage of community empowerment-based, comprehensive HIV prevention held constant among female sex workers (2011–16)	5.0%
	ART held constant among total population[a] (2011–16)	62.7%
Scenario 1:	Interpolated scale-up of community empowerment-based, comprehensive HIV prevention coverage from 2011 to additional 30% by 2016	35.0%
	ART held constant among total population[a] (2011–16)	62.7%
Scenario 2:	Interpolated scale-up of community empowerment-based, comprehensive HIV prevention coverage from 2011 to additional 60% by 2016	65.0%
	ART held constant among total population[a] (2011–16)	62.7%

(continued next page)

Table 4.5   *(continued)*

Scenario		Coverage reached by 2016
Scenario 3:	Interpolated scale-up of community empowerment-based, comprehensive HIV prevention coverage from 2011 to reach 100% by 2016	100.0%
	ART held constant among total population[a] (2011–16)	62.7%

Source: Authors.
Note: ART = antiretroviral therapy.
a. Baseline ART and scale-up among adults based on county UNAIDS projections estimates.

Figure 4.12 (Table 4.B.7) presents the number and trends of new HIV infections among female sex workers in Kenya when the community empowerment-based, comprehensive HIV prevention is brought to scale from a baseline coverage level of 5% to 35%, 65%, and 100% by 2016. A total of 17,000 new infections may be averted between 2012 and 2016 among female sex workers when the intervention reaches a maximum, 100% coverage, compared to the status quo- an 18% reduction. Even when the intervention reaches 65% coverage by 2016, a total of 10,800 new infections are averted between 2012 and 2016 when compared to status quo (11% reduction). Comparing all scale-up scenarios to Status Quo, in which both ART and community empowerment-based, comprehensive HIV prevention are held constant, there is an observed change in the trajectory of the epidemic among sex workers with the increased coverage of the community empowerment-based, comprehensive HIV prevention among female sex workers.

Figure 4.12   Modeling Scale-up of the Community Empowerment-based, Comprehensive HIV Prevention in Kenya: Number of New HIV Infections among Sex Workers

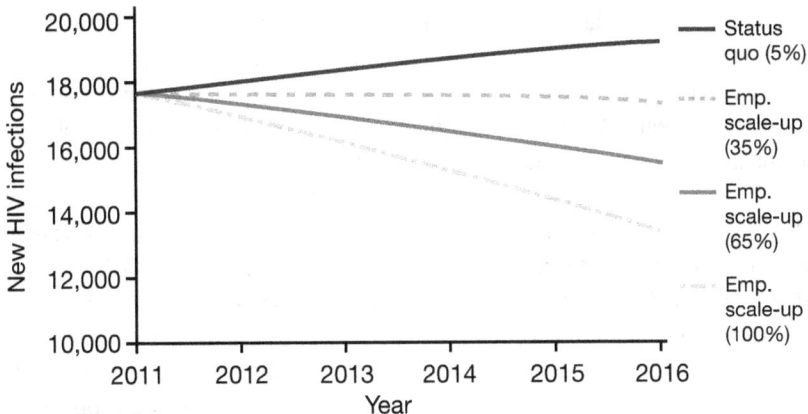

Source Authors.
Note: Emp. = empowerment

Figure 4.13 (Table 4.B.8) display the prevalence of HIV infection among female sex workers. While the overall prevalence is declining among sex workers, evidenced by the reduction from 34% to 29% in 2016 that occurs during the Status Quo scenario; bringing the community empowerment-based, comprehensive HIV prevention to 65% coverage, effects a further decrease in prevalence to 26% among female sex workers.

Figure 4.13   Modeling Scale-up of the Community Empowerment-based, Comprehensive HIV Prevention in Kenya: Annual HIV Prevalence among Sex Workers

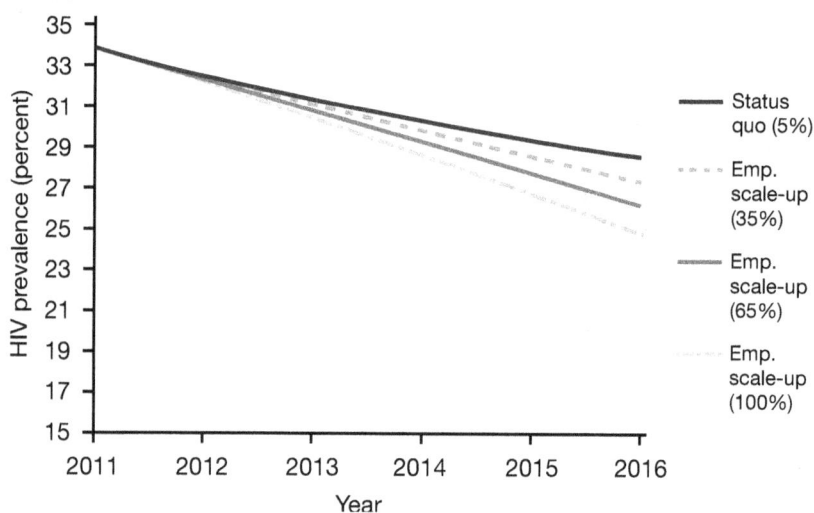

Source: Authors.
Note: Emp. = empowerment

Figure 4.14 (Table 4.B.9) depict the number of new infections among the adult population when the community empowerment-based, comprehensive HIV prevention is increased to 35%, 65%, and 100% among the female sex work population. When ART coverage is held constant from 2011 levels, the number of new adult infections in Kenya will increase. Increasing the coverage of the community empowerment-based, comprehensive HIV prevention demonstrates fewer new infections among adults when empowerment is brought to scale among female sex workers. Reaching 35%, 65%, and 100% coverage demonstrates 2%, 4%, and 6% reductions in the number of new infections among the general population, between 2012 and 2016. Thus, when the community empowerment-based, comprehensive HIV prevention reaches coverage of 65% among sex workers, a total of 20,683 new infections among the adult population may be averted between 2012 and 2016. Even a coverage of 35% demonstrated great impact, averting more than 10,000 infections among the adult population.

Figure 4.14   Modeling Scale-up of the Community Empowerment-based, Comprehensive HIV Prevention in Kenya: New Infections among the Adult Population

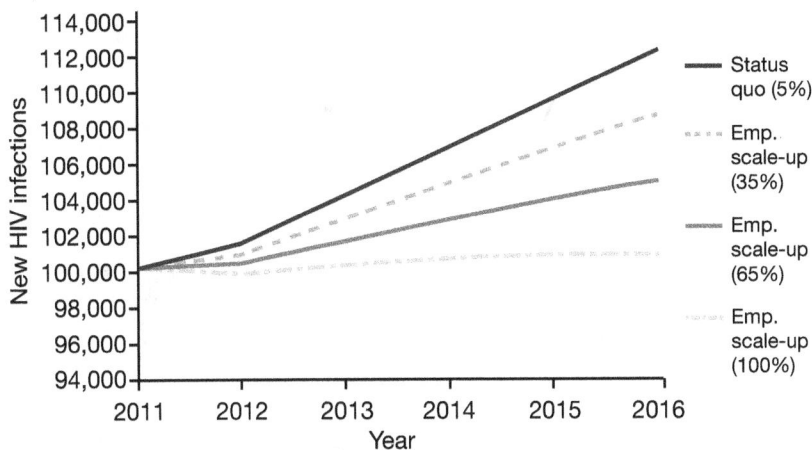

Source: Authors.
Note: Emp. = empowerment; ART = antiretroviral therapy.

Kenya: Population-wide ART scale-up and combination with the community empowerment-based, comprehensive HIV prevention for female sex workers

Table 4.6 displays the scenarios used to model the scale-up of ART among adults and the combination of ART and the community empowerment-based, comprehensive HIV prevention for female sex workers in Kenya.

Table 4.6   ART[a] Modeling Scenarios

ART modeling scenarios		Coverage by 2016
Status quo	ART held constant among total population[a] (2011–16)	62.7%
	Baseline coverage of community empowerment-based, comprehensive HIV prevention held constant among female sex workers	5.0%
Scenario 1:	Scale-up in coverage of ART by 2016 according to country estimations	85.0%
	Baseline coverage of community empowerment-based, comprehensive HIV prevention held constant among female sex workers	5.0%
Scenario 2:	Scale-up in coverage of ART by 2016 according to country estimations	85.0%
	Interpolated scale-up of community empowerment-based, comprehensive HIV prevention coverage from 2011 by additional 60%	65.0%

Source: Authors.
Note: ART = antiretroviral therapy.
a. Baseline ART and scale-up among adults based on country UNAIDS projections estimates (percent coverage).

Figure 4.15   ART Expansion among the Adult Population and Combination with Community Empowerment-based, Comprehensive HIV Prevention for Sex Workers in Kenya: Trends in New Infections among Female Sex Workers

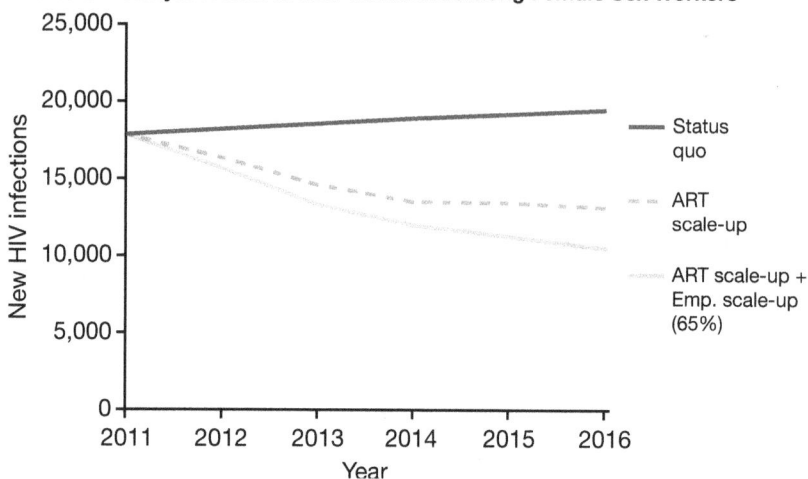

Source: Authors.
Note: Emp. = empowerment; ART = antiretroviral therapy.

Figure 4.15 (Table 4.B.10) presents the number of new HIV infections and trends of these infections among female sex workers in Kenya when ART is expanded among eligible adults, according to national estimates, by 2016. An additional scenario depicts the impact when the expansion of ART is combined with expanded coverage of the community empowerment-based, comprehensive HIV prevention , reaching 65% among female sex workers by 2016. These scenarios are compared against that Status Quo, which represents maintained coverage levels of ART and community empowerment-based, comprehensive HIV prevention from 2011 through 2016. More than 23,200 new infections among female sex workers may be averted between 2012 and 2016 when ART expands among the adult population, compared to the status quo. This represents a 25% reduction in new infections among female sex workers. With the addition of the community empowerment-based, comprehensive HIV prevention, a total of 31,200 new infections may be averted, resulting in a 33% reduction in new infections between 2012 and 2016. In the presence of ART expansion, the community empowerment-based, comprehensive HIV prevention averts an additional 8,000 infections among female sex workers during this time period.

Figure 4.16 (Table 4.B.11) displays the prevalence of HIV infection among female sex workers. The HIV prevalence among female sex workers is declining; a trend that is evident during the Status Quo scenario. Expanding ART initiates a decline in the prevalence to 27% in 2016, compared with Status Quo. This decline is enhanced with the addition of the community empowerment-based, comprehensive HIV prevention, bringing the prevalence to 25% in 2016.

Figure 4.16   ART Expansion among the Adult Population and Combination with Scale-up of the Community Empowerment-based, Comprehensive HIV Prevention for Sex Workers in Kenya: Trends in HIV Prevalence among Female Sex Workers

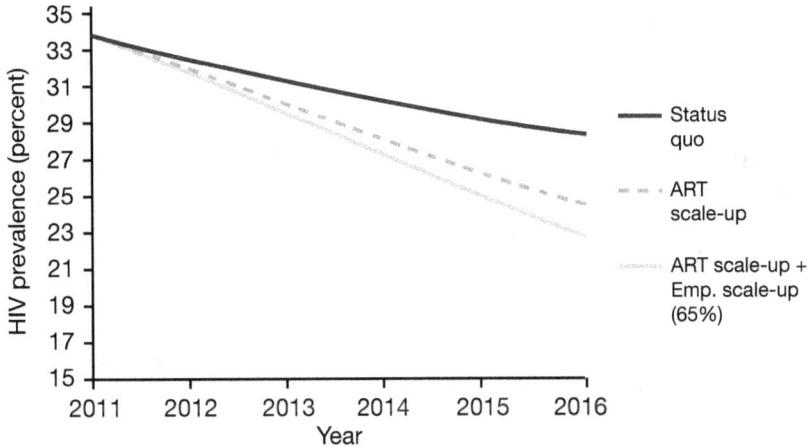

Source: Authors.
Note: Emp. = empowerment; ART = antiretroviral therapy.

Figure 4.17   ART Expansion among the Adult Population and Combination with Community Empowerment-based, Comprehensive HIV Prevention for Sex Workers in Kenya: Trends in New HIV Infections among Adults

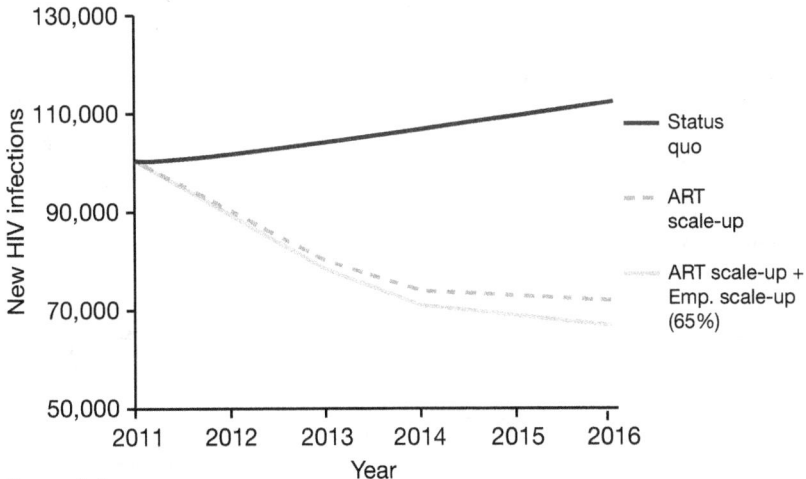

Source: Authors.
Note: Emp. = empowerment; ART = antiretroviral therapy.

Figure 4.17 (Table 4.B.12) present the number and trends of new HIV infections among the adult population in Kenya, between 2011 to 2016, when ART is expanded among eligible adults, according to national estimates. An additional scenario depicts the impact when the expansion of ART is combined when the coverage of the community empowerment-based, comprehensive HIV prevention expands from 5% to 65% of the female sex worker population by 2016. Among adults, more than 145,00 new infections may be averted between 2012 and 2016 when ART expands, compared to the status quo. This represents a 23% reduction in new infections among the adult population, between 2012–2016. With the addition of the community empowerment-based, comprehensive HIV prevention, a total of 160,000 new infections may be averted, resulting in a 30% reduction in new infections between 2011 and 2016. Thus, the addition of the community empowerment-based, comprehensive HIV preventions averts an additional 14,600 infections beyond the benefits observed with only ART scale-up.

Thailand (ART initiation at CD<350): Community empowerment-based, comprehensive HIV prevention among female sex workers

Table 4.7 displays the scenarios used to model the scale-up of the community empowerment-based, comprehensive HIV prevention among female sex workers in Thailand while ART coverage is maintained from 2011 levels through 2016 and ART initiation occurs at CD4<350.

Table 4.7   Community Empowerment-based, Comprehensive HIV Prevention Modeling Scenarios[a]

Scenario		Coverage
Status quo	Baseline coverage of community empowerment-based, comprehensive HIV prevention held constant among female sex workers (2011–16)	10.0%
	ART held constant among total population (2011–16)[b]	53.0%
Scenario 1:	Interpolated scale-up of community empowerment-based, comprehensive HIV prevention coverage from 2011 to additional 30% by 2016	40.0%
	ART held constant among total population (2011–16)[b]	53.0%
Scenario 2:	Interpolated scale-up of community empowerment-based, comprehensive HIV prevention coverage from 2011 to additional 60% by 2016	70.0%
	ART held constant among total population (2011–16)[b]	53.0%

(Continued next page)

Table 4.7   *(continued)*

Scenario		Coverage
Scenario 3:	Interpolated scale-up of community empowerment-based, comprehensive HIV prevention coverage from 2011 to reach 100% by 2016	100.0%
	ART held constant among total population (2011–16)[b]	53.0%

Source: Authors.
a. Second Thailand analysis with ART initiation at CD4 200 included in Modeling Annex 3.
b. Baseline ART and scale-up among adults based on county UNAIDS projections estimates.

Figure 4.18   Modeling Scale-Up of the Community Empowerment-based, Comprehensive HIV Prevention in Thailand: Trends in Number of New HIV Infections among Female Sex Workers

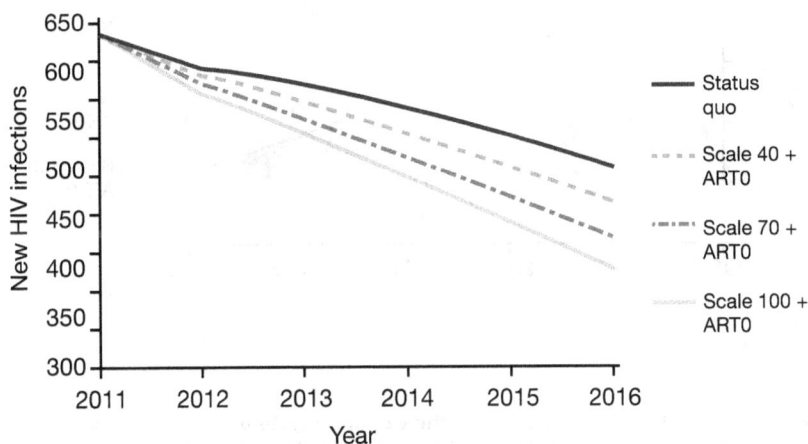

Source: Authors.
Note: ART = antiretroviral therapy.

Figure 4.18 (Table B.13) presents the number of new HIV infections and trends of these infections among female sex workers in Thailand when the community empowerment-based, comprehensive HIV prevention is brought to scale from a baseline coverage level of 10% to 40%, 70%, and 100% by 2016. More than 300 new infections are averted between 2012 and 2016 among female sex workers when the intervention reaches a maximum 100% coverage, compared to the status quo- a 12% reduction. At 70% coverage, a figure that is perhaps more feasible in this time period, more than 200 new infections are averted between 2012 and 2016 when compared to Status Quo.

Figure 4.19 (Table B.14) displays the prevalence of HIV infection among female sex workers. The HIV epidemic among female sex workers, as well as the adult population is declining overall; a trend that is evident during the

Status Quo scenario. Bring the community empowerment-based, comprehensive HIV prevention to scale, however, effects a further decrease in prevalence from 1.82% to 1.76% within a five year period, when the community empowerment-based, comprehensive HIV prevention reaches 70% by 2016.

Figure 4.19   Modeling Scale-up of the Community Empowerment-based, Comprehensive HIV Prevention in Thailand: Trends in Prevalence of HIV Infection among Female Sex Workers

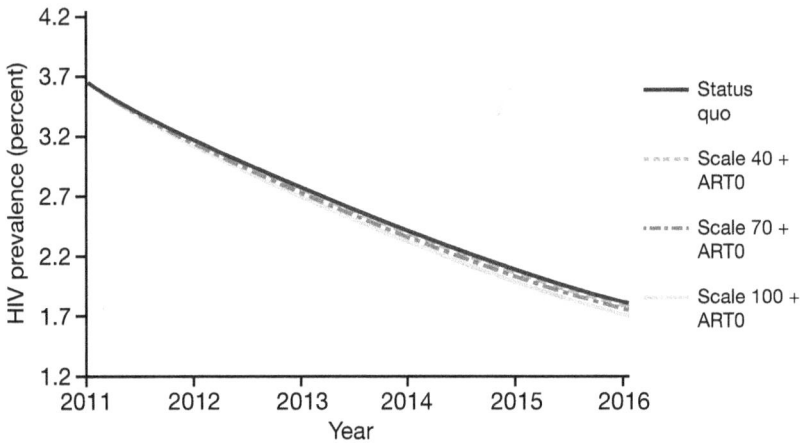

Source: Authors.
Note: ART = antiretroviral therapy.

Figure 4.20   Modeling Scale-up of the Community Empowerment-based, Comprehensive HIV Prevention in Thailand: Annual Number of New HIV Infections among the Adult Population

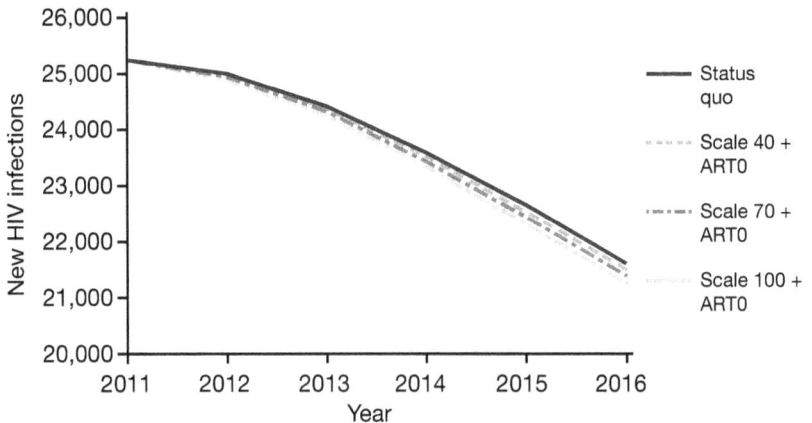

Source: Authors.
Note: ART = antiretroviral therapy.

Figure 4.20 (Table B.15) depicts the number of new infections among the adult population when the community empowerment-based, comprehensive HIV prevention is increased to 40%, 70%, and 100% among the female sex work population. When coverage of ART and the community empowerment-based, comprehensive HIV prevention do not increase (Status Quo), the number of new infections among the adult population totals approximately 117,000 in Thailand between 2012 and 2016. Increasing the coverage of the community empowerment-based, comprehensive HIV prevention to 70% among sex workers, while ART coverage is maintained, reduces then number of new infections among the adult population, averting over 700 new infections between 2012 and 2016, a 1% reduction. Even greater impact is observed when coverage reaches 100%.

Thailand: *Population-wide ART scale-up and combination with the community empowerment-based, comprehensive HIV prevention for sex workers*

Table 4.8 displays the scenarios used to model the scale-up of ART among adults, when initiation occurs at CD4<350, and the combined expansion of ART among adults with an expansion of the community empowerment-based, comprehensive HIV prevention for female sex workers.

Table 4.8   ART[a] Modeling Scenarios

Scenarios		Coverage by 2016
Status quo	ART held constant among total population (2011–16)	53.0%
	Baseline coverage of community empowerment-based, comprehensive HIV prevention held constant among female sex workers	10.0%
Scenario 1:	Scale-up in coverage of ART by 2016 according to country estimations	227,722
	Baseline coverage of community empowerment-based, comprehensive HIV prevention held constant among female sex workers	10.0%
Scenario 2:	Scale-up in coverage of ART by 2016 according to country estimations	227,722
	Interpolated scale-up of community empowerment-based, comprehensive HIV prevention coverage from 2011 of additional 60%	70.0%

Source: Authors.
Note: ART = antiretroviral therapy.
a. Baseline ART and scale-up among adults based on country UNAIDS projections estimate, absolute numbers and ART initiation at CD4<350.

Figure 4.21 (Table 4.B.16) presents the number of new HIV infections and trends of these infections among female sex workers in Thailand when ART is expanded among eligible adults, according to national estimates, by 2016. An additional scenario depicts the impact when the expansion of ART is combined with expanded coverage of the community empowerment-based, comprehensive HIV prevention among sex workers, reaching 70% by 2016. These scenarios are compared against the Status Quo, which represents maintained coverage levels of ART and community empowerment-based, comprehensive HIV prevention from 2011 through 2016. A total of 600 new infections among sex workers are averted between 2012 and 2016 when ART expands among the adult population, as compared to the status quo. This represents a 22% reduction in new infections among female sex workers. With the addition of the community empowerment-based, comprehensive HIV prevention, almost 800 new infections are averted, resulting in a 28% reduction in new infections among sex workers between 2012 and 2016. In the presence of ART expansion, the community empowerment-based, comprehensive HIV prevention averts almost 200 infections.

Figure 4.21   Expansion of ART among Adult Population in Combination with Community Empowerment-based, Comprehensive HIV Prevention: Trends in New HIV Infections among Female Sex Workers

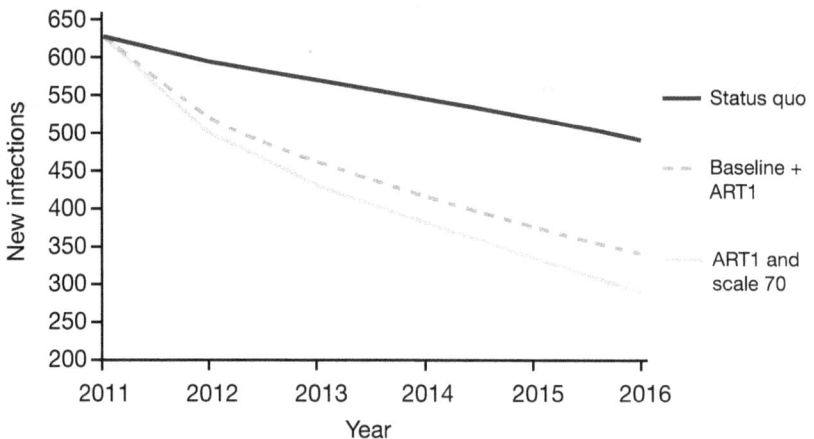

Source: Authors.
Note: ART = antiretroviral therapy.

Figure 4.22 (Table 4.B.17) display the prevalence of HIV infection among female sex workers. The HIV epidemic among female sex workers, as well as the adult population is declining; a trend that is evident with the Status Quo scenario. The slightly higher prevalence observed with the expansion of

ART is likely related to the fact that ART saves lives; therefore the proportion of people living with HIV will actually begin to increase as ART improves longevity of the population living with HIV. Further decline in HIV prevalence to 1.79% by 2016 is observed when ART expansion among adults is combined with the community empowerment-based, comprehensive HIV prevention that reaches a coverage of 70% of female sex workers in 2016.

Figure 4.22   ART expansion among the adult population and combination with community empowerment-based, comprehensive HIV prevention for sex workers in Thailand: prevalence of HIV (%) among female sex workers

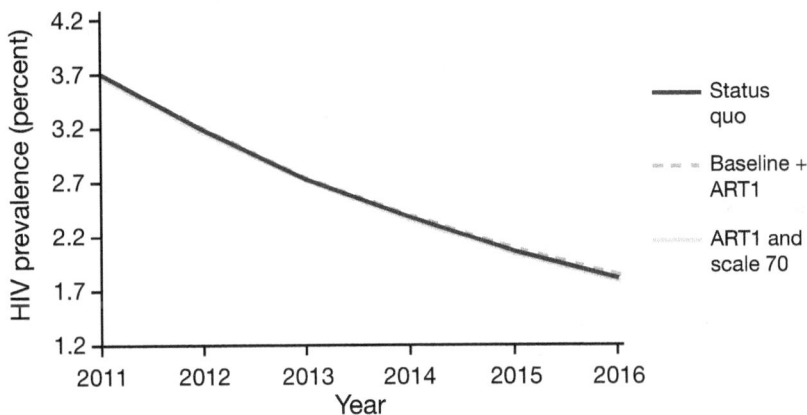

Source: Authors.
Note: ART = antiretroviral therapy.

Figure 4.23 (Table 4.B.18) presents the number and trends of new HIV infections among the adult population in Thailand, between 2011 to 2016, when ART is expanded among eligible adults, according to national estimates. An additional scenario depicts the impact when the expansion of ART is combined with expanded coverage of the community empowerment-based, comprehensive HIV prevention, expands from 10% to 70% coverage of the female sex worker population by 2016. Among adults, approximately 24,900 new infections may be averted between 2012 and 2016 when ART expands, when compared to the status quo. This represents a 21% reduction in new infections among the adult population, between 2012–2016. With the addition of the community empowerment-based, comprehensive HIV prevention, a total of 25,400 new infections are averted, resulting in a 22% reduction in new infections between 2011 and 2016. Thus, in addition ot the benefits observed with ART expansion, the expansion of the community empowerment-based, comprehensive HIV prevention averts an additional 500 infections among the adult population during this time period.

Figure 4.23   ART Expansion among the Adult Population in Combination with Community Empowerment-based, Comprehensive HIV Prevention for Sex Workers in Thailand: Number of New Infections among the Adult Population

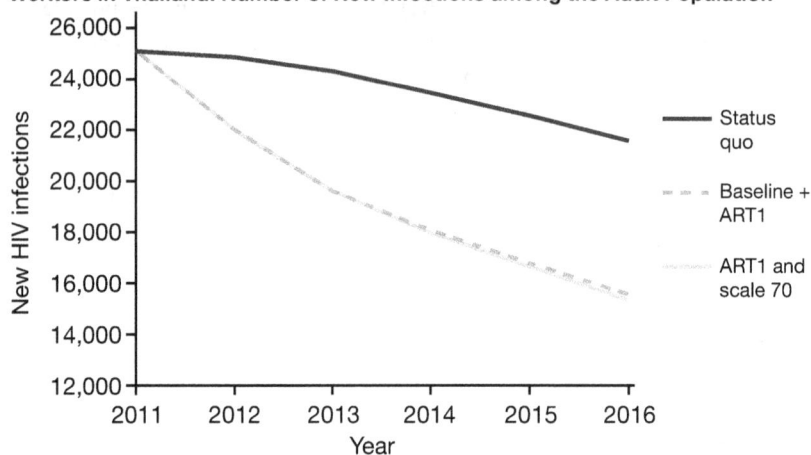

Source: Authors.
Note: ART = antiretroviral therapy.

Ukraine: Community empowerment-based, comprehensive HIV prevention among female sex workers

Table 4.9 displays the scenarios used to model the scale-up of the community empowerment-based, comprehensive HIV prevention among female sex workers in Ukraine.

Table 4.9   Community Empowerment-based, Comprehensive HIV Prevention Modeling Scenarios

Scenario		Coverage by 2016
Status quo	Baseline coverage of community empowerment-based, comprehensive HIV prevention held constant among female sex workers (2011–16)	5.0%
	ART held constant among total population (2011–16)	12.0%
Scenario 1:	Interpolated scale-up of community empowerment-based, comprehensive HIV prevention coverage from 2011 to additional 30% by 2016	35.0%
	ART held constant among total population (2011–16)	12.0%
Scenario 2:	Interpolated scale-up of community empowerment-based, comprehensive HIV prevention coverage from 2011 to additional 60% by 2016	65.0%
	ART held constant among total population (2011–16)	12.0%

(continued next page)

Table 4.9   *(continued)*

Scenario		Coverage by 2016
Scenario 3:	Interpolated scale-up of community empowerment-based, comprehensive HIV prevention coverage from 2011 to reach 100% by 2016	100.0%
	ART held constant among total population (2011–16)	12.0%

Source: Authors.
Note: ART = antiretroviral therapy.

Figure 4.24 (Table 4.B.19) and present the number of new HIV infections and trends of these infections among female sex workers in Ukraine when the community empowerment-based, comprehensive HIV prevention is brought to scale from a baseline coverage level of 5% to reach 35%, 65%, and 100% by 2016. Approximately 3,500 new infections are averted between 2012 and 2016 among female sex workers when the intervention reaches a maximum, 100% coverage, compared to the status quo- an 18% reduction in new infections within five years. At a more feasible 65% coverage, a total of 2,200 new infections are averted between 2011 and 2016 when compared to status quo (12% reduction).

Figure 4.24   Modeling Scale-up of the Community Empowerment-based, Comprehensive HIV Prevention in Ukraine: Number of New HIV Infections among Sex Workers

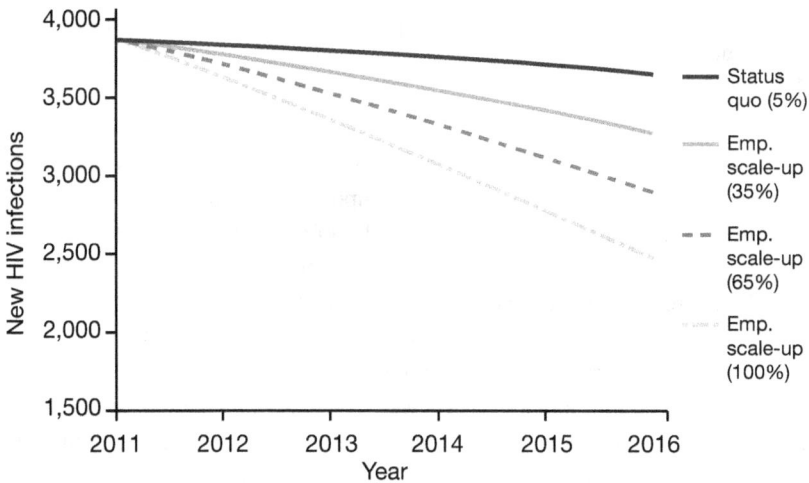

Source: Authors.
Note: Emp. = empowerment.

Figure 4.25 (Table 4.B.20) display the prevalence of HIV infection among female sex workers. While the overall prevalence is steady among sex workers, around 16% from 2011 to 2016, during the Status Quo, bringing the community empowerment-based, comprehensive HIV prevention to scale begins to effect a decrease in the epidemic. Thus, prevalence proportions among sex workers in Ukraine decline to 15.4%, 14.5% and 13.5% by 2016 when community empowerment-based, comprehensive HIV prevention reaches 35%, 65%, and 100% coverage by 2016.

Figure 4.25   Modeling the Scale-up of the Community Empowerment-based, Comprehensive HIV Prevention in Ukraine: Trends in HIV Prevalence among Female Sex Workers

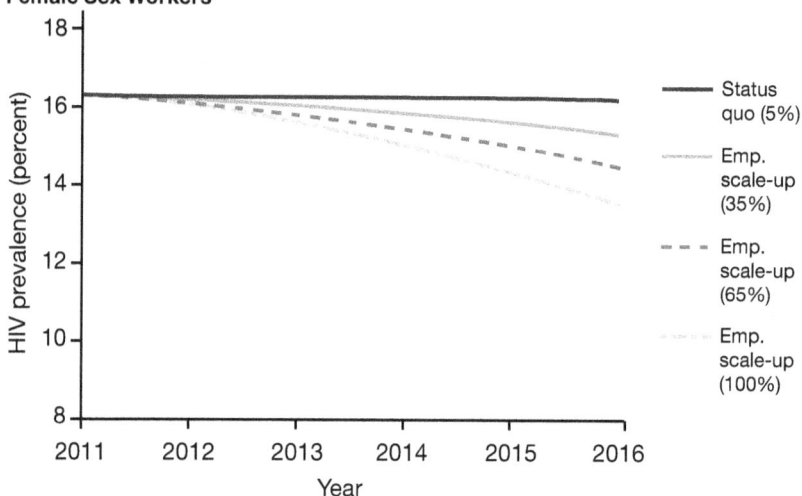

Source: Authors.
Note: Emp. = empowerment.

Figure 4.26 (Table 4.B.21) depicts the number of new infections among the adult population when the community empowerment-based, comprehensive HIV prevention is increased to 35, 65, and 100% among the female sex work population. When ARTs and the community empowerment-based, comprehensive HIV prevention are held constant from 2011 levels, the adult annual incidence in Ukraine will remain relatively stable between 2012 and 2016. Increasing the coverage of the community empowerment-based, comprehensive HIV prevention demonstrates fewer new infections among adults when community empowerment-based, comprehensive HIV prevention is brought to scale among female sex workers. Reaching 65% and 100% coverage by 2016 demonstrably reduces the number of new infections by 3% and 4% among adults, between 2012 and 2016. Though the percent reduction may apprear low, the absolute numbers are high: reaching coverage of 65% of sex workers, averts almost 7,000 infections among the adult population within a five year period.

Figure 4.26 Mo eling the Scale-up of the Community Empowerment-based, Comprehensive HIV Prevention in Ukraine: Trends in New HIV Infections among the Adult Population

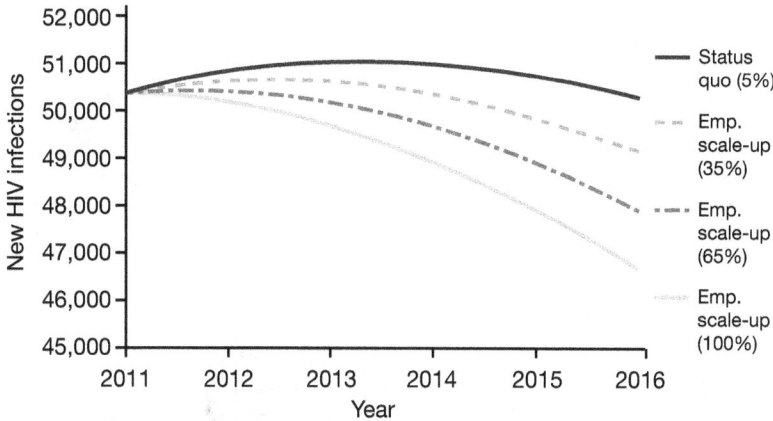

Source: Authors.
Note: Emp. = empowerment.

Ukraine: Population-wide ART scale-up and combination with the community empowerment-based, comprehensive HIV prevention for female sex workers

Table 4.10 displays the scenarios used to model the scale-up of ART among adults and the combination of ART and the community empowerment-based, comprehensive HIV prevention for female sex workers in Ukraine.

Table 4.10 ART[a] Modeling Scenarios

ART modeling scenarios		Coverage by 2016
Status quo	ART held constant among total population, 2011–16	12.0%
	Baseline coverage of community empowerment-based, comprehensive HIV prevention held constant among female sex workers	5.0%
Scenario 1:	Scale-up in coverage of ART by 2016 according to country estimations	58,000
	Baseline coverage of community empowerment-based, comprehensive HIV prevention held constant among female sex workers	5.0%
Scenario 2:	Scale-up in coverage of ART by 2016 according to country estimations	58,000
	Interpolated scale-up of community empowerment-based, comprehensive HIV prevention coverage from 2011 by additional 60% by 2016	65.0%

Source: Authors.
Note: ART = antiretroviral therapy.
a. Baseline ART and scale-up among adults based on county UNAIDS projections estimates (absolute numbers).

Figure 4.27   ART Expansion among the Adult Population and Combination with Community Empowerment-based, Comprehensive HIV Prevention for Sex Workers in Ukraine: New Infections among Female Sex Workers, 2011–16

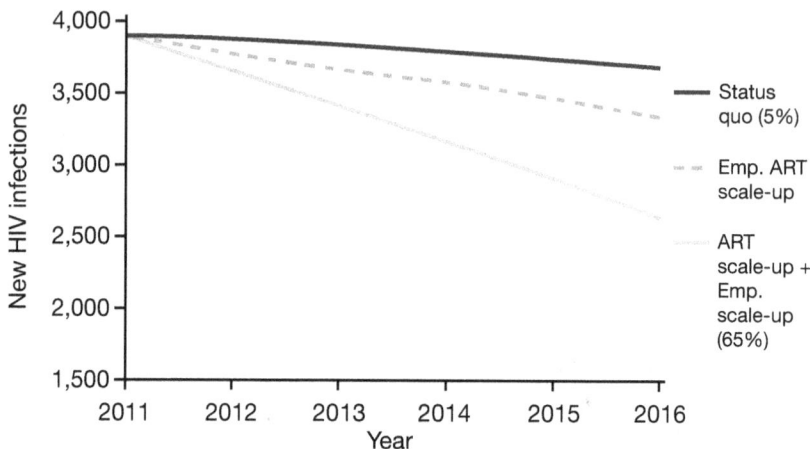

Source: Authors.
Note: Emp. = empowerment; ART = antiretroviral therapy.

Figure 4.27 (Table 4.B.22) present the number of new HIV infections and trends of these infections among female sex workers in Ukraine when ART is expanded among eligible adults, according to national estimates, by 2016. An additional scenario depicts the impact when the expansion of ART is combined with expanded coverage of the community empowerment-based, comprehensive HIV prevention, reaching 65% coverage by 2016. These scenarios are compared against that Status Quo, which represents maintained coverage levels of ART and community empowerment-based, comprehensive HIV prevention from 2011 through 2016. More than 1,000 infections among female sex workers are averted between 2012 and 2016 when ART expands among the adult population, compared to the status quo. This represents almost a 6% reduction in new infections among female sex workers during this time period. With the addition of the community empowerment-based, comprehensive HIV prevention, more than 3,100 new infections are averted, resulting in a 17% reduction in new infections between 2012 and 2016. Thus, in addition to benefits obseved with ART expansion, the expansion of community empowerment-based, comprehensive HIV prevention averts another 2,100 infections among the sex worker population.

Figure 4.28 (Table 4.B.23) displays the prevalence of HIV infection among female sex workers. While the prevalence is steady around 16% when ARTs and the community empowerment-based, comprehensive HIV prevention are constant, expanding ART to the adult population initiates a slight decrease in the prevalence observed in 2016, compared with Status Quo. This decline is augmented with the addition of the community empowerment-based, comprehensive HIV prevention, which may bring the prevalence down to 14% in 2016. In this case, the fact that ART saves lives, may prevent the prevalence from declining further within this five year timeframe.

Figure 4.28   ART Expansion among the Adult Population and Combination with Community Empowerment-based, Comprehensive HIV Prevention for Sex Workers in Ukraine: Trends in HIV Prevalence (%) among Female Sex Workers, 2011–16

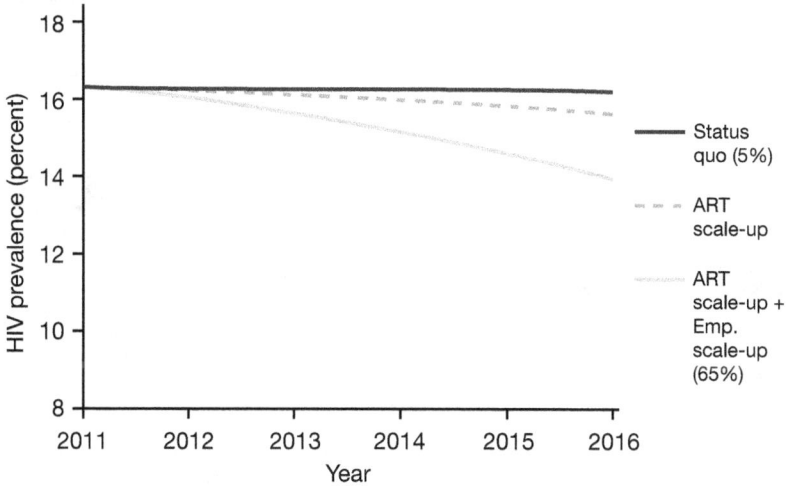

Source: Authors.
Note: Emp. = empowerment; ART = antiretroviral therapy.

Figure 4.29 (Table 4.B.24) presents the number and trends of new HIV infections among the adult population in Ukraine, between 2011 to 2016, when ART is expanded among eligible adults, according to national estimates. An additional scenario depicts the impact when the expansion of ART is combined with expanded coverage of the community empowerment-based, comprehensive HIV prevention, expands from 5% to 65% coverage of the female sex worker population by 2016. Among adults, a total of 15,900 new infections are averted between 2012 and 2016 when ART expands, compared to the status quo. This represents a 6% reduction in new infections among the adult population, between 2012–2016. With the addition of the community empowerment-based, comprehensive HIV prevention, a total of 22,300 new infections are averted, resulting in almost a 9% reduction in new infections between 2012 and 2016. Thus, the expansion of the community empowerment-based, comprehensive HIV prevention averts an additional 6,400 infections among adults, in addition to those averted by ART.

Figure 4.29   ART Expansion among the Adult Population and Combination with Community Empowerment-based, Comprehensive HIV Prevention for Sex Workers in Ukraine: Trends in New HIV Infections among the Adult Population

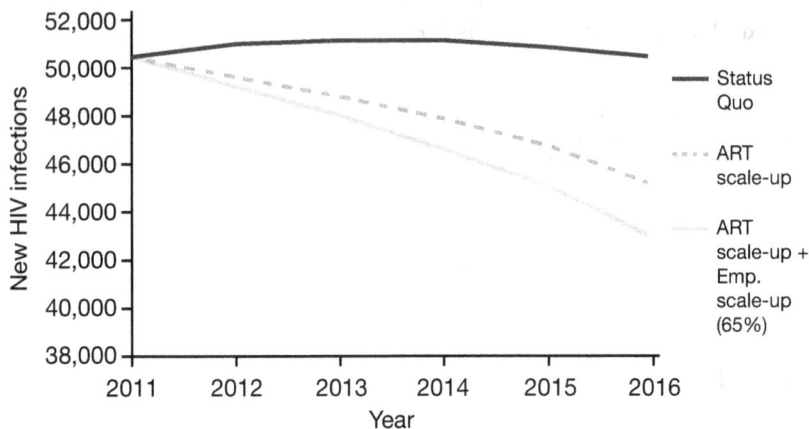

Source: Authors.
Note: Emp. = empowerment; ART = antiretroviral therapy.

Uncertainty Analyses

Table 4.11   Range of Cumulative Infections Averted among Adults Between 2012–16 When the Community Empowerment-based, Comprehensive HIV Prevention is Expanded to a Maximum, Feasible Coverage among Female Sex Workers by 2016

Infections averted	Brazil	Kenya	Thailand	Ukraine
Low range	3,991	16,661	580	5,913
Median	5,103	21,242	745	7,507
High range	6,976	28,828	1,021	10,135
Goals	4,741	20,683	725	6,920

Source: Authors.
Note: ART = antiretroviral therapy. Early initiation of ART occurs at CD4<350 for all countries.

Table 4.11 and Figure 4.30 display the number and range of adult infections averted in each country when the uncertainty analysis is applied to model scenario in which the community empowerment-based, comprehensive HIV prevention reaches the maximum feasible coverage level by 2016. The vertical line in Figure 4.30 depicts a 95% plausibility range around the median uncertainty estimate. For Kenya and Ukraine, coverage of the community empowerment-based, comprehensive HIV prevention increases from 5% to 65% from 2011 to 2016 and for Thailand and Brazil coverage of the community empowerment-based, comprehensive HIV prevention increases from 10% in 2011 to 70% in 2016 as ART coverage is maintained at 2011 levels. The median uncertainty estimate is also compared against the Goals for further validation.

Across these epidemics, the community empowerment-based, comprehensive HIV prevention may avert between 700 adult infections, as observed in Thailand, and 20,700 infections, as in Kenya, within the five year time span. Even at the lowest range of impacts, we see that the expansion of the community empowerment-based, comprehensive HIV prevention may cumulatively avert between 600 and 16,700 adult infections across the epidemics.

Figure 4.30   Cumulative Infections Averted among Adults Between 2012 and 2016 When the Community Empowerment-based, Comprehensive HIV Prevention is Expanded to a Maximum, Feasible Coverage among Female Sex Workers by 2016

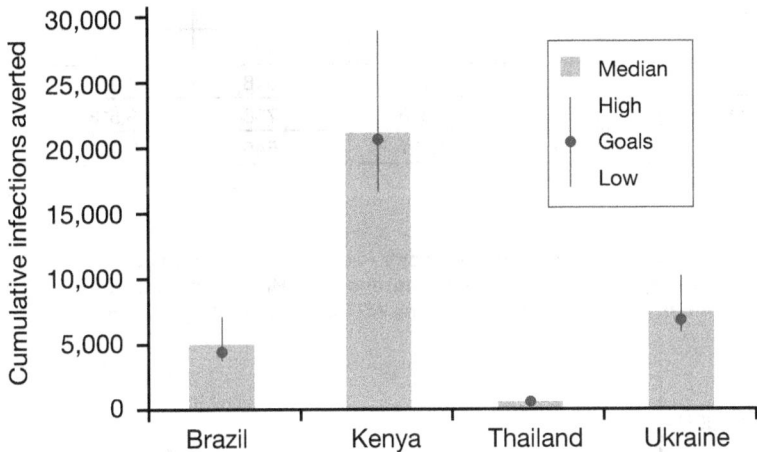

Source: Authors.

Table 4.12 and Figure 4.31 display the number and range of adult infections averted in each country when the uncertainty analysis when the community empowerment-based, comprehensive HIV prevention is scaled up among sex workers simultaneously with ART among adults. Specific focus is on the infections averted by the community empowerment-based, comprehensive HIV prevention in this context; the total infections averted by the combination of both interventions are not included in the table (the country results sections provide these combined values). For these estimates, coverage of the community empowerment-based, comprehensive HIV prevention in Kenya and Ukraine again increase from 5% in 2011 to 65% in 2016 and for Thailand and Brazil coverage increases from 10% in 2011 to 70% in 2016, in addition to reaching country estimates for ART coverage and initiation at CD4<350.

Across these epidemics, the community empowerment-based, comprehensive HIV prevention may cumulatively avert between 550 adult infections, as observed in Thailand, and approximately 14,800 infections, as in Kenya, in addition to the number of infections averted by ART within the five year time span. Even at the lowest range of impacts, we see that the expansion of the community empowerment-based, comprehensive HIV prevention may cumulatively avert between 400 and 12,000 adult infections across the epidemics.

Table 4.12   Cumulative Adult Infections Averted by the Expansion of the Community Empowerment-based, Comprehensive HIV Prevention, in the Context of Early Initiation and Expanding ART among Adults, 2012–16

Infections averted	Brazil	Kenya	Thailand	Ukraine
Low range	2,286	11,989	427	5,547
Median	3,046	15,340	548	7,045
High range	4,194	20,816	758	9,513
Goals	2,806	14,751	545	6,424

Source: Authors.

Figure 4.31   Cumulative Adult Infections Averted by the Expansion of the Community Empowerment-based, Comprehensive HIV Prevention, in the Context of Early Initiation and Expanding ART among Adults, 2012–16

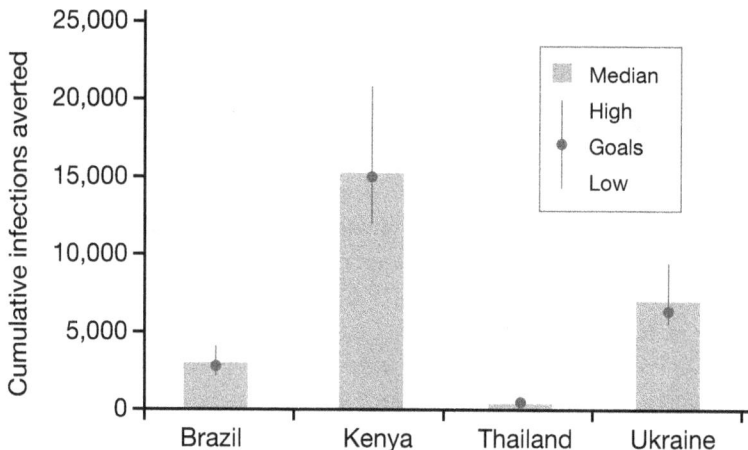

Source: Authors.

These analyses demonstrate the range of impacts associated with the community empowerment-based, comprehensive HIV prevention. In the environment in which ART does not expand among adults, a greater number of adult infections are averted as there are more infections for the community empowerment-based, comprehensive HIV prevention to avert.

Discussion

These modeling combinations are informative and acknowledge that female sex workers and the general adult population are not isolated from each other. These scenarios demonstrate the impact and community empowerment-based, comprehensive HIV prevention for female sex workers and the early initiation of ART among adults on infections among both the female sex work population and the general adult population of HIV prevention programs for both populations.

Expanding the empowerment HIV prevention intervention among sex workers has demonstrable impact on the HIV epidemics among female sex workers, cumulatively averting between 220 and 10,800 infections among sex workers across epidemic scenarios. Similarly, the expansion of this community empowerment-based, comprehensive HIV prevention demonstrates additional impact on the adult population, cumulatively 700 to 20,700 infections among adults within five years. Impacts of the community empowerment-based, comprehensive HIV prevention are greatest in countries, such as Kenya, where the prevalence of HIV is high among adults as well as female sex workers. These intervention impacts are particularly important in light of possible synergies that exist between the community empowerment-based, comprehensive HIV prevention and provision of ART to those in need. Furthermore, these impacts are important to note for countries where there may be limited access to ART drugs or other resources, but where community empowerment-based, comprehensive HIV prevention-based interventions may be more feasibly implemented. Countries, such as Brazil and Thailand, which have made great headway to decrease HIV transmission, still demonstrate impact when the community empowerment-based, comprehensive HIV prevention is scaled-up. Though lower than other countries, impacts are observed, and highlight the need for continued support of such interventions for sex workers to further reduce the number of new infections.

Both interventions rely on outreach to the affected populations and, particularly for more hidden populations, successful access to these populations may be realized through a community-based approach, such as that which is employed by the community empowerment-based, comprehensive HIV prevention. Early initiation and expansion of ART among the adult populations, reduces mortality and morbidity. It reduces HIV incidence among female sex workers through reducing HIV infectiousness among their clients. Such impacts are only possible among sex workers, however, if a good outreach program is in place to find sex workers in need of treatment and if they subsequently have equal access to HIV testing and treatment services. Built on an enabling outreach program, the community empowerment-based, comprehensive HIV prevention may cumulatively avert between 550 adult infections, as observed in Thailand, and almost 14,800 infections, as in Kenya, within the five-year time span, even as ART coverage increases.

These results do not imply that the intervention is less effective; rather, when ART coverage increases there are fewer adult infections for the community empowerment-based, comprehensive HIV prevention to avert. Moreover, early initiation of ART among sex workers benefits mostly their clients, while an community empowerment-based, comprehensive HIV prevention can prevent infections among sex workers directly and the general population, indirectly. It should also not be interpreted that early initiation of ART alone should be implemented for HIV prevention; consideration should be given to the fact that ART treatment of HIV infected individuals prevents transmission between discordant couples. The community empowerment-based, comprehensive HIV prevention works among both those with and without HIV infection, as well as those undiagnosed infections, to prevent HIV transmission and transmission of other STIs. The community empowerment-based, comprehensive HIV prevention has the added benefit of averting other morbidity and mortality associated with HIV and STI infection. As the Network of Sex Worker Projects indicated, condom use is considered the most important form of protection during sex work (personal communication, September. 2011).

These findings must be viewed in light of several limitations. First, sex work populations are heterogeneous groups in most countries and, as this report's case studies attest, sex workers demonstrate an array of behaviors, risk exposures, and HIV prevalence that vary across geography and contexts. Thus, a limitation to the Goals model is the need to assess the sex workers as a single population with a specified behavior and risk. To meet this need, we conducted pooled analyses when faced with multiple and varied estimates, and readers should thus take this into consideration when reviewing the results. Furthermore, the Goals model currently assumes that all sexual transmission of HIV among female sex workers is via vaginal sex and does not account for any anal intercourse or associated condom use.

We estimated the impacts of early initiation of ART and scale-up of ART among sex workers as well as the adult population. Early initiation is a new intervention and most countries have adopted this policy only as recently as 2010. Therefore, it is important to recognize that ART coverage among people in need of ART in 2011 may be lower than earlier years, when ART was initiated at a CD4 < 200 and fewer people were classified as 'in need of ART'. This is particularly reflected when comparing the impacts of the ART scenarios in Thailand (see the Thailand Modeling results for initiation at CD4<350 and the Modeling appendix for initiation at CD4<200). Because ART coverage is based on a country's ability to provide treatment to a certain population size, with early initiation, there is a lower baseline coverage (53%) of treatment for people in need of ART when compared to estimates when initiation begins at CD4<200 (coverage was estimated at 68% among those in need of ART). As a result of differences in baseline coverage, there were no major differences in impacts observed between the two different initiation criteria in Thailand within this short, five year time span, as would have been expected with early initiation.

Related to the impacts of ART among sex workers, it is important to note that the model does not link voluntary HIV counseling and testing that is associated with community empowerment to ART, as ART is allocated based on CD4 count. Additionally, CD4 count and the populations within each risk group who are in need of and covered by ART are influenced by disease progression and the length of time in the risk group; hence, sex workers who are living with HIV may 'move out' of the sex work population (so not captured as this group by Goals, but rather as medium risk individuals) before progressing to the disease stage in which they would require ART. Finally, the effects of discrimination and criminalization on access to treatment are not accounted for with this model. Thus, the estimates of the sex work population in need of and receiving ART may be optimistic, if sex workers do not have equal access to testing and ART services, as other studies have highlighted (Thuy, Nhung et al. 1998; Chakrapani and Newman 2009; Beattie and Bhattacharjee 2012).

Modeling Annex 4.A   Goals Model Description

Goals Model Description

The Goals model is widely used to support national (Forsythe, Stover et al. 2011) and international planning for HIV programs (Stover, Walker et al. 2002; Stover, Bertozzi et al. 2006; Stover, Bollinger et al. 2007) by projecting the expected impact and cost of combinations of prevention and treatment programs. It contains a transmission model that calculates the number of new HIV infections over time as a result of sexual and injecting drug transmission.

T he Goals model is implemented within Spectrum's suite of policy tools and interacts with other Spectrum models. The demographic projection module, DemProj, performs demographic calculations and provides information on the size of the adult population and the number of people becoming adults, aging out of the 15–49 age group and dying from non-HIV causes. Demographic data are drawn from the United Nations Population Division estimates of historical trends from 1970–2010 and projections to 2015. This includes the distribution of the population by age and sex in the base year and trends in fertility, mortality and migration.

The AIM (AIDS Impact model) module projects the consequences of changes in incidence, including the number of people living with HIV, number of new infections, number of pregnant women infected with HIV, and mortality due to AIDS. It is widely used to forecast national near-term treatment and PMTCT needs (Stover, Johnson et al. 2010). The Goals model works in tandem with AIM, and in this modeling project it uses official ART program statistics from national Spectrum/AIM projection models.

Model Structure and Internal Validity of Modeling Assumptions

The Goals model simulates an HIV epidemic in an adult population aged 15–49. The adult population is disaggregated by sex and risk group. Although people enter the model at age 15, they are assumed not to be sexually active until they reach the median age at first sex for a particular country.

Individuals are allocated into one of five risk categories, chosen partly because they are epidemiologically important and partly because information about three of the categories (stable couples, multiple partners, sex workers and clients) is available from national surveys. The risk categories are: stable couples (men and women reporting a single partner in the last year), multiple partners (men and women who report more than one partner in the last year), female sex workers and clients, men who have sex with men and injecting drug users.

Risk groups are defined by the behaviors specified in each application, so almost any risk structure might be modeled. While any individual may belong to more than one group, people are classified according to their highest risk. Once a person joins a risk group he or she remains in that risk group until aging out at age 50, dying from non-HIV causes, dying from AIDS or changing behavior.

Behavior change allows people to move from one risk group to the next lower risk group. Duration in a risk group may be specified as a lifetime or as an average number of years. For example, duration in sex work might be set to

5 or 10 years. Those leaving the highest risk groups (sex work, men who have sex with men, injecting drug users) move to the medium risk group (multiple partners) and those leaving the multiple partners group move to the stable couples risk group.

Sexual Transmission of HIV

Transmission of HIV from an infected partner to an uninfected partner depends on many factors. For the susceptible partner the important characteristics are: the number of partners he or she has, if male, whether he is circumcised and whether new prevention methods, such as PrEP or vaccines, are used.

Transmission from the infected partner is affected by: stage of infection (primary, asymptomatic, or symptomatic), whether he or she is receiving ART, whether he or she has received an HIV vaccine that reduces infectiousness.

The following characteristics of the partnership influence transmission: number of sex acts per partner per year, whether either partner has a sexually transmitted infection and condom use.

HIV Transmission Equation

The probability of transmission to an uninfected partner during one year is given by the following equation,

$$\text{where: } 1 - [P_{s,k,t} \times (1 - r \times R_t \times MC_{k,t} \times C_{k,t} \times V_{k,t} \times S_{k,t} \times \Pr_{k,t})^a + (1 - P_{s,k,t})]^n$$

$P_{s,k,t}$	=	HIV prevalence in the partner population of risk group **k** at time **t**
r	=	Base probability of HIV transmission per act
R_t	=	Multiplier for the effect of stage of infection
$C_{k,t}$	=	Multiplier for effect of condom use
$MC_{k,t}$	=	Multiplier for effect of male circumcision
$S_{k,t}$	=	Multiplier for effect of sexually transmitted infections
$\Pr_{k,t}$	=	Multiplier for effect of PrEP
$V_{k,t}$	=	Multiplier for effect of HIV vaccines
a	=	Number of acts per partner per year
n	=	Number of partners per year

New infections are calculated as the susceptible population multiplied by the probability of becoming infected.

Progression of HIV Positive Individuals

The model structure has seven CD4 compartments, selected on the basis of eligibility criteria and mortality patterns. Many HIV-related parameters vary as a function of CD4 count: progression to lower CD4 counts, HIV-related mortality, probability of initiating ART and infectiousness. The probability of HIV-related death, but also ART enrollment, increases as CD4 counts decrease. An assumption is made that most newly infected people start with CD4 counts above 500 CD4 cells/uL, although some portion, p, can start at 350–499 CD4 cells /uL.

ART Allocation

The number of people on ART in each year is an input into Spectrum/AIM. It is used to determine the number of people newly starting ART in each year in order to achieve the specified number of patients. Loss to follow up (LTFU) is indirectly captured by maintaining a specified number of coverage of those on treatment. The CD4 count threshold for ART eligibility can also be specified by the user. Following recent WHO guidelines, this study assumed ART eligibility of CD4< 350 cells/mm^3. New ART patients are allocated according to two equally weighted criteria. Firstly, the same proportion of patients from each eligible CD4 category are started on ART. Secondly, new ART patients are allocated on the basis of expected HIV-related mortality without ART.

Impact of Behavior Change Interventions

The impact of behavior change is captured in the calculation of HIV transmission through adjusted values for key transmission parameters: condom use, number of partners, age at first sex, needle sharing among injecting drug users.

The impact of interventions on each of these behaviors is determined by an impact matrix that describes the impact of each intervention on each behavior for each risk group. Several interventions, ranging from community based to those prioritized to vulnerable populations are included in the matrix. Their impact on sexual behavior is based extensive literature search [5].

The impact on condom use is calculated as a reduction in the non-use of condoms in order to allow for the aggregation of impacts when several interventions are present. Thus, condom use is calculated as one minus the non-use of condoms in the base year multiplied by the product across all interventions of the increase in coverage of each intervention and its impact on condom non-use.

In this application we used the following formula to relate the pooled risk ratio for increased condom use after exposure to the community empowerment-based, comprehensive HIV prevention intervention, to the relative decrease in condom non-use: D=(RR-1) x (1-cl)/cl in which cl was the pooled condom use at baseline of the intervention.

Modeling Annex 4.B   Tables of Annual New Infections Observed and Trends in Prevalence with Scale-up of Interventions per Modeled Country

Table 4.B.1   Modeling Scale-Up of the Community Empowerment-based, Comprehensive HIV Prevention in Brazil: Number of New HIV Infections among Female Sex Workers

Year	Status quo (10%)	Emp. scale-up (40%)	Emp. scale-up (70%)	Emp. scale-up (100%)
2011	3,670	3,670	3,670	3,670
2012	3,680	3,620	3,561	3,502
2013	3,660	3,539	3,418	3,298
2014	3,612	3,428	3,246	3,066
2015	3,543	3,296	3,053	2,815
2016	3,460	3,150	2,850	2,557
Cumulative (2012–16)	17,955	17,033	16,128	15,238
Reduction	(Ref.)	5.1%	10.2%	15.1%
Infections averted	(Ref.)	922	1,827	2,717

Source: Authors.
Note: Emp. = empowerment; Ref. = reference.

Table 4.B.2   Modeling Scale-up of the Community Empowerment-based, Comprehensive HIV Prevention in Brazil: Annual HIV Prevalence (%) among Female Sex Workers

Year	Status quo (10%)	Emp. scale-up (40%)	Emp. scale-up (70%)	Emp. scale-up (100%)
2011	4.84	4.84	4.84	4.84
2012	4.61	4.60	4.59	4.58
2013	4.39	4.36	4.33	4.30
2014	4.20	4.14	4.08	4.02
2015	4.01	3.92	3.83	3.74
2016	3.84	3.71	3.58	3.45

Source: Authors.
Note: Emp. = empowerment.

Table 4.B.3   Modeling Scale-up of the Community Empowerment-based, Comprehensive HIV Prevention in Brazil: Annual Number of New HIV Infections among the Adult Population

Year	Status quo (10%)	Emp. scale-up (40%)	Emp. scale-up (70%)	Emp. scale-up (100%)
2011	28,932	28,932	28,932	28,932
2012	30,164	30,021	29,879	29,737
2013	31,291	30,989	30,690	30,393
2014	32,273	31,801	31,337	30,881
2015	33,133	32,483	31,851	31,238
2016	33,921	33,085	32,284	31,518
Cumulative (2012–16)	160,782	158,379	156,041	153,767
Reduction	(Ref.)	1.5%	2.9%	4.4%
Infections averted	(Ref.)	2,403	4,741	7,015

Source: Authors.
Note: Emp. = empowerment; Ref. = reference.

Table 4.B.4   ART Expansion among the Adult Population and Combination with Community Empowerment-based, Comprehensive HIV Prevention for Sex Workers in Brazil: Number of New Infections among Female Sex Workers

Year	Status quo (10%)	ART scale-up	ART scale-up + Emp. scale-up (70%)
2011	3,762	3,762	3,762
2012	3,670	3,670	3,670
2013	3,680	3,078	2,979
2014	3,660	2,636	2,461
2015	3,612	2,325	2,089
2016	3,543	2,052	1,768
Cumulative (2012–16)	17,955	11,953	10,832
Reduction	(Ref.)	33.4%	39.7%
Infections averted	(Ref.)	6,002	7,123

Source: Authors.
Note: ART = antiretroviral therapy; Emp. = empowerment; Ref. = reference.

Table 4.B.5   ART Expansion among the Adult Population and Combination with Community Empowerment-based, Comprehensive HIV Prevention for Sex Workers in Brazil: Prevalence (%) of HIV among Female Sex Workers

Year	Status quo	ART scale-up	Art scale-up + Emp. scale-up (70%)
2011	4.84	4.84	4.84
2012	4.61	4.56	4.54
2013	4.39	4.25	4.21
2014	4.20	3.96	3.88
2015	4.01	3.67	3.56
2016	3.84	3.41	3.25

Source: Authors.
Note: ART = antiretroviral therapy; Emp. = empowerment.

Table 4.B.6   ART Expansion among the Adult Population and Combination with Community Empowerment-based, Comprehensive HIV Prevention for Sex Workers in Brazil: Number of New Infections among the Adult Population

Year	Status quo	ART scale-up	Art scale-up + Emp. scale-up (70%)
2011	28,932	28,932	28,932
2012	30,164	25,376	25,139
2013	31,291	22,650	22,222
2014	32,273	20,794	20,207
2015	33,133	19,086	18,370
2016	33,921	17,981	17,143
Cumulative (2012–16)	160,782	105,887	103,081
Reduction	(Ref.)	34.1%	35.9%
Infections averted	(Ref.)	54,895	57,701

Source: Authors.
Note: ART = antiretroviral therapy; Emp. = empowerment; Ref. = reference.

Table 4.B.7   Modeling Scale-Up of the Community Empowerment-based, Comprehensive HIV Prevention in Kenya: Number of New HIV Infections among Sex Workers

Year	Status quo (5%)	Emp. scale-up (35%)	Emp. scale-up (65%)	Emp. scale-up (100%)
2011	17,856	17,856	17,856	17,856
2012	17,779	17,779	17,779	17,779
2013	18,019	17,685	17,351	16,961
2014	18,396	17,708	17,020	16,216
2015	18,741	17,682	16,621	15,384
2016	19,046	17,593	16,142	14,451
Cumulative (2012–16)	93,515	88,111	82,715	76,432
Reduction	(Ref.)	5.8%	11.5%	18.3%
Infections averted	(Ref.)	5,404	10,800	17,083

Source: Authors.
Note: Emp. = empowerment; Ref. = reference.

Table 4.B.8   Modeling Scale-up of the Community Empowerment-based, Comprehensive HIV Prevention in Kenya: Annual HIV Prevalence (%) among Sex Workers

Year	Status quo (5%)	Emp. scale-up (35%)	Emp. scale-up (65%)	Emp. scale-up (100%)
2011	33.75	33.75	33.75	33.75
2012	32.42	32.33	32.23	32.12
2013	31.29	31.02	30.75	30.43
2014	30.31	29.79	29.27	28.67
2015	29.44	28.62	27.80	26.85
2016	28.65	27.49	26.32	24.96

Source: Authors.
Note: Emp. = empowerment.

Table 4.B.9   Modeling Scale-up of the Community Empowerment-based, Comprehensive HIV Prevention in Kenya: New HIV Infections among the Adult Population

Year	Status quo (5%)	Emp. scale-up (35%)	Emp. scale-up (65%)	Emp. scale-up (100%)
2011	100,002	100,002	100,002	100,002
2012	101,468	100,873	100,279	99,587
2013	104,129	102,851	101,576	100,095
2014	106,908	104,887	102,882	100,561
2015	109,650	106,827	104,040	100,838
2016	112,283	108,593	104,978	100,860
Cumulative (2012–16)	534,438	524,031	513,755	501,941
Reduction	(Ref.)	1.9%	3.9%	6.1%
Infections averted	(Ref.)	10,407	20,683	32,497

Source: Authors.
Note: Emp. = empowerment; Ref. = reference.

Table 4.B.10   ART Expansion among the Adult Population and Combination with Community Empowerment-based, Comprehensive HIV Prevention for Sex Workers in Kenya: Number of New Infections among Female Sex Workers

Year	Status quo	ART scale-up	ART scale up + Emp. scale-up (65%)
2011	17,856	17,856	17,856
2012	17,779	17,779	17,779
2013	18,019	16,139	15,536
2014	18,396	14,361	13,265
2015	18,741	13,411	11,853
2016	19,046	13,299	11,220
Cumulative (2012–16)	93,515	70,273	62,356
Reduction	(Ref.)	25%	33%
Infections averted	(Ref.)	23,242	31,159

Source: Authors.
Note: ART = antiretroviral therapy; Emp. = empowerment; Ref. = reference.

Table 4.B.11   ART Expansion among the Adult Population and Combination with Community Empowerment-based, Comprehensive HIV Prevention for Sex Workers in Kenya: HIV Prevalence (%) among Female Sex Workers

Year	Status quo	ART scale-up	ART scale up + Emp. scale-up (65%)
2011	35.28	35.28	35.28
2012	33.75	33.75	33.75
2013	32.42	32.03	31.86
2014	31.29	30.11	29.66
2015	30.31	28.22	27.42
2016	29.44	26.55	25.33

Source: Authors.
Note: ART = antiretroviral therapy; Emp. = empowerment.

Table 4.B.12   ART Expansion among the Adult Population and Combination with Community Empowerment-based, Comprehensive HIV Prevention for Sex Workers in Kenya: New HIV Infections among Adults

Year	Status quo	ART scale-up	ART scale up + Emp. scale-up (65%)
2011	100,002	100,002	100,002
2012	101,468	90,564	89,494
2013	104,129	80,051	78,033
2014	106,908	74,123	71,220
2015	109,650	73,014	69,123
2016	112,283	71,460	66,591
Cumulative (2012–16)	534,438	389,212	374,461
Reduction	(Ref.)	27%	30%
Infections averted	(Ref.)	145,226	159,977

Source: Authors.
Note: ART = antiretroviral therapy; Emp. = empowerment; Ref. = reference.

Table 4.B.13   Modeling Scale-up of the Community Empowerment-based, Comprehensive HIV Prevention in Thailand: Number of New HIV Infections among Female Sex Workers

Year	Status quo	Scale 40 + ART0	Scale 70 + ART0	Scale 100 + ART0
2011	629	629	629	629
2012	596	588	580	572
2013	578	562	546	531
2014	553	530	507	485
2015	524	495	466	438
2016	494	460	426	392
Cumulative (2012–16)	2,745	2,635	2,525	2,418
Reduction	(Ref.)	4.0%	8.0%	11.9%
Infections averted	(Ref.)	110	220	327

Source: Authors.
Note: ART = antiretroviral therapy; Ref. = reference.

Table 4.B.14   Modeling Scale-up of the Community Empowerment-based, Comprehensive HIV Prevention in Thailand: Annual HIV Prevalence (%) among Female Sex Workers

Year	Status quo	Scale 40 + ART0	Scale 70 + ART0	Scale 100 + ART0
2011	3.66	3.66	3.66	3.66
2012	3.14	3.14	3.14	3.13
2013	2.71	2.70	2.70	2.69
2014	2.35	2.34	2.33	2.31
2015	2.06	2.04	2.02	1.99
2016	1.82	1.79	1.76	1.73

Source: Authors.
Note: ART = antiretroviral therapy.

Table 4.B.15   Modeling Scale-up of the Community Empowerment-based, Comprehensive HIV Prevention in Thailand: Annual Number of New HIV Infections among the Adult Population

Year	Status quo	Scale 40 + ART0	Scale 70 + ART0	Scale 100 + ART0
2011	25,188	25,188	25,188	25,188
2012	24,933	24,904	24,875	24,846
2013	24,347	24,293	24,238	24,184
2014	23,531	23,455	23,379	23,304
2015	22,592	22,497	22,404	22,312
2016	21,606	21,495	21,387	21,280
Cumulative (2012–16)	117,009	116,644	116,283	115,926
Reduction	(Ref.)	0.3%	0.6%	0.9%
Infections averted	(Ref.)	365	726	1,083

Source: Authors.
Note: ART = antiretroviral therapy; Ref. = reference.

Table 4.B.16   ART Expansion among the Adult Population in Combination with Community Empowerment-based, Comprehensive HIV Prevention for Sex Workers in Thailand: Number of New Infections among Female Sex Workers

Year	Status quo	Baseline and ART1	ART1 and scale 70
2011	629	629	629
2012	596	524	509
2013	578	463	437
2014	553	419	385
2015	524	383	341
2016	494	347	299
Cumulative (2012–16)	2,745	2,136	1,971
Reduction	(Ref.)	22.2%	28.2%
Infections averted	(Ref.)	609	774

Source: Authors.
Note: ART = antiretroviral therapy; Ref. = reference.

Table 4.B.17   ART Expansion among the Adult Population in Combination with Community Empowerment-based, Comprehensive HIV Prevention for Sex Workers in Thailand: Prevalence (%) of HIV among Female Sex Workers

Year	Status quo	Baseline and ART1	ART1 and scale 70
2011	3.66	3.66	3.66
2012	3.14	3.15	3.15
2013	2.71	2.73	2.72
2014	2.35	2.38	2.36
2015	2.06	2.09	2.05
2016	1.82	1.84	1.79

Source: Authors.
Note: ART = antiretroviral therapy.

Table 4.B.18   ART Expansion among the Adult Population in Combination with Community Empowerment-based, Comprehensive HIV Prevention for Sex Workers in Thailand: Number of New Infections among the Adult Population

Year	Status quo	Baseline and ART1	ART1 and scale 70
2011	25,188	25,188	25,188
2012	24,933	22,046	21,994
2013	24,347	19,700	19,613
2014	23,531	18,106	17,990
2015	22,592	16,798	16,661
2016	21,606	15,507	15,354
Cumulative (2012–16)	117,009	92,157	91,612
Reduction	(Ref.)	21.2%	21.7%
Infections averted	(Ref.)	24,852	25,397

Source: Authors.
Note: ART = antiretroviral therapy; Ref. = reference.

Table 4.B.19   Modeling Scale-up of the Community Empowerment-based, Comprehensive HIV Prevention in Ukraine: New HIV Infections among Sex Workers

Year	Status quo (5%)	Emp. scale-up (35%)	Emp. scale-up (65%)	Emp. scale-up (100%)
2011	3,866	3,866	3,866	3,866
2012	3,846	3,776	3,706	3,625
2013	3,812	3,669	3,526	3,361
2014	3,766	3,546	3,328	3,078
2015	3,713	3,412	3,118	2,783
2016	3,655	3,270	2,898	2,480
Cumulative (2012–16)	18,792	17,673	16,576	15,327
Reduction	(Ref.)	6.0%	11.8%	18.4%
Infections averted	(Ref.)	1,119	2,216	3,465

Source: Authors.
Note: Emp. = empowerment; Ref. = reference.

Table 4.B.20   Modeling Scale-up of the Community Empowerment-based, Comprehensive HIV Prevention in Ukraine: Annual HIV Prevalence (%) among Female Sex Workers

Year	Status quo (10%)	Emp. scale-up (35%)	Emp. scale-up (65%)	Emp. scale-up (100%)
2011	16.31	16.31	16.31	16.31
2012	16.27	16.20	16.14	16.06
2013	16.26	16.06	15.87	15.64
2014	16.26	15.88	15.50	15.06
2015	16.27	15.64	15.03	14.33
2016	16.26	15.36	14.47	13.47

Source: Authors.
Note: Emp. = empowerment.

Table 4.B.21   Modeling the Scale-up of the Community Empowerment-based, Comprehensive HIV Prevention in Ukraine: Number of New Infections among the Adult Population

Year	Status quo (5%)	Emp. scale-up (35%)	Emp. scale-up (65%)	Emp. scale-up (100%)
2011	50,430	50,430	50,430	50,430
2012	50,886	50,683	50,480	50,244
2013	51,099	50,663	50,232	49,735
2014	51,040	50,355	49,685	48,921
2015	50,767	49,813	48,894	47,863
2016	50,313	49,072	47,895	46,603
Cumulative (2012–16)	254,105	250,586	247,186	243,366
Reduction	(Ref.)	1.4%	2.7%	4.2%
Infections averted	(Ref.)	3,519	6,9191	10,739

Source: Authors.
Note: Emp. = empowerment; Ref. = reference.

Table 4.B.22   ART Expansion among the Adult Population and Combination with Community Empowerment-based, Comprehensive HIV Prevention for Sex Workers in Ukraine: Number of New Infections among Female Sex Workers

Year	Status quo	ART scale-up	ART scale up + Emp. scale-up (65%)
2011	3,866	3,866	3,866
2012	3,846	3,754	3,617
2013	3,812	3,650	3,377
2014	3,766	3,555	3,142
2015	3,713	3,458	2,906
2016	3,655	3,321	2,637
Cumulative (2012–16)	18,792	17,738	15,679
Reduction	(Ref.)	5.6%	16.6%
Infections averted	(Ref.)	1,054	3,113

Source Authors.
Note: ART = antiretroviral therapy; Emp. = empowerment; Ref. = reference.

Table 4.B.23   ART Expansion among the Adult Population and Combination with Community Empowerment-based, Comprehensive HIV Prevention for Sex Workers in Ukraine: Prevalence (%) of HIV Infection among Female Sex Workers

Year	Status quo	ART scale-up	ART scale up + Emp. scale-up (65%)
2011	16.31	16.31	16.31
2012	16.27	16.21	16.08
2013	16.26	16.09	15.71
2014	16.26	15.97	15.24
2015	16.27	15.83	14.67
2016	16.26	15.66	14.01

Source: Authors.
Note: ART = antiretroviral therapy; Emp. = empowerment.

Table 4.B.24   ART Expansion among the Adult Population and Combination with Community Empowerment-based, Comprehensive HIV Prevention for Sex Workers in Ukraine: New HIV Infections among the Adult Population

Year	Status quo	ART scale-up	ART scale-up + Emp. scale-up (65%)
2011	50,430	50,430	50,430
2012	50,886	49,609	49,213
2013	51,099	48,759	47,931
2014	51,040	47,869	46,595
2015	50,767	46,861	45,125
2016	50,313	45,150	42,960
Cumulative (2012–16)	254,105	238,248	231,824
Reduction	(Ref.)	6.2%	8.8%
Infections averted	(Ref.)	15,857	22,281

Source: Authors.
Note: ART = antiretroviral therapy; Emp. = empowerment; Ref. = reference.

Modeling Annex 4.C   Thailand (ART initiation with CD4<200)

Thailand: Community empowerment-based, comprehensive HIV prevention among female sex workers

Table 4.C.1 (adapted from Table 4.2) displays the scenarios used to model the scale-up of the community empowerment-based, comprehensive HIV prevention among female sex workers in Thailand while ART coverage is maintained from 2011 levels through 2016 and ART initiation occurs at CD4<200.

Table 4.C.1   Community Empowerment-based, Comprehensive HIV Prevention Modeling Scenarios

Scenario		Coverage
Status quo	Baseline coverage of community empowerment-based, comprehensive HIV prevention held constant among female sex workers, 2011–16	10.0%
	ART held constant among total population, 2011–16	68.0%
Scenario 1:	Interpolated scale-up of community empowerment-based, comprehensive HIV prevention coverage from 2011 to additional 30% by 2016	40.0%
	ART held constant among total population, 2011–16	68.0%
Scenario 2:	Interpolated scale-up of community empowerment-based, comprehensive HIV prevention coverage from 2011 to additional 60% by 2016	70.0%
	ART held constant among total population, 2011–16	68.0%
Scenario 3:	Interpolated scale-up of community empowerment-based, comprehensive HIV prevention coverage from 2011 to reach 100% by 2016	100.0%
	ART held constant among total population, 2011–16	68.0%

Source: Authors.
Note: ART = antiretroviral therapy.

Table 4.C.2 and Figure 4.C.1 present the number of new HIV infections and trends of these infections among female sex workers in Thailand when the community empowerment-based, comprehensive HIV prevention is brought to scale from a baseline coverage level of 10% to reach 40%, 70%, and 100% by 2016. A total of 327 new infections are averted between 2012 and 2016 among female sex workers when the intervention reaches a maximum, 100% coverage, compared to the status quo- a 12% reduction. At a 70% coverage, a figure that is perhaps more feasible in this time period, a total of 220 new infections are averted between 2012 and 2016 when compared to status quo.

Table 4.C.2   Modeling Scale-up of the Community Empowerment-based, Comprehensive HIV Prevention in Thailand: Number of New HIV Infections among Female Sex Workers

Year	Status quo	Scale 40 + ART0	Scale 70 + ART0	Scale 100 + ART0
2011	622	622	622	622
2012	598	590	581	573
2013	577	561	545	529
2014	548	526	503	481
2015	519	490	462	433
2016	490	456	422	389
Cumulative (2012–16)	2,732	2,623	2,513	2,405
Reduction	(Ref.)	4.0%	8.0%	12.0%
Infections averted	(Ref.)	109	219	327

Source: Authors.
Note: ART = antiretroviral therapy; Ref. = reference.

Figure 4.C.1   Modeling Scale-up of the Community Empowerment-based, Comprehensive HIV Prevention in Thailand: Trends in Number of New HIV Infections among Female Sex Workers

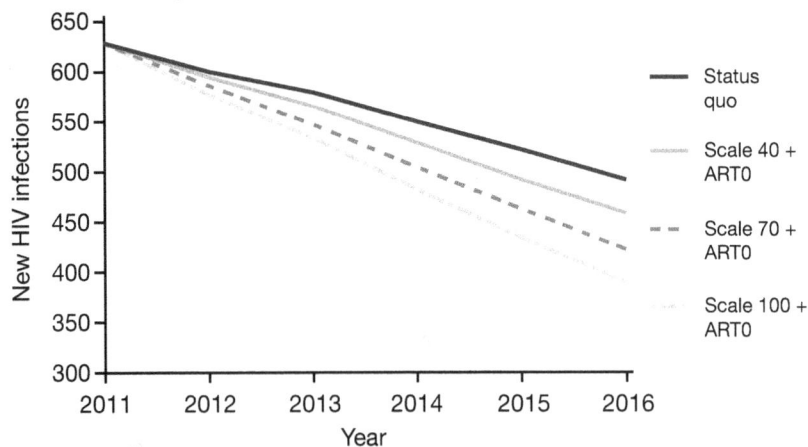

Source: Authors.
Note: ART = antiretroviral therapy.

Table 4.C.3   Modeling Scale-up of the Community Empowerment-based, Comprehensive HIV Prevention in Thailand: Annual HIV Prevalence among Female Sex Workers

Year	Status quo	Scale 40 + ART0	Scale 70 + ART0	Scale 100 + ART0
2011	3.67	3.67	3.67	3.67
2012	3.15	3.15	3.15	3.14
2013	2.72	2.71	2.70	2.70
2014	2.36	2.35	2.33	2.32
2015	2.07	2.05	2.02	2.00
2016	1.82	1.79	1.76	1.73

Source: Authors.
Note: ART = antiretroviral therapy.

Table 4.C.3 and Figure 4.C.2 display the prevalence of HIV infection among female sex workers. The HIV epidemic among female sex workers, as well as the adult population is declining overall; a trend that is evident during the Status Quo scenario. Bring the empowerment intervention to scale, however, effects a further decrease in prevalence from 1.82% to 1.76% within a five year period, when the community empowerment-based, comprehensive HIV prevention reaches 70% by 2016.

Figure 4.C.2   Modeling Scale-Up of the Community Empowerment-based, Comprehensive HIV Prevention in Thailand: Trends in Prevalence of HIV Infection among Female Sex Workers

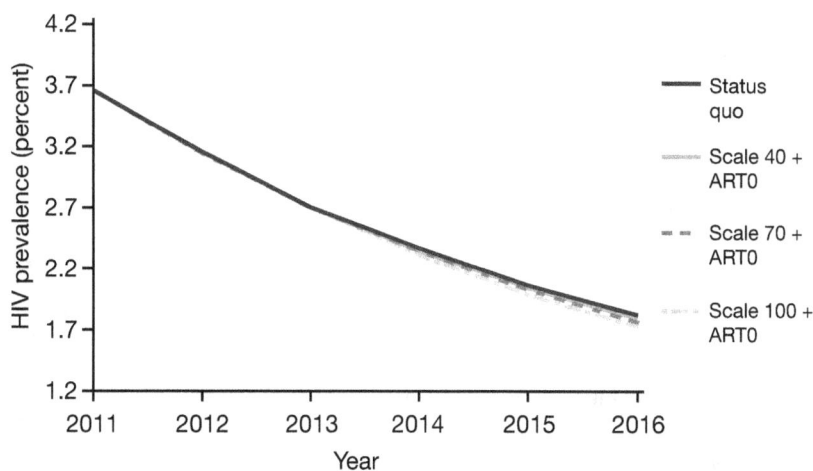

Source: Authors.
Note: ART = antiretroviral therapy.

Table 4.C.4   Modeling Scale-up of the Community Empowerment-based, Comprehensive HIV Prevention in Thailand: Annual Number of New HIV Infections among the Adult Population

Year	Status quo	Scale 40 + ART0	Scale 70 + ART0	Scale 100 + ART0
2011	25,003	25,003	25,003	25,003
2012	25,010	24,980	24,951	24,922
2013	24,301	24,247	24,192	24,138
2014	23,338	23,262	23,187	23,113
2015	22,384	22,292	22,200	22,109
2016	21,447	21,339	21,232	21,127
Cumulative (2012.16)	116,480	116,120	115,762	115,409
Reduction	(Ref.)	0.3%	0.6%	0.9%
Infections averted	(Ref.)	360	718	1,071

Source: Authors.
Note: ART = antiretroviral therapy; Ref. = reference.

Figure 4.C.3   Modeling Scale-up of the Community Empowerment-based, Comprehensive HIV Prevention in Thailand: Annual Number of New HIV Infections among the Adult Population

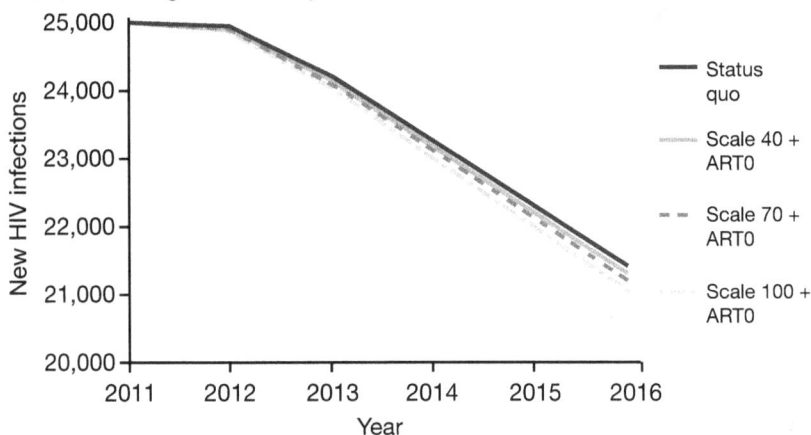

Source: Authors.
Note: ART = antiretroviral therapy.

Table 4.C.4 and Figure 4.C.3 depict the number of new infections among the adult population when the community empowerment-based, comprehensive HIV prevention is increased to 40%, 70%, and 100% among the female sex work population. When coverage of ART and the community empowerment-based, comprehensive HIV prevention do not increase, the number of new infections among the adult population totals almost 117,000 in Thailand between 2012 and 2016. Increasing the coverage of the community empowerment-based, comprehensive HIV prevention to 70% among sex workers, while ART coverage is maintained, reduces then number of new infections among the adult population, averting over 700 new infections between 2012 and 2016. Even greater impact is observed when coverage reaches 100%.

Thailand: Population-wide ART scale-up and combination with the community empowerment-based, comprehensive HIV prevention for female sex workers

Table 4.C.5 (adapted from Table 4.C.2 above) displays the scenarios used to model the scale-up of ART among adults, when initiation occurs at CD4<200, and the combined expansion of ART among adults with an expansion of the community empowerment-based, comprehensive HIV prevention for female sex workers. National estimates assume a total of 227,722 individuals can be covered by ART in 2016.

Table 4.C.5   ART[a] Modeling Scenarios

Scenarios		Coverage
Status quo	ART held constant among total population (2011–16)	68.0%
	Baseline coverage of community empowerment-based, comprehensive HIV prevention held constant among female sex workers	10.0%
Scenario 1:	Scale-up in coverage of ART by 2016 according to country estimations	227,722
	Baseline coverage of community empowerment-based, comprehensive HIV prevention held constant among female sex workers	10.0%
Scenario 2:	Scale-up in coverage of ART by 2016 according to country estimations	227,722
	Interpolated scale-up of community empowerment-based, comprehensive HIV prevention coverage from 2011 of additional 60% by 2016	70.0%

Source: Authors.
Note: ART = antiretroviral therapy.
a. Baseline ART and scale-up among adults based on county UNAIDS projections estimate, absolute numbers and ART initiation at CD4 < 200.

Table 4.C.6   ART Expansion among the Adult Population and Combination with Empowerment for Sex Workers in Thailand: Number of New Infections among Female Sex Workers, 2011–16

Year	Status quo	Baseline and ART1	ART and scale 70
2011	622	622	622
2012	598	503	489
2013	577	451	426
2014	548	419	384
2015	519	390	347
2016	490	356	307
Cumulative (2012–16)	2,732	2,119	1,953
Reduction	(Ref.)	22.4%	28.5%
Infections averted	(Ref.)	613	779

Source: Authors.
Note: ART = antiretroviral therapy; Ref. = reference.

Figure 4.C.4   Expansion of ART among Adult Population and Combination with Community Empowerment-based, Comprehensive HIV Prevention: Trends in New HIV Infections among Female Sex Workers

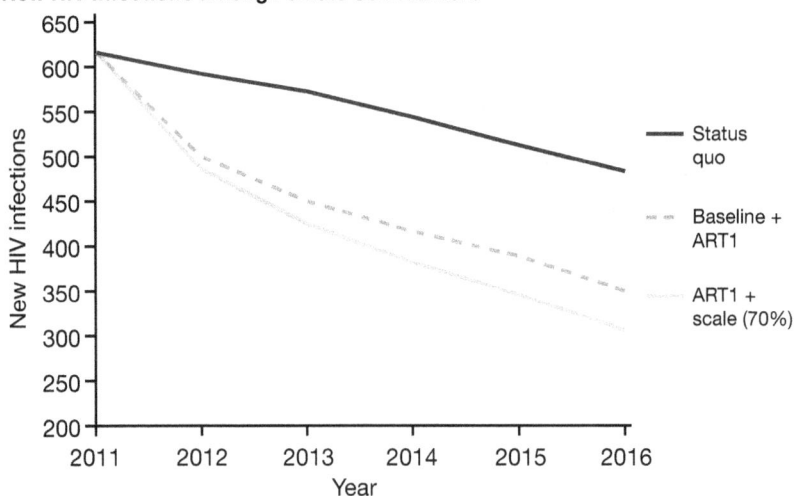

Source: Authors.
Note: ART = antiretroviral therapy.

Table 4.C.6 and Figure 4.C.4 present the number of new HIV infections and trends of these infections among female sex workers in Thailand when

ART is expanded among eligible adults, according to national estimates, by 2016. An additional scenario depicts the impact when the expansion of ART is combined with expanded coverage of the community empowerment-based, comprehensive HIV prevention among sex workers, reaching 70% by 2016. These scenarios are compared against the Status Quo, which represents maintained coverage levels of ART and Empowerment from 2011 through 2016. A total of 613 new infections among sex workers are averted between 2012 and 2016 when ART expands among the adult population, as compared to the status quo. This represents a 22% reduction in new infections among female sex workers. With the addition of the Empowerment Intervention, a total of 779 new infections are averted, resulting in a 29% reduction in new infections among sex workers between 2012 and 2016. In the presence of ART expansion, the Empowerment Intervention averts an additional 166 infections among female sex workers.

Table 4.C.7 and Figure 4.C.5 display the prevalence of HIV infection among female sex workers. The HIV epidemic among female sex workers, as well as the adult population is declining; a trend that is evident during the Status Quo scenario. The slightly higher prevalence observed with the expansion of ART is likely related to the fact that ART saves lives; therefore the proportion of people living with HIV will actually begin to increase as ART improves longevity of the population living with HIV. A decrease in HIV prevalence to 1.83% by 2016 is observed when ART expansion among adults is combined with the Empowerment Intervention that reaches a coverage of 70% of female sex workers in 2016.

Table 4.C.7   ART Expansion among the Adult Population and Combination with Empowerment for Sex Workers in Thailand: Prevalence of HIV among Female Sex Workers

Year	Status quo	Baseline and ART1	ART and scale 70
2011	3.67	3.67	3.67
2012	3.15	3.17	3.17
2013	2.72	2.76	2.75
2014	2.36	2.41	2.39
2015	2.07	2.12	2.09
2016	1.82	1.87	1.83

Source: Authors.
Note: ART = antiretroviral therapy.

Figure 4.C.5   ART Expansion among the Adult Population and Combination with Empowerment for Sex Workers in Thailand: Prevalence of HIV among Female Sex Workers

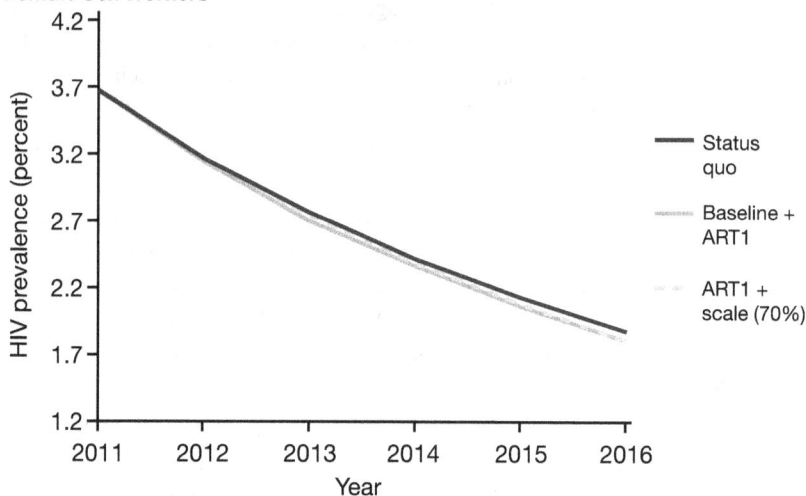

Source: Authors.
Note: ART = antiretroviral therapy.

Table 4.C.8 and Figure 4.C.6 present the number and trends of new HIV infections among the adult population in Thailand, between 2011 to 2016, when ART is expanded among eligible adults, according to national estimates. An additional scenario depicts the impact when the expansion of ART is combined with expanded coverage of the Empowerment Intervention, expands from 10% to 70% coverage of the female sex worker population by 2016. Among adults, a total of 24,784 new infections are averted between 2012 and 2016 when ART expands, when compared to the status quo. This represents a 21% reduction in new infections among the adult population, between 2012–2016. With the addition of the Empowerment Intervention, a total of 25,327 new infections are averted, resulting in a 22% reduction in new infections between 2011 and 2016. Thus, in addition ot the benefits observed with ART expansion, the expansion of the community empowerment-based, comprehensive HIV prevention for female sex workers averts an additional 543 infections among the adult population.

Table 4.C.8   ART Expansion among the Adult Population and Combination with Empowerment for Sex Workers in Thailand: Number of New Infections among the Adult Population

Year	Status quo	Baseline and ART1	ART1 and scale 70
2011	25,003	25,003	25,003
2012	25,010	21,267	21,217
2013	24,301	19,289	19,204
2014	23,338	18,137	18,023
2015	22,384	17,101	16,963
2016	21,447	15,902	15,746
Cumulative (2012–16)	116,480	91,696	91,153
Reduction	(Ref.)	21.3%	21.7%
Infections averted	(Ref.)	24,784	25,327

Source: Authors.
Note: ART = antiretroviral therapy; Ref. = reference.

Figure 4.C.6   ART Expansion among the Adult Population and Combination with Empowerment for Sex Workers in Thailand: Trends New Infections among the Adult Population

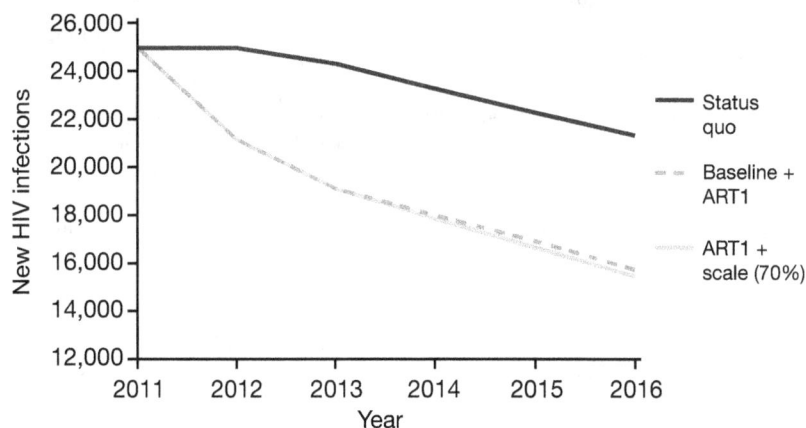

Source: Authors.
Note: ART = antiretroviral therapy.

References

AIDS Alliance Ukraine. (2011). *"Publications of the HIV/AIDS Alliance in Ukraine."* 2011. http://www.aidsalliance.org.ua/cgi-bin/index.cgi?url=/en/library/our/index.htm.

Beattie, T. S. and P. Bhattacharjee (2012). "Personal, interpersonal and structural challenges to accessing HIV testing, treatment and care services among female sex workers, men who have sex with men and transgenders in Karnataka state, South India." *Journal of Epidemiology and Community Health.* http://jech.bmj.com/content/early/2012/04/10/jech-2011-200475. full

Chakrapani, V. and P. Newman (2009). "Barriers to free antiretroviral treatment access for female sex workers in Chennai, India." *AIDS Patient Care and STDs* 23 (11): 973–980.

Chersich, M. F., S. M. Luchters, et al. (2007). "Heavy episodic drinking among Kenyan female sex workers is associated with unsafe sex, sexual violence and sexually transmitted infections." *International Journal of STD & AIDS* 18 (11): 764–769.

Eshleman, S. H., S. E. Hudelson, et al. (2011). "Analysis of genetic linkage of HIV from couples enrolled in the HIV Prevention Trials Network 052 trial." *Journal of Infectious Diseases* 204 (12): 1918–1926.

Forsythe, S., J. Stover, et al. (2011). *"The past, present, and future of HIV, AIDS, and Resource Allocation."* http://www.biomedcentral.com/1471-2458/9/S1/S4

Hirbod, T., R. Kaul, et al. (2008). "HIV-neutralizing immunoglobulin A and HIV-specific proliferation are independently associated with reduced HIV acquisition in Kenyan sex workers." *AIDS* 22 (6): 727–735.

Kerrigan, D., L. Moreno, et al. (2006). "Environmental-structural interventions to reduce HIV/STI risk among female sex workers in the Dominican Republic." *American Journal of Public Health* 96 (1): 120–125.

Kerrigan, D., P. Telles, et al. (2008). "Community development and HIV/STI-related vulnerability among female sex workers in Rio de Janeiro, Brazil." *Health Education Research* 23 (1): 137–145.

Lacap, P. A., J. D. Huntington, et al. (2008). "Associations of human leukocyte antigen DRB with resistance or susceptibility to HIV-1 infection in the Pumwani Sex Worker Cohort." *AIDS* 22 (9): 1029–1038.

Lippman, S. A., M. Chinaglia, et al. (2012). "Findings from Encontros: a multilevel STI/HIV intervention to increase condom use, reduce STI, and change the social environment among sex workers in Brazil." *Sexually Transmitted Diseases* 39 (3): 209–216.

Lippman, S. A., A. Donini, et al. (2010). "Social-environmental factors and protective sexual behavior among sex workers: the Encontros intervention in Brazil." *American Journal of Public Health* 100 Suppl 1: S216–223.

Luchters, S. M., D. Vanden Broeck, et al. (2010). "Association of HIV infection with distribution and viral load of HPV types in Kenya: a survey with 820 female sex workers." *BMC Infectious Diseases* 10: 18.

Malta, M., M. M. Magnanini, et al. (2010). "HIV prevalence among female sex workers, drug users and men who have sex with men in Brazil: a systematic review and meta-analysis." *BMC Public Health* 10: 317.

McClelland, R. S., B. A. Richardson, et al. (2011). "Association between participant self-report and biological outcomes used to measure sexual risk behavior in human immunodeficiency virus-1-seropositive female sex workers in Mombasa, Kenya." *Sexually Transmitted Diseases* 38 (5): 429–433.

Medley, A., C. Kennedy, et al. (2009). "Effectiveness of peer education interventions for HIV prevention in developing countries: a systematic review and meta-analysis." *AIDS Educ Prev* 21 (3): 181–206. http://d.yimg.com/kq/groups/13416053/.../effectiveness_peer_edu.pdf

NSWP. (2011). *"Female, Male and Transgender Sex Workers' Perspectives on HIV & STI Prevention and Treatment Services: a global sex worker consultation."* http://www.nswp. org/resource/nswp-who-community-consultation-report-archived.

Stover, J., S. Bertozzi, et al. (2006). "The global impact of scaling up HIV/AIDS prevention programs in low- and middle-income countries." *Science* 311 (5766): 1474–1476.

Stover, J., L. Bollinger, et al. (2007). "The impact of an AIDS vaccine in developing countries: a new model and initial results." *Health Affairs* 26 (4): 1147–1158.

Stover, J., P. Johnson, et al. (2010). "The Spectrum projection package: improvements in estimating incidence by age and sex, mother-to-child transmission, HIV progression in children and double orphans." *STI* 86 (Suppl 2): ii16–21.

Stover, J., N. Walker, et al. (2002). "Can we reverse the HIV/AIDS pandemic with an expanded response?" *The Lancet* 360 (9326): 73–77.

Thuy, N. T., V. T. Nhung, et al. (1998). "HIV infection and risk factors among female sex workers in southern Vietnam." *AIDS* 12 (4): 425–432.

Tovanabutra, S., E. J. Sanders, et al. (2010). "Evaluation of HIV type 1 strains in men having sex with men and in female sex workers in Mombasa, Kenya." *AIDS Research and Human Retroviruses* 26 (2): 123–131.

UNAIDS (2009). *Report of the UNAIDS HIV Prevention Reference Group Meeting.* Glion, Switzerland: UNAIDS.

UNAIDS (2010). "Brazil, Epidemiological Fact Sheet on HIV/AIDS and Sexually Transmitted Infections." http://data.unaids.org/Publications/Fact-Sheets01/brazil_en.pdf

UNAIDS and Ministry of Health of Ukraine (2008). *Ukraine: National report on monitoring progress toward the UNGASS Declaration of Commitment on HIV/AIDS.* Reporting period: January 2006–December 2007. Kiev.

van der Elst, E. M., H. S. Okuku, et al. (2009). "Is audio computer-assisted self-interview (ACASI) useful in risk behaviour assessment of female and male sex workers, Mombasa, Kenya?" *PLoS ONE* 4 (5): e5340.

WHO (2010). *Antiretroviral therapy for HIV infection in adults and adolescents: 2010 revision.* Geneva: WHO.

WHO, UNFPA, et al. (2012). *Prevention and Treatment of HIV and other Sexually Transmitted Infections for Sex Workers. Recommendations for a public health approach.* World Heath Organization, Geneva: WHO

CHAPTER 5

Cost-effectiveness Analyses

Introduction

Key Themes

- The cost per participant for the community empowerment-based comprehensive HIV prevention intervention ranges from $102 to $184, with Ukraine having the lowest and Brazil the highest cost per participant. Labor costs are the major expense, and account for the majority of variation across countries.

- Total national 5-year program cost for the community empowerment intervention is highest in Brazil with an average cost of $167M – $170M, and lowest in Ukraine at $14M – $15M (2011 USD). The size of the sex worker population and labor costs account for the majority of the variation.

- When averted HIV-related treatment costs are removed the net 5-year national cost of the community empowerment intervention is significantly reduced. For example, in Brazil net program costs are $93M, and in Thailand $45M. In Ukraine and Kenya net costs show cost savings of $39M and $8.6M respectively.

- The cost per HIV infection averted is lowest in Ukraine ($1,990) and Kenya ($3,813) and highest in Thailand ($66,128) and Brazil ($32,773). Higher costs are driven largely by lower base rates of HIV prevalence, and higher labor costs.

- When the community empowerment prevention intervention is conducted in the context of enhanced ART provision the cost-effectiveness is reduced modestly. For example, in Ukraine the cost per DALY saved is increased from $85 to $93. This effect is explained by reductions in population-level HIV prevalence driven by the ART program.

(continued next page)

Key Themes   *(continued)*

- The cost per DALY saved by the empowerment intervention is high compared to many other HIV prevention interventions, but below others that have been deemed important to support. For example: 1) 50% coverage of School-Based Sex Education at $530; 2) HAART (simple) + Directly Observed Treatment Strategy for TB at $596.
- As a percentage of the national health expenditure on HIV programs the empowerment intervention would consume 4.6% in Brazil, 16% in Kenya, and 4.8% in Thailand. In Ukraine it would reduce net HIV expenditure by 9.6% due to averted care costs.

The objectives of this section are to estimate the cost-effectiveness of implementation and expansion of the community empowerment-based comprehensive HIV prevention intervention for sex workers described earlier in the modeling section. We explore the potential impact of the empowerment intervention in Brazil, Kenya, Thailand, and Ukraine under two scenarios: 1) assuming static provision of ART programs at current levels; and 2) in the context of large-scale expansion of ART delivery. These analyses are intended to assist policy makers and program managers in identifying optimal allocation of HIV prevention funds, and provide results in a metric that will allow comparisons of the utility of the intervention to other allocation options, both for HIV prevention and alternative health interventions.

Methods

Establishing a Base-Case Cost Estimate

For the sex worker community empowerment-based, comprehensive HIV prevention intervention we first did a detailed costing of a model program in Brazil (the *Encontros* project) that has high fidelity to the proposed intervention of interest using a micro-costing methodology. This intervention was selected as it closely matches the inclusion criteria of those studies included in the meta-analysis used to derive the efficacy estimates, has been well studied, and is located in one of the target countries for this analysis (Brazil). In addition, none of the other selected countries had to date conducted a similar intervention with the necessary evaluation and micro-costing data available. Detailed micro-costing worksheets were completed by staff in Brazil who implemented the *Encontros* project (Lippman, Donini et al. 2010). A series of queries and revisions were made to refine the estimates, and consultations were made with a study team that earlier evaluated the efficacy of *Encontros*.

Data collected include a range of costs for each item, with high, low, average costs recorded. Cost data were converted from local currency to 2011 US dollars. We also collected the number of units utilized for each expenditure, and the proportion of discrete expenses used expressly for the intervention – with high, low and average values estimated for these for sensitivity analyses. The time horizon utilized was one year with 1000 sex workers. Categories of cost that were collected include: 1) Conversion rate of local currency to US dollars; 2) estimated buying power of the currency based on the World Bank's Purchasing Power Parity Index (UN Statistics Division Millennium Development Indicators Unit 2012); 3) startup costs; 4) commodities used in the intervention; 5) labor costs for intervention workers; 6) promotional and advertising costs; 7) rent; 8) maintenance; 9) incentives; 10) volunteer activities; 11) user fees; 12) value of donated goods and services; and 13) other relevant costs. We then multiplied the number of resources units used by the monetary value, and removed non-intervention expenses to derive a cost per participant. The analytic perspective used was the donor perspective, examining the cost of adding mobilization, risk reduction counseling, peer education, and enhancing access to STI and ART services provided at government clinics which was also consistent with the *Encontros* model as it was implemented in partnership with the Ministry of Health and local and state municipal AIDS programs, which meant that STI and HIV prevention, testing, care, and service costs were covered through the local public health services.

There are challenges inherent in developing a cost-base of a comprehensive HIV prevention related to the ways in which the breadth and content of activities developed to mobilize sex worker communities vary across contexts. In the *Encontros* experience, it was key that the types of community activities developed to promote sex worker human rights and health and mobilize the sex worker community were defined in partnership with sex workers and in accordance with the context of the intervention in a small, border town with high levels of stigma where a sex worker organization did not exist at the beginning of the project but rather was founded as an outcome of the intervention (Murray, Lippman et al 2010). The involvement of the government in the project was also distinct as per the Brazil case study, where there has been a long history of a partnership forged around concepts of citizenship and human rights between sex worker organizations and the government in Brazil. Thus, the focus of the cost-analysis is thus to inform the optimal allocation of HIV prevention funds in categories of cost while also allowing emphasizing that the types of activities to be developed in each category should be in accordance with the needs of sex workers, the social, cultural and political context in which they work, and the principles of a community-empowerment based intervention as defined in this report.

To generate cost estimates for Kenya, Thailand, and Ukraine we used the base case cost analysis from the Brazilian micro-costing exercise to establish model program implementation parameters, and adapted the values to each country. To do this we first adjusted the Brazilian values to current 2011 U.S. Dollars, and weighted the results by the Purchasing Power Parity (PPP) index (UN Statistics Division Millennium Development Indicators Unit 2012) for each country. The resulting values were then reviewed and adjusted as needed by comparison results to available labor statistics (International Labor Organization 2012), comparisons to other available micro-costing results conducted previously by the study team, and expert consultation with colleagues who have implemented field projects in these settings.

Once reasonable estimated base-case scenarios were established for each country we then incorporated other required adjustments to the cost data, including discounting, annuitization and distribution of startup costs over the life of project, and calculation of net program costs for a separate analysis which subtracts the estimated lifetime treatment costs from total program costs. We also developed a model to convert HIV infections averted (from the Goals model) to Disability Adjusted Life Years (DALY) saved, and conducted sensitivity analyses on the cost data from Brazil with a stochastic model. These are described below.

Time Preference

An important consideration in any cost-effectiveness analysis is the value given to present versus distant benefits of the interventions being considered. Even with zero inflation there is a societal preference for intervention benefits incurred sooner over those realized later in time. To account for this it is necessary to discount the future costs and benefits of the interventions under consideration. Following recommendations set by the U.S. Panel on Cost-Effectiveness in Health and Medicine (Gold 1996) we harmonized the discount rate used for costs with those used for benefits, and utilize a 3% discount rate, with sensitivity analysis conducted with a 0%, 3%, and 6% discount rate. We also utilized these same discount rates in the annuity function for one-time capital expenditures, and to discount the future health benefits. Startup costs were distributed over the life of the intervention (3 years) using an annuity function with results discounted at 0%, 3% and 6%. For calculation of Disability Adjusted Life Years saved per HIV infection averted, and lifetime ART treatment costs we utilized a 3% discount rate.

Calculation of Net Program Costs and Base Case Ratios

To examine net intervention costs and benefits we also developed scenarios that removed the medical cost for HIV treatment saved from the intervention from the gross program cost. This was based on an estimated of cost of medical care available in the Goals Model for each country, which was multiplied by the number of HIV infections averted. These were discounted, summed, and subtracted from the total program costs to generate net program costs. In Brazil the estimated cost per person of lifetime HIV/AIDS-related treatment is $14,520; in Kenya $4,220; Thailand $5,590, and Ukraine $7,170.

We conducted sensitivity analysis on all categories of cost inputs to allow us to fully convey any uncertainty in study results, and identify parameters that are most highly associated with cost-effective intervention implementation. We applied a stochastic model to the cost values using the software program @Risk™ and subjected the results across model iterations to multivariate analysis to identify the independent effects of each cost category on the overall program cost. Samples for each value in model runs were generated with a Latin Hypercube estimation, and we used a triangular distribution function for model parameters, which specifies low, most likely, and high values. In any iteration of the model each input parameter was assigned a value randomly, but constrained by the likelihood of occurring as specified by the probability distribution function. The resulting model output was calculated, and the inputs and outputs saved. By determining the percent change in the outcome that results from repeated model iterations it was possible to track when additional iterations make no additional meaningful impacts, and the model was stopped—which is the process of achieving model convergence. Convergence was set to occur when the addition of model iterations changes the average and standard deviation of the output by less than 1.5%. The ultimate result of this process was a dataset of inputs (varied across the distribution function constraints) and associated outputs. With this dataset it was then possible to conduct multivariate analysis, and identify the independent relationship between changes in model parameters and the outcome of interest. As well, and importantly, the output can also now be conveyed as a distribution rather than a single value, which helps to express the uncertainty inherent in the model, and the likelihood of different outcomes occurring.

For the Brazilian sensitivity analysis we utilized actual variations in each cost category recorded in the micro-costing we conducted, and included variation on the number of units, the cost per unit, and the allocation of each unit cost to intervention-related activities. For Kenya, Thailand, and Ukraine we subjected each summary cost value to variation of +/- 30% of the base-case value, and conducted multivariate sensitivity analyses on the results generated across model iterations, regressing cost inputs on the total program cost. The efficacy data were also subjected to sensitivity analyses in a separate process using a stochastic model with triangular probability distribution functions. Results from the cost and efficacy analyses were combined for presentation to generate the range of values presented, with low, median, and high values included in summary tables and figures.

Calculating Disability Adjusted Life Years

We assessed the intervention's impact on health outcomes in terms of quality, quantity, and age adjusted societal impact in terms of the number of HIV infections averted and the Disability Adjusted Life Year. The advantage of the DALY over direct measures of HIV cases averted is that it accounts for the quality and duration of the life saved due to the intervention. While the QALY applies disability weights to stages of illness, adjusting for the resulting quality of life with each stage of illness, the DALY goes one step further and applies an additional age weight associated with the estimates contribution to society contributed by an individual at different stages of life. It is reasonable to examine these factors as there may be a societal value placed on targeting interventions toward those who have the potential for longer and higher quality lives (in the case of QALYs), and also will contribute more to societal goals (in the case of DALYs).

We used methodology developed by Holtgrave and Qualls (Holtgrave, Qualls et al. 1996) to calculate DALY's which involves deriving estimates of the average age of persons infected, and the duration of the sequelae of several stages of AIDS. The weights for DALYs are found in Murray & Lopez's "The Global Burden of Disease" (Murray, Lopez et al. 1996) which we adopted to allow for consistency in comparisons to other cost-effectiveness analyses which have used these same assumptions. We assumed that death occurs 11 years after infection, and disability occurs 8 years after infection and lasts for 3 years. Disability states were assigned a value of 0.5 life-years. We assumed that age of infection occurred on average at 22 years, and for each country we used demographic life tables available at the WHO Global Health Observatory Data Repository (The World Health Organization) to identify female life expectancy at age 22 (Brazil at 58.7 years; Kenya at 48.2 years; Thailand at 55.1 years, and Ukraine at 54.9 years). As described earlier, a 3% discount rate was applied to future benefits in the DALY calculation. From this process we estimated that for every HIV infection averted there are 23.5 DALYs saved in Brazil, 22.7 DALYs saved in Kenya, and 23.3 DALYs saved in both Thailand and Ukraine.

Results

Intervention Cost per Participant by Country

Table 5.2 shows the detailed distribution of estimated cost of the sex worker empowerment intervention by country. The overall gross total annual program cost in Brazil is estimated to be $179,950 to reach 1,000 sex workers. This results in a cost per participant of $180. With adjustment made for price parity, 3% discounting, and distribution of startup costs over a 3-year life of program the cost per participant in Brazil is $184. In Ukraine the gross annual total program costs to reach 1,000 participants is estimated to be $101,708 with cost per participant of $102. In Thailand the gross annual total program costs to reach 1,000 participants is estimated to be $106,395 with cost per participant of $106. In Kenya the gross annual total program costs to reach 1,000 participants is estimated to be $139,635 with cost per participant of $140.

Figure 5.1 shows the distribution of the annual program costs by category for Brazil, where we had the greatest level of detail. The vast majority of expenses are for personnel, followed by overhead (at 10% of total program cost), training and events, and community mobilization efforts. Small levels of funding are dedicated to local travel, office operations, monitoring, and capital costs for equipment and furniture.

In Figure 5.2 results are shown for the probability density of values for the estimated cost per participant in Brazil produced across model iterations. This graph depicts the likelihood of cost values occurring as a probability, accounting for variation in model inputs across 50,000 model iterations. When all parameters are set at their lowest (least expensive) value, the minimum cost per participant is $149. The highest value for cost per participant was $227. The average and most likely result was $184 per participant. Note that the high and low values are very unlikely, and the 5th percentile value is $168 and the 95th percentile value $201.

In Figure 5.3 sensitivity analysis results are shown with the relative contribution of model parameters shown in rank order for Brazil. The majority of the uncertainty in the model is explained by variations in the percent of time dedicated to intervention by counselors. Counselor and community coordinator salary, the number and salary of peer educators, and the number counselors also explain significant variation across model iterations. Smaller effects are identified for other personnel items and the administrative overhead rate (varied in the model at +/- 20% from the base case estimate of 10% of total program costs). The full detailed sensitivity results for Brazil, where we had the most costing detail, are shown in Table 5.3.

Figures 5.4, 5.6, and 5.8 show the probability density of values across model iterations for the estimated cost per participant in Kenya, Thailand, and Ukraine respectively. Given that cost estimates were collapsed by category there are fewer input parameters, resulting in much more rapid model convergence with approximately 4,900 iterations of the stochastic model needed to achieve convergence in each of the Kenya, Thailand, and Ukraine analyses.

For Kenya (Figure 5.4) when all parameters are set at their lowest (least expensive) value, the minimum cost per participant was $108. The highest value for cost per participant was $170. The average and most likely result was $140 per participant. Note that the high and low values are very unlikely, and the 5th percentile value is $119 and the 95th percentile value $160.

For Thailand (Figure 5.6) when all parameters are set at their lowest (least expensive) value, the minimum cost per participant was $83. The highest value for cost per participant was $130. The average and most likely result was $106 per participant. Note that the high and low values are very unlikely, and the 5th percentile value is $91 and the 95th percentile value of $122.

For Ukraine (Figure 5.8) when all parameters are set at their lowest (least expensive) value, the minimum cost per participant was $79. The highest value for cost per participant was $126. The average and most likely result was $102 per participant. Note that the high and low values are very unlikely, and the 5th percentile value is $87 and the 95th percentile value $116.

Figures 5.5, 5.7 and 5.9 show the sensitivity analysis for cost per participant by category for Kenya, Thailand, and Ukraine respectively. The standardized regression coefficients shown allow for rank ordering of how sensitive the cost per participant is to discrete items. Note that given that the composition of each country program in Kenya, Thailand, and Ukraine were based on the micro-costing from Brazil, the pattern of effects is quite similar across these three programs. The vast majority of expenses in all sites is for personnel, followed by overhead (at 10% of total program cost), and community mobilization efforts. Variation in the cost of other discrete items has minimal effects on the cost per participant.

Cost per HIV Infection Averted

Two scenarios were modeled with regard to the estimated cost per HIV infection averted and associated analyses (total program cost, net program cost, and cost per DALY saved) resulting from the community empowerment intervention. These two scenarios are: 1) in the context of status quo static ART provision in each country, and 2) in the context of early initiation of ART provision together with expanded access to ART. The assumptions for the two scenarios are summarized in Table 5.1, and are described previously in the modeling section in greater detail. As noted in the modeling section, within Goals, behavioral interventions may be applied and brought to scale among specified risk groups, though ART coverage is applied to the adult population and is not specific to subgroups such as female sex workers. Thus, the cost analyses contrast scale up of the Empowerment intervention by variation in these two scenarios.

Table 5.1   Estimated Associated Costs per HIV Infection Averted: Two Scenarios

ART modeling scenarios		Brazil	Kenya	Thailand	Ukraine
Status quo	ART held constant among total population[a] (2011–16)	45%	62.7%	53.0%	12.0%
	Baseline coverage of community empowerment-based prevention intervention held constant among female sex workers (2011–16)	10.0%	5.0%	10.0%	5.0%
Scenario 2:	Scale-up in coverage of ART by 2016 according to country estimations (% coverage or number)[a]	270,000	85.0%	227,722	58,000
	Interpolated scale-up of community empowerment-based prevention intervention coverage from 2011 to additional 60% by 2016	70.0%	65.0%	70.0%	65.0%

Source: Authors.
Note: ART = antiretroviral therapy.
a. Baseline ART and scale-up among adults based on county UNAIDS projections estimates.

Cost per HIV Infection Averted with Static ART Provision

Figure 5.10 summarizes the cost per HIV infection averted from the community empowerment intervention under the context of static provision of ART provision by country. The lowest cost per HIV infection averted was found in Ukraine with a median value of $1,990 (range $1,374–$2,756), followed by Kenya with median value of $3,813 (range $2,597–$5,261). Values were much higher for Brazil and Thailand with median values of $32,773 (range $23,213–$43,818) and $66,128 (range $42,947–$90,001) respectively.

Cost per HIV Infection Averted with Enhanced ART Provision

Figure 5.11 summarizes the cost per HIV infection averted from the community empowerment intervention under the context of enhanced provision of ART provision by country. The lowest cost per HIV infection averted was found in Ukraine with a median value of $2,168 (range $1,502–$2,963), followed by Kenya with median value of $5,291 (range $3,624–$7,463). Values were much higher for Brazil and Thailand with median values of $55,761 (range $38,552–$75,943) and $89,908 (range $59,110– $127,416) respectively.

Total Community Empowerment Program Cost with Static ART Provision

Figure 5.12 summarizes the total program cost estimated for each country for the Empowerment intervention under a static, status quo, provision of ART among adults. Brazil has the highest cost with a median value of $167M (range $93M–$306M), followed by Kenya with $81M (range $43–$152), Thailand with $49M (range $25M–$92M), and Ukraine with $15M (range $8M–$28M).

Total Community Empowerment Program Cost with Enhanced ART Provision

Figure 5.13 summarizes the total program cost estimated for each country for the Empowerment intervention under a static, status quo, provision of ART among adults. Brazil has the highest cost with a median value of $170M (range $88M–$319M), followed by Kenya with $81M (range $43–$155), Thailand with $49M (range $25M–$96M), and Ukraine with $15M (range $8M–$28M).

Net Program Cost (Subtracting Averted Medical Costs) with Static ART Provision

Figure 5.14 shows the effect of subtracting lifetime averted medical costs from AIDS-related illnesses from gross program costs. In Ukraine the resulting value indicates a cost savings of $39M in the median calculation (range $34M – $45M). Similarly in Kenya the median estimate indicates cost savings of $9M (range $27M savings - $30M expense). In Brazil and Thailand net program cost did not show cost savings with values of $93M (range $35M – $204M) and $45M (range $22M – $86M) respectively.

Net Program Cost (Subtracting Averted Medical Costs) with Enhanced ART Provision

Figure 5.15 shows the effect of subtracting lifetime averted medical costs from AIDS-related illnesses from gross program costs, but under a scenario of background levels of enhanced ART provision. In Ukraine the resulting value indicates a cost savings of $35M in the median calculation (range $31M–$40M). In no other countries are cost savings found. For example, in Kenya the median estimate shows expense of $16M (range $7M savings–$67M expense). In Brazil and Thailand net program cost show expense of $126M (range $55M–$258M) and $46M (range $23M–$92M) respectively. It should be noted that the slight increase in net costs for these scenarios in contrast to the static ART provision models shown in the prior figure (Figure 5.14) is likely driven by the fact the much more substantial ART program lowers incidence and prevalence significantly, and thus the Empowerment program is operating in an environment with lower prevalence. Thus, the expenditures on the community empowerment program stay the same, while the impact in terms of reductions in incidence are reduced given lower prevalence of HIV driven by the enhanced ART program.

Cost per DALY Saved with Static ART Provision

In Figure 5.16 the cost per Disability Adjusted Life Years saved from the Empowerment intervention in the context of static, status quo, provision of ART are shown for each country. In Ukraine and Kenya the cost per DALY saved are the lowest, at $85 (range $59–$118) and $168 (range $114–$232) respectively. Brazil and Thailand have much less cost-effective programs by comparison; with values of $1,395 (range $988–$1,865) and $2,838 (range $1,843–$3,863) respectively.

Cost per DALY Saved in the Context of Enhanced ART Provision

In Figure 5.17 the cost per Disability Adjusted Life Years saved from the empowerment intervention in the context of enhanced provision of ART are shown for each country. A similar pattern to the previous estimates are found, with Ukraine and Kenya programs yielding the cost per DALY saved which are the lowest, at $93 (range $64–$1278) and $233 (range $159–$329) respectively. Brazil and Thailand again have much less cost-effective programs by comparison; with values of $2,373 (range $1,641–$3,232) and $3,859 (range $2,537–$5,469) respectively.

Discussion

These analyses help to frame the potential utility of the community empowerment-based comprehensive HIV prevention intervention for female sex workers under scenarios of both static national provision of ART and enhanced ART provision. Examining the utility of the intervention in terms of the cost per HIV infection averted and cost per Disability Adjusted Life Year Saved (DALY) allows policy makers and program managers concerned with comparative effectiveness and maximizing impact to directly compare program options. These costing exercises also allow us to generate national program costs for scale up, and when coupled with estimations of averted medical care cost, allow for improved long term planning in establishing national priorities by considering the net value of the intervention in terms of both the expense of the intervention, but also the potential cost savings over time. In general, the analyses presented herein indicate that the cost-effectiveness of the program is highly sensitive to epidemiologic factors associated with the geographic setting, and to a lesser degree the cost of labor across sites.

Care was taken to collect the best available data and use the most realistic assumptions available for these analyses, yet there are some important limitations that should be highlighted. One important limitation is that across those countries selected for the modeling study, only Brazil had a community empowerment-based HIV prevention project with the necessary intervention evaluation data available for micro-costing. Thus, we took great care to generate highly detailed cost estimates from this site and worked closely with project staff from Brazil to generate estimates. This was important, as it formed the base-case analysis for cost estimations in Kenya, Thailand, and Ukraine. As a result, there is a greater degree of cost detail from Brazil that was used in the sensitivity analyses, and there is also the risk that some values estimated for other countries may be different in an actual implementation. The specific activity costs included were also those related to the intervention designed in the Brazilian context, which in keeping with the core principles of a community empowerment-based intervention model, would necessarily have to be adapted for the local context where the intervention would be implemented and take into account the extent to which existing public health services provide the necessary supplies for a comprehensive HIV prevention intervention, such as condoms and HIV/STI-relatedclinical services. To mitigate this risk we cross-checked our estimated values with a variety of other costing exercises that have been conducted in target settings, and examined the literature for labor cost estimates by country. We thus used a larger range of input values for cost items from Kenya, Thailand, and Ukraine for the sensitivity analyses to convey the increased uncertainty from these sites, and in the report present the range of values we identified. Another limitation is found in the estimation of Disability Adjusted Life Years per HIV infection averted.

We drew from established methods for the calculations, which will enhance comparative examination with other interventions examined in the literature. Yet it should be recognized that with ever evolving treatment advances it is possible that longer life and higher quality life while on treatment may happen with future medical advances. Such enhancements would affect the veracity of our estimates, and they should thus be considered as reflecting the state of the current art in treatment. The meta-analysis used to establish the efficacy estimates for the analysis also have some degree of uncertainty. In this regard the model incorporated the 95% confidence interval around the point estimate for use in sensitivity analysis, and in establishing ranges of values for use in analyses. Finally, an important limitation is found in the modeled results used in the analyses which come from the Goals model. As with any model there are a host of assumptions that underpin the modeling analysis, and there are no doubt challenges to culling such a large set of data across multiple countries. Thus, any limitations found in the modeling work convey to the cost-effectiveness analysis. Regardless, sensitivity analysis was conducted with the Goals model, and we adopted the range of model outputs, which allowed for us to communicate the uncertainty inherent in the modeling and costing calculations.

The cost per participant for the community empowerment intervention ranged from $102 to $184, with Ukraine having the lowest cost, and Brazil the highest cost per participant. Labor costs are the major expense, and also account for the majority of variation across countries. However, in general the cost of the program per participant is modest given the intensity of the interactions. Total national 5-year program cost for the Empowerment intervention was found to be highest in Brazil with an average cost of $167M–$170M, and lowest in Ukraine at $14M–$15M (2011 USD). The size of the sex worker population in each country, as well as differences in labor costs across countries, account for the majority of the variation in the cost per participant. For example, in Brazil there is a much larger population in general, and thus a larger number of sex workers than in Ukraine. In addition, labor costs are marginally higher in Brazil as compared to Ukraine as well.

One important finding was that when averted HIV-related treatment costs are removed, the net 5-year national cost of the community empowerment intervention is significantly reduced. For example, in Brazil net program costs are $93M, and in Thailand $45M. In Ukraine and Kenya net costs show cost savings of $39M and $8.6M respectively. Interpretation of the overall cost of the programs should be consider with this in mind, as both Ukraine and Kenya investment in these program not only saves lives and enhances the quality of life, but also over time results in reductions in medical care costs that exceed the cost of the intervention.

The cost per HIV infection averted is lowest in Ukraine ($1,990) and Kenya ($3,813) and highest in Thailand ($66,128) and Brazil ($32,773). Higher costs are driven largely by lower base rates of HIV prevalence, and higher labor costs. When the Empowerment intervention is conducted in the context of enhanced ART provision the cost-effectiveness is reduced modestly. For example, in Ukraine the cost per DALY saved is increased from $85 to $93. This effect is explained by reductions in population-level HIV prevalence driven by the ART program. It is interesting, and perhaps counterintuitive, that addition of an expanded ART program would weaken the cost-effectiveness of the community empowerment intervention. But in reality intervention programs do affect one another, and in this case the benefits of the ART program in reducing HIV incidence over time render the benefits of the community empowerment program less effective. Caution should be taken in interpretation of this interrelationship, as the community empowerment intervention would continue to provide important prevention benefits even with lowered HIV prevalence, and there are strong theoretical arguments for a sustained combination of intervention strategies to get the best population outcomes.

An important consideration is also how the results obtained in this study compare to other interventions in terms of the cost per DALY saved. We estimate that the cost per DALY saved from the empowerment intervention, independent of ART program enhancements, ranges in the median scenario from $85 in Ukraine to $2,838 in Thailand. How does this compare to other HIV-related interventions? A 2005 report in the British Medical Journal summarized the cost per DALY for a host of HIV intervention programs, and identified some very cost-effective interventions (Hogan, Baltussen et al. 2005). For example, a variety of peer education programs for sex workers result in a cost per DALY of less than $4. However, the nature, extent and intensity of the peer intervention for sex workers were not detailed in the analyses presented in the paper. Such limited costs suggest a very superficial intervention that has not been supported in the literature to date to be effective in reducing HIV. Prevention of mother to child HIV transmission programs were approximately $310 per DALY saved, and ART programs averaged from $542 to $1,280 per DALY saved.

Another important consideration is the comparative cost-effectiveness with regard to other non-HIV-related health issues confronting the health systems in settings where these interventions would be implemented. The World Health Organization report comparisons to other non-HIV interventions are summarized (The World Health Organization [WHO-Choice] 2012). Highlighting some of the most cost-effective interventions we find that in

Kenya, the community empowerment intervention examined herein results in an estimated cost per DALY saved of $168, which compares to $41 for insecticide treated bed nets, $79 for measles vaccination (at 50% coverage), and $8 for a community delivered new born health care program. In Thailand the empowerment intervention costs $2,838 per DALY saved—compared to $333 for measles vaccination, and $34 for community new born health care. In Brazil community new born health care is $87 per DALY saved compared to the empowerment intervention which yielded $1,395 per DALY saved. For Ukraine the empowerment intervention was $84 per DALY saved versus $2,491 for measles vaccination programs.

Finally, the cost burden to the overall health system of the community empowerment intervention needs to be considered for the interventions examined, both in terms of the proportion of the overall health budget, and the HIV-specific budget. Let us compare these to both the HIV—and non-HIV—related national health care expenditures in a multi-country study provide a point of comparison (Amico, Aran et al. 2010). We estimated that 5-year net program cost of Empowerment intervention to be $125M in Brazil, $16M in Kenya, and $46M in Thailand. In Ukraine we estimated a net cost saving of the intervention of $35m. These compare to total 5-year national health care expenditure on HIV of $2.7B in Brazil, $1.9B in Kenya, $965M in Thailand, and $365M in Ukraine. Comparing to total national 5-year heath care spending of $245M in Brazil, $3.2B in Kenya, $34B in Thailand, and $29B in Ukraine. As a percent of the total HIV-related health care expenditure per country, the empowerment intervention would be 4.6% for Brazil, 16% for Kenya, and 4.8% for Thailand. In Ukraine the program would have a net cost reduction of 9.6%.

It has been noted that the allocation of national prevention funding is frequently grossly mismatched to the distribution of new infections that could be averted, and this is especially true for sex workers(Commission on AIDS in Asia 2008). Prior analyses of Round 8 (2008) investments in Key Populations by the Global Fund to Fight AIDS, Tuberculosis and Malaria for example suggestion that only 3% of funding in that round went to prevention programs targeting sex workers through that mechanism (Global Fund, 2011). There is thus a good justification based on the analyses presented herein to more equitably allocate HIV prevention funding to interventions focused on sex workers such as the comprehensive community empowerment intervention described herein.

Thus, in terms of comparative effectiveness alone, the community empowerment intervention compares well to other widely utilized interventions, especially when considering the values we obtained from Ukraine and Kenya. In addition, as a percentage of national expenditures on HIV the empowerment intervention is a modest proportion in most countries we examined, and actually reduces the net costs in Ukraine. However, allocation of health resources should never be made solely on the basis of cost-effectiveness, as there are important ethical and human rights principles that supersede the raw comparison of cost-effectiveness results. Importantly, how the intervention fits within an overall prevention program, and the human right to effective and lifesaving interventions are imperative considerations that much be considered.

Lastly, it is also important to note that as interventions such as the community-empowerment-based comprehensive HIV prevention in the context of sex worker, as modeled here, are taken to scale and implemented over time additional cost-savings may be generated, and in turn the costs reflected here may be reduced in this process. Underestimating the cost of effective HIV prevention among sex workers, as has often been the case historically, however, does not serve the sex worker community or the field of HIV prevention if the ultimate goal is to equitably allocate resources to interventions which are both rights-based and cost-effective.

Table 5.2   Cost of Community Empowerment-based Comprehensive HIV Prevention by Country

Personnel	Brazil	Ukraine	Thailand	Kenya
Project Coordinator (about 2/3 time effort)	$23,890	$13,503	$14,125	$18,538
5 Counselors (pre and post test counseling) at about 1/3 time of effort	$27,850	$15,741	$16,466	$21,610
Community activities coordinator	$19,891	$11,242	$11,760	$15,434
3 Interns to assist in organizing activities each at about 1/3 time effort	$7,419	$4,193	$4,387	$5,757
NGO Coordinator at 1/5 effort	$10,503	$5,936	$6,210	$8,150
8 Peer educators each at 90% effort each	$29,648	$16,757	$17,529	$23,006
Workshop Assistant	$5,043	$2,850	$2,982	$3,913
Local Travel	**Brazil**	**Ukraine**	**Thailand**	**Kenya**
Misc. transportation costs for community activities - taxi fare	$1,867	$1,055	$1,104	$1,449
Misc. transportation costs for community activities -mototaxi fare	$1,332	$753	$788	$1,034

(continued next page)

Table 5.2 *(continued)*

Office Operations	Brazil	Ukraine	Thailand	Kenya
Office supplies (paper, staples, Xerox, etc.)	$883	$499	$522	$685
Internet and Telephone	$2,486	$1,405	$1,470	$1,929

Mobilization[a]	Brazil	Ukraine	Thailand	Kenya
Collective cultural activities with sex workers including weekly film screenings, fashion workshops, arts workshops such as candle making and erotic soaps, and bi-monthly community parties	$7,488	$4,232	$4,427	$5,810
Documentary about project implementation to disseminate project experience	$6,100	$3,448	$3,607	$4,734
Mobilization Activities: Examples include paper for signs, balloons to decorate car	$60	$34	$35	$46

Monitoring	Brazil	Ukraine	Thailand	Kenya
Monitoring visits from the national sex worker association (Approx 2 visits)	$1,392	$787	$823	$1,081

Equipment / Furniture	Brazil	Ukraine	Thailand	Kenya
Projector (used for showing movies)	$522	$295	$309	$405

Equipment / Furniture	Brazil	Ukraine	Thailand	Kenya
Office furniture, painting the clinic, etc.	$1,194	$ 675	$706	$926
Computers	$1,343	$759	$794	$1,042
Truck rental for International AIDS Day	$50	$28	$29	$39
Equipment for trainings	$159	$90	$94	$123

HIV Counseling Training (3 days)	Brazil	Ukraine	Thailand	Kenya
Travel cost for staff from Sao Paulo to attend training for three days	$935	$528	$ 553	$725
Coffee Breaks and lunch for participants	$363	$205	$214	$281

Organizational Training workshop with National Network of Sex Workers (2 days)	Brazil	Ukraine	Thailand	Kenya
Airfare and lodging for two people	$2,763	$1,562	$1,634	$2,144
Food for participants for two days	$497	$281	$294	$386
Room rental	$276	$156	$163	$214

(continued next page)

Treatment Center Management Training (2 days)	Brazil	Ukraine	Thailand	Kenya
Travel cost for one person for three days	$614	$347	$ 363	$477
Coffee Breaks and lunch for participants	$376	$213	$222	$292
Citizenship, STIs, and HIV/AIDS for sex workers (3 days for entire staff)	Brazil	Ukraine	Thailand	Kenya
Travel and Lodging	$995	$562	$588	$772
Coffee Breaks and lunch for participants	$1,019	$576	$602	$791
Quality of care in STI management and sexual and reproductive rights (1 week for entire staff)	Brazil	Ukraine	Thailand	Kenya
Consultancy fees for trainers	$394	$223	$233	$306
Hotel and Lodging for trainers	**$1,868**	**$1,056**	**$1,104**	**$1,449**
Coffee Breaks and lunch for participants	$1,104	$624	$653	$857
Training of Community Health Care workers	Brazil	Ukraine	Thailand	Kenya
Coffee Breaks and Snacks for participants	$172	$97	$101	$133
Workshop for the development of IEC materials	**$887**	**$501**	**$525**	**$688**
Design and Production of IEC materials - ANNUAL–approx. 5000 pieces	$2,210	$1,249	$1,307	$1,715
Subtotal	**$163,591**	**$92,462**	**$96,723**	**$126,941**
Overhead	$16,359	$9,246	$9,672	$12,694
Annual Total	**$179,950**	**$101,708**	**$106,395**	**$139,635**
Cost per Participant in 2011 USD	**$180**	**$102**	**$106**	**$140**
After Adjustment for Discounting & Distribution of Startup Costs (Standard Deviation)	$102 ($8.7)	$106 ($9.2)	$140 ($9.8)	$184 ($9.8)

Source: Authors

a. A key component of the moblization activities in the *Encontros* project was using social and cultural spaces for discussions on issues related to citizenship, rights, and HIV prevention in a border town context with high levels of stigma towards sex workers. Thus, in addition to peer education, condom distribution, and clinical services, the project also promoted collective activities with sex workers including fashion workshops, weekly screenings and discussions of films about sexuality, and arts workshops including painting the public clinic, candle making, and erotic soap making. Fashion designs and other products made were then showcased in a weekly community market and by-monthly fashion shows at parties open to the entire community to engage the public in dialogue about sex worker rights, reduce stigma surrounding sex work, disseminate HIV and STI prevention and service information, and form partnerships with other government and community organizations.

Figure 5.1   Distribution of Costs by Category, Brazil (Annual Cost per 1000 Sex Workers, in US$)

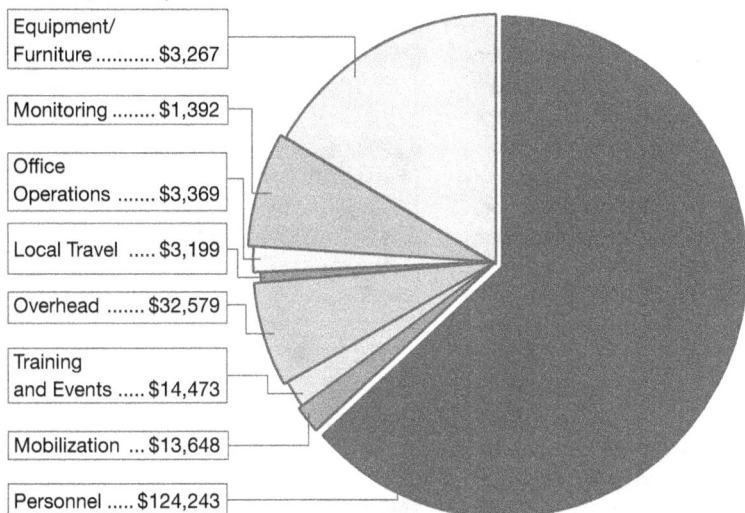

Equipment/
Furniture $3,267

Monitoring $1,392

Office
Operations $3,369

Local Travel $3,199

Overhead $32,579

Training
and Events $14,473

Mobilization ... $13,648

Personnel $124,243

Source: Authors.

Figure 5.2   Cost per Participant for Empowerment Intervention in Brazil: Probability Distribution across 50,000 Model Iteration

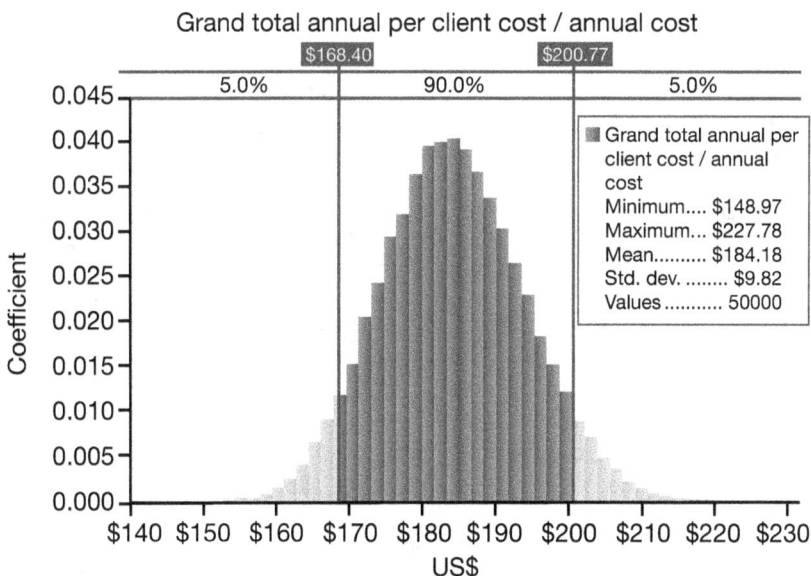

Grand total annual per client cost / annual cost

$168.40 $200.77

5.0%   90.0%   5.0%

Grand total annual per
client cost / annual
cost
Minimum.... $148.97
Maximum... $227.78
Mean.......... $184.18
Std. dev. $9.82
Values 50000

Coefficient (y-axis): 0.000, 0.005, 0.010, 0.015, 0.020, 0.025, 0.030, 0.035, 0.040, 0.045

US$ (x-axis): $140 $150 $160 $170 $180 $190 $200 $210 $220 $230

Source: Authors.
Note: Std. dev. = standard development.

Figure 5.3   Multivariate Sensitivity Analysis Results: Cost per Participant for Empowerment Intervention in Brazil

Grand total annual per client cost / Annual cost (regression coefficient)

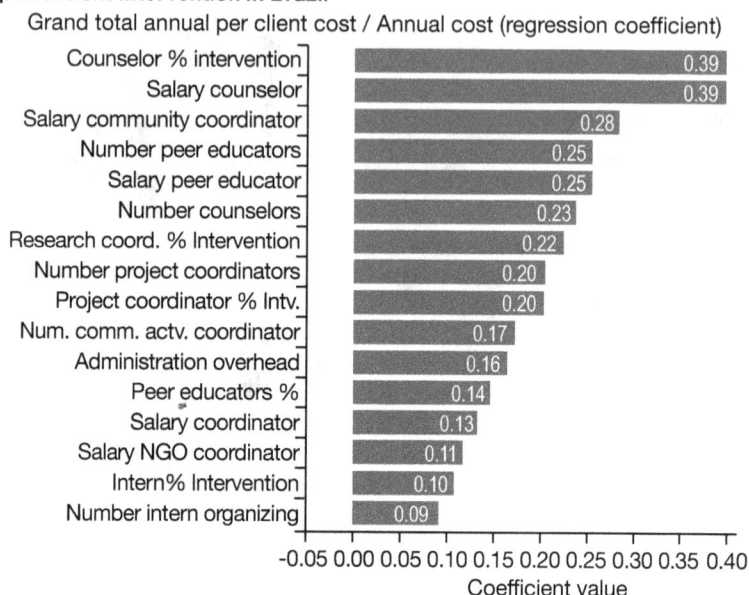

Source: Authors.
Note: comm. = community; coord. = coordinator; intv. = intervention; actv. = activity; num. = number.

Table 5.3   Full Rank Order Multivariate Sensitivity Analysis Results (Regression Coefficients > 0.10) for Cost per Participant of Community Empowerment in Brazil

Regression and Rank Information for Grand Total Annual per Participant Cost / Annual Cost			
Rank	Name	Regression	Correlation
1	Counselor % intervention	0.388	0.419
2	Salary counselor	0.386	0.414
3	Salary community coordinator	0.276	0.308
4	Number peer educators	0.247	0.270
5	Salary peer educator	0.246	0.267
6	Number counselors	0.231	0.244
7	Research coordinator % intervention	0.219	0.235
8	Number project coordinators	0.199	0.211
9	Project Coordinator % intervention	0.198	0.215
10	Number community activity coordinators	0.165	0.168
11	Administration overhead	0.161	0.660
12	Peer educators %	0.137	0.146
13	Salary coordinator	0.129	0.141
14	Salary NGO coordinator	0.109	0.108

Source: Authors.

Figure 5.4   Distribution of Cost per Participant across Model Iterations—Kenya

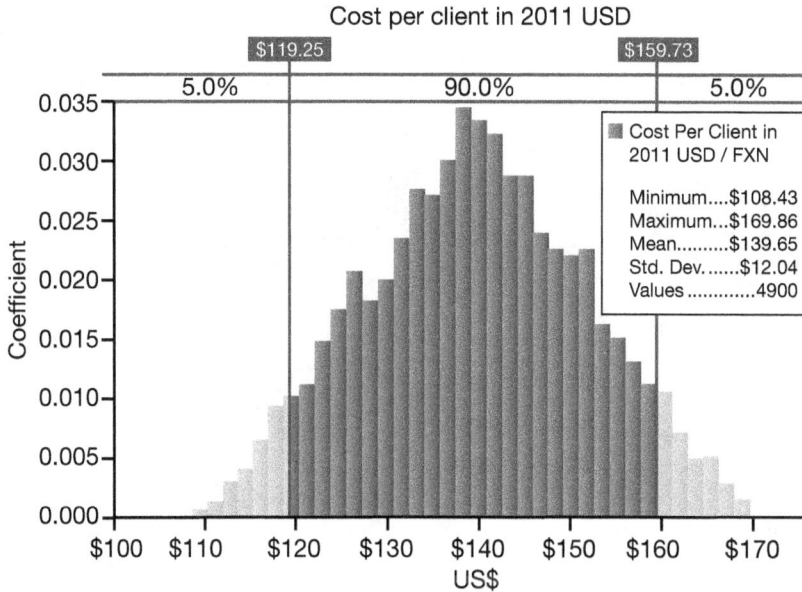

Cost per client in 2011 USD

Source: Authors.
Note: Std. dev. = standard development; FXN = function.

Figure 5.5   Sensitivity Analysis—Kenya

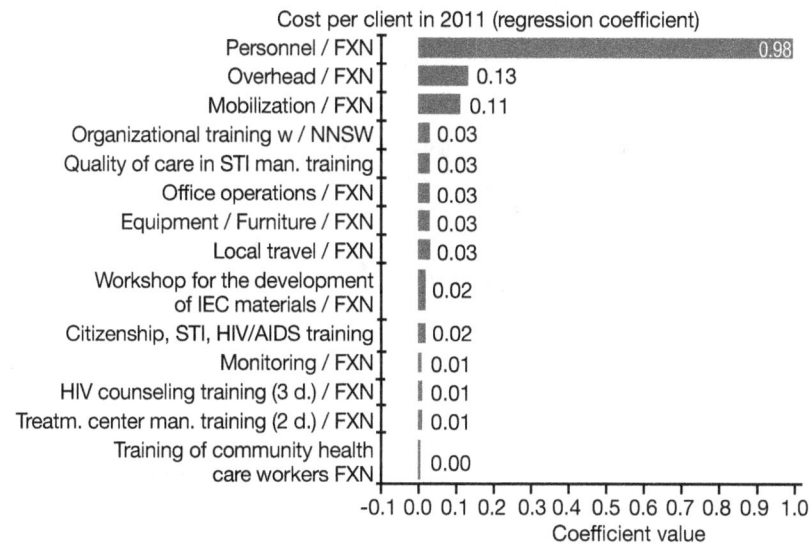

Cost per client in 2011 (regression coefficient)

Source: Authors.
Note: d. = days; FXN = function; man. = management; treatm. = treatment; NNSW = national network of sex workers; STI = sexually transmitted infections; w = with.

Figure 5.6   Distribution of Cost per Participant across Model Iterations—Thailand

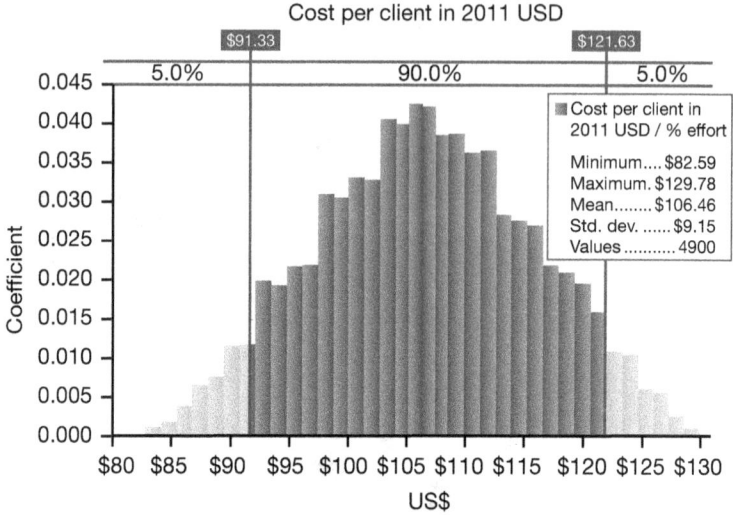

Cost per client in 2011 USD

| | $91.33 | | $121.63 |
| 0.045 | 5.0% | 90.0% | 5.0% |

Cost per client in 2011 USD / % effort

Minimum.... $82.59
Maximum. $129.78
Mean....... $106.46
Std. dev. $9.15
Values 4900

Source: Authors.
Note: Std. dev. = standard development.

Figure 5.7   Sensitivity Analysis–Thailand

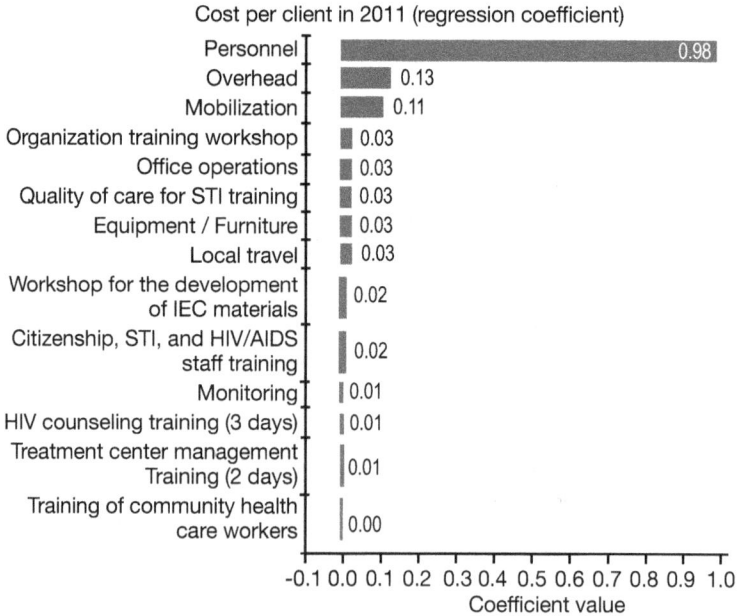

Cost per client in 2011 (regression coefficient)

Personnel	0.98
Overhead	0.13
Mobilization	0.11
Organization training workshop	0.03
Office operations	0.03
Quality of care for STI training	0.03
Equipment / Furniture	0.03
Local travel	0.03
Workshop for the development of IEC materials	0.02
Citizenship, STI, and HIV/AIDS staff training	0.02
Monitoring	0.01
HIV counseling training (3 days)	0.01
Treatment center management Training (2 days)	0.01
Training of community health care workers	0.00

Coefficient value

Source: Authors.
Note: STI = sexually transmitted infections.

Figure 5.8   Distribution of Cost per Participant across Model Iterations—Ukraine

Cost per client in 2011 USD

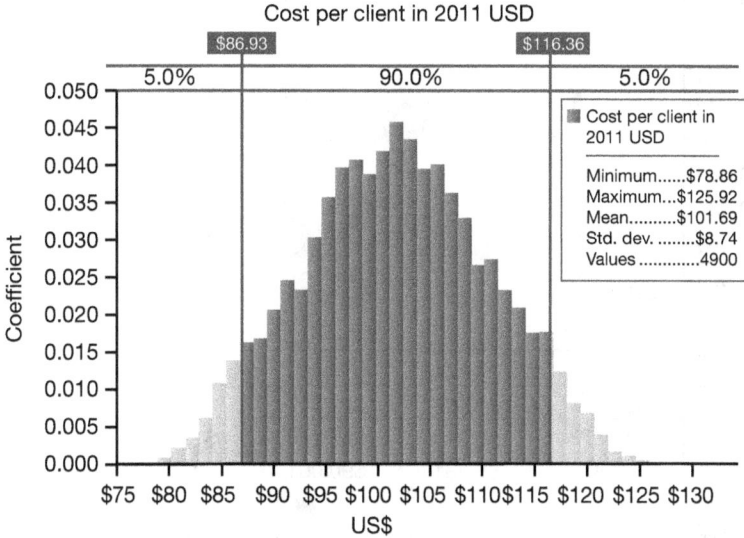

Source: Authors.
Note: Std. dev. = standard development.

Figure 5.9   Sensitivity Analysis–Ukraine

Cost per client in 2011 (regression coefficient)

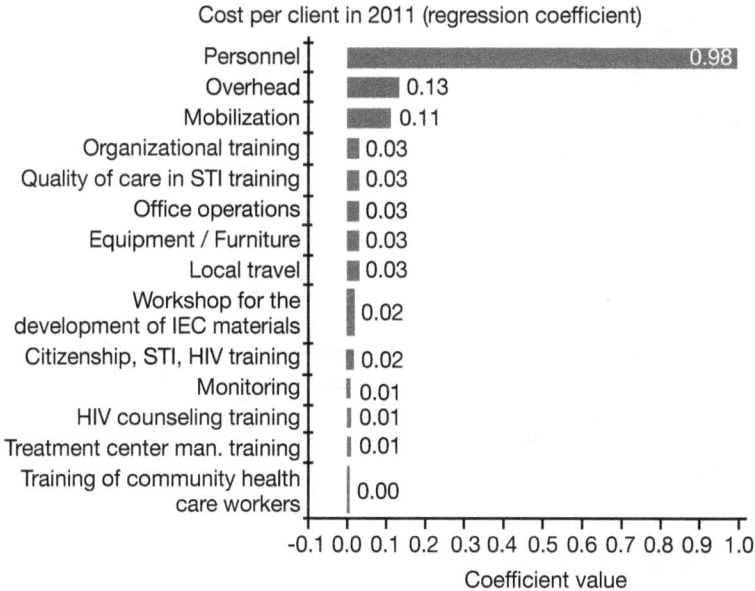

Source: Authors.
Note: man. = management; STI = sexually transmitted infections.

Figure 5.10   Cost per HIV Infection Averted with Static ART Provision[a]

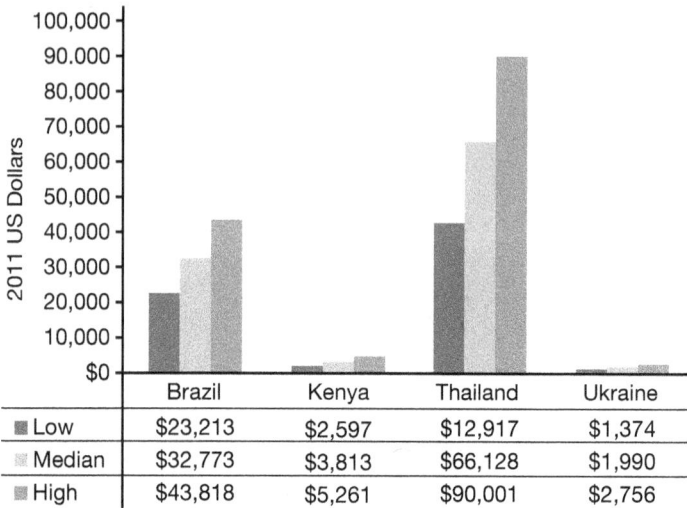

	Brazil	Kenya	Thailand	Ukraine
Low	$23,213	$2,597	$12,917	$1,374
Median	$32,773	$3,813	$66,128	$1,990
High	$43,818	$5,261	$90,001	$2,756

Source: Authors.
Note: ART = antiretroviral therapy.
a. Cumulative among adults between 2012 and 2016 when the empowerment intervention is expanded to a maximum, feasable coverage among female sex workers by 2016.

Figure 5.11   Cost per HIV Infection Averted in Context of Enhanced ART[a] Provision

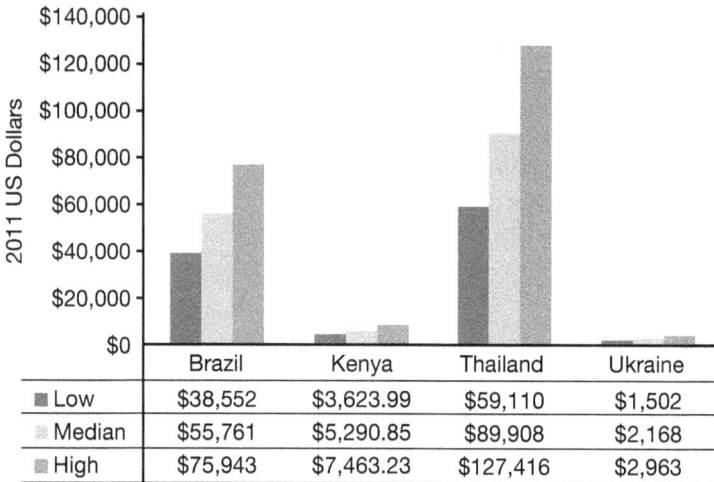

	Brazil	Kenya	Thailand	Ukraine
Low	$38,552	$3,623.99	$59,110	$1,502
Median	$55,761	$5,290.85	$89,908	$2,168
High	$75,943	$7,463.23	$127,416	$2,963

Source: Authors.
Note: ART = antiretroviral therapy.
a. Cumulative due to expansion of empowerment intervention, in the context of early initiation and expanding ART among adults, 2012–16

Figure 5.12 Total Empowerment Program Cost with Static ART Provision[a]

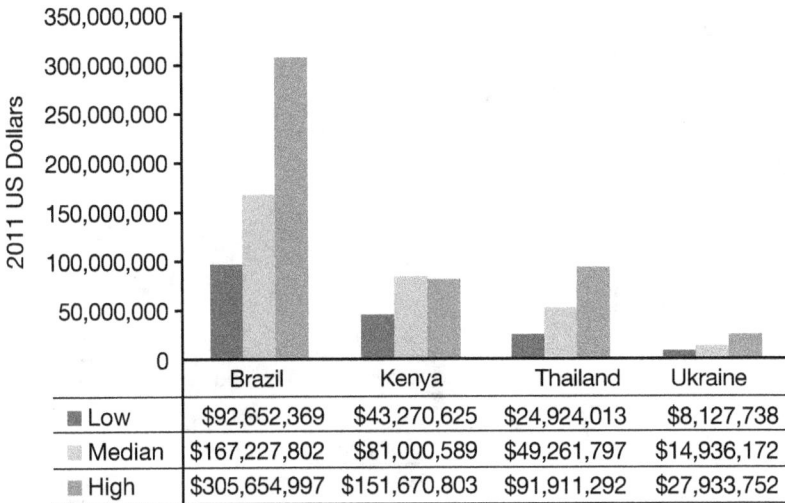

	Brazil	Kenya	Thailand	Ukraine
■ Low	$92,652,369	$43,270,625	$24,924,013	$8,127,738
Median	$167,227,802	$81,000,589	$49,261,797	$14,936,172
High	$305,654,997	$151,670,803	$91,911,292	$27,933,752

Source: Authors.
Note: ART = antiretroviral therapy.
a. Cumulative among adults between 2012 and 2016 when the empowerment intervention is expanded to a maximum, feasable coverage among female sex workers by 2016.

Figure 5.13 Total Empowerment Program Cost in Context of Enhanced ART Provision[a]

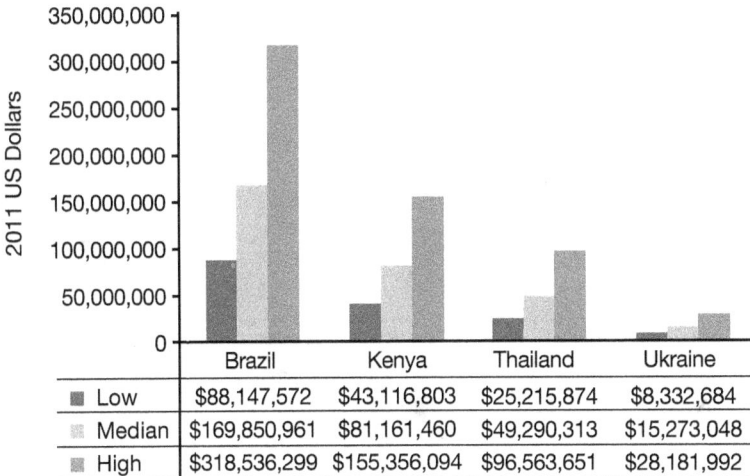

	Brazil	Kenya	Thailand	Ukraine
■ Low	$88,147,572	$43,116,803	$25,215,874	$8,332,684
Median	$169,850,961	$81,161,460	$49,290,313	$15,273,048
■ High	$318,536,299	$155,356,094	$96,563,651	$28,181,992

Source: Authors.
Note: ART = antiretroviral therapy.
a. Cumulative due to the expansion of empowerment intervention, in the context of early initiation and expanding ART among adults, 2012–16

Figure 5.14   Net Program Cost (Subtracting Averted Medical Costs) with Static ART Provision[a]

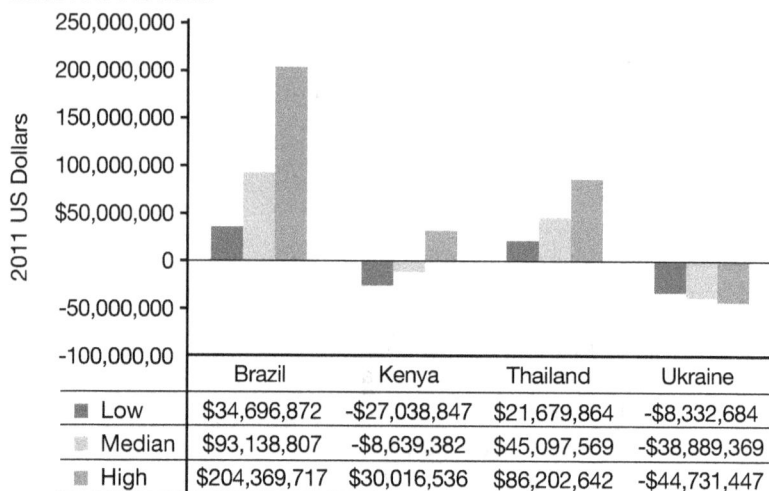

	Brazil	Kenya	Thailand	Ukraine
■ Low	$34,696,872	-$27,038,847	$21,679,864	-$8,332,684
▧ Median	$93,138,807	-$8,639,382	$45,097,569	-$38,889,369
▨ High	$204,369,717	$30,016,536	$86,202,642	-$44,731,447

Source: Authors.
Note: ART = antiretroviral therapy.
a. Culmulative among adults between 2012 and 2016 when the empowerment intervention, is expanded to a maximum, feasable coverage among female sex workers.

Figure 5.15   Net Program Cost (Subtracting Averted Medical Costs) with Enhanced ART Provision[a]

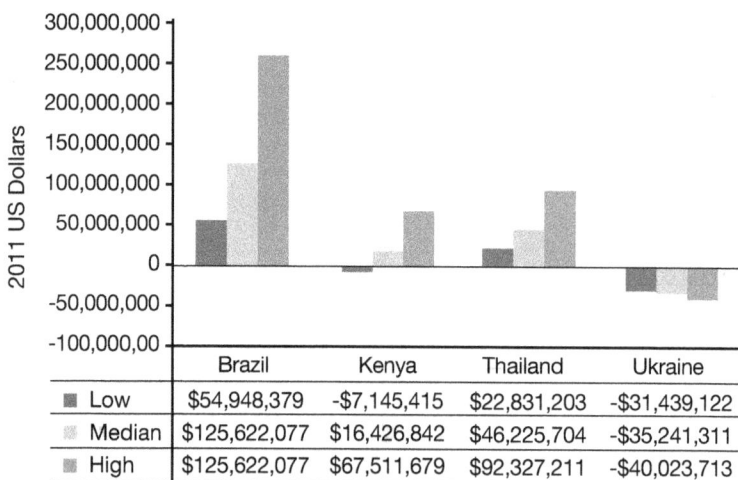

	Brazil	Kenya	Thailand	Ukraine
■ Low	$54,948,379	-$7,145,415	$22,831,203	-$31,439,122
▧ Median	$125,622,077	$16,426,842	$46,225,704	-$35,241,311
▨ High	$125,622,077	$67,511,679	$92,327,211	-$40,023,713

Source: Authors.
Note: ART = antiretroviral therapy.
a. Net program costs: culmulative due to expansion of empowerment intervention, in the context of early initiation and expanding ART among adults, 2012–16

Figure 5.16   Cost per DALY with Static ART Provision[a]

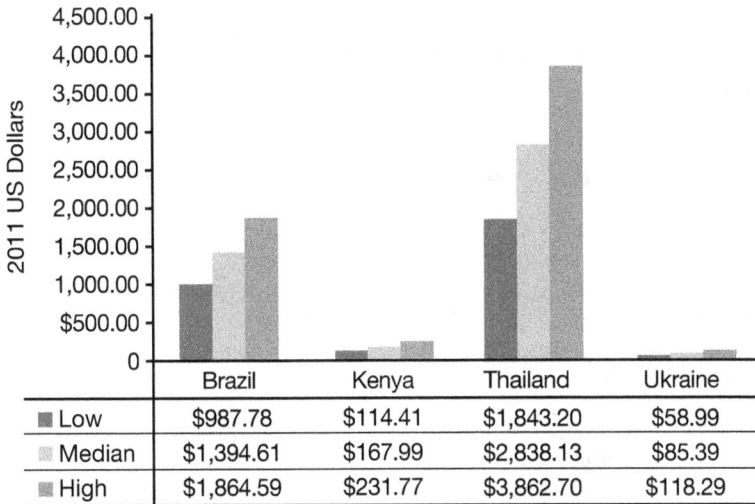

	Brazil	Kenya	Thailand	Ukraine
▣ Low	$987.78	$114.41	$1,843.20	$58.99
▨ Median	$1,394.61	$167.99	$2,838.13	$85.39
▣ High	$1,864.59	$231.77	$3,862.70	$118.29

Source: Authors.
Note: ART = antiretroviral therapy.
a. Culmulative among adults between 2012 and 2016 when the empowerment intervention is expanded to a maximum, feasable coverage among female sex workers by 2016.

Figure 5.17   Cost per DALY in Context of Enhanced ART Provision[a]

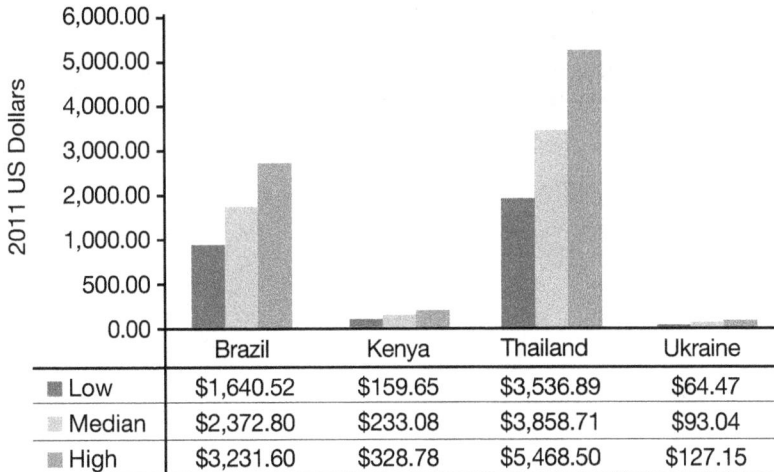

	Brazil	Kenya	Thailand	Ukraine
▣ Low	$1,640.52	$159.65	$3,536.89	$64.47
▨ Median	$2,372.80	$233.08	$3,858.71	$93.04
▣ High	$3,231.60	$328.78	$5,468.50	$127.15

Source: Authors.
Note: ART = antiretroviral therapy.
a. Culmulative due to the expansion of empowerment intervention, in the context of early initiation and expanding ART among adults, 2012–16

References

Amico, P., C. Aran, et al. (2010). "HIV spending as a share of total health expenditure: an analysis of regional variation in a multi-country study." *PLoS One* 5 (9): e12997.

Commission on AIDS in Asia (2008). *Redefining AIDS in Asia: Crafting an Effective Response.* http://data.unaids.org/pub/Report/2008/20080326_report_commission_aids_en.pdf . New Delhi.

Gold, M. R. (1996). *Cost-effectiveness in health and medicine.* New York: Oxford University Press.

Hogan, D. R., R. Baltussen, et al. (2005). "Cost effectiveness analysis of strategies to combat HIV/AIDS in developing countries." *BMJ* 331 (7530): 1431–1437.

Holtgrave, D. R., N. L. Qualls, et al. (1996). "Economic evaluation of HIV prevention programs." *Annual Review of Public Health* 17: 467–488.

International Labor Organization. (2012). *"Wages and hours of work in 159 occupations"*, 2012. http://laborsta.ilo.org/.

Lippman, S. A., A. Donini, et al. (2010). "Social-environmental factors and protective sexual behavior among sex workers: the Encontros intervention in Brazil." *American Journal of Public Health* 100 Suppl 1: S216–223.

Murray, C. J. L., A. D. Lopez, et al. (1996). *The global burden of disease: a comprehensive assessment of mortality and disability from diseases, injuries, and risk factors in 1990 and projected to 2020.* Cambridge, Mass., Published by the Harvard School of Public Health on behalf of the World Health Organization and the World Bank ; Distributed by Harvard University Press.

UN Statistics Division *Millennium Development Indicators Unit.* (2012). "Purchasing power parities (PPP) conversion factor, local currency unit to international dollar." from http://mdgs.un.org/unsd/mdg/SeriesDetail.aspx?srid=699

World Health Organization. *"Global Health Observatory Data Repository / Life Tables."* http://apps.who.int/ghodata/?vid=720.

World Health Organization (WHO-Choice) (2012). *Choosing Interventions that are Cost-Effective.* Geneva. http://www.who.int/choice/results/en/.

CHAPTER 6

Modeling Violence and HIV among Sex Workers

Introduction

Key Themes

- A growing body of evidence demonstrates a high prevalence of violence against sex workers and related risk for HIV infection.

- Violence is often not considered in HIV prevention strategies; however, based on emerging evidence, it has to be.

- We used mathematical modeling to study the impact of reducing violence against female sex worker on HIV infection among sex workers and the adult population.

- The models illustrate that reducing violence against sex workers can impart significant reductions in HIV incidence and prevalence among sex workers, as well as among the adult population, even in the context of expanded ART coverage.

- In Ukraine, characterized by a concentrated epidemic, reductions in violence could avert over 1,400 new HIV infections among sex workers, and over 4,000 in the adult population within a 5 year time span.

- In Kenya, home to a generalized epidemic, reductions in violence against sex workers could avert over 5,300 new infections among sex workers and 10,000 among all adults over the next 5 years.

The past three decades of research on HIV among sex workers overwhelmingly confirms the relevance of structural risk factors, many of which are beyond the immediate control of sex workers. Structural risk factors that include criminalization as well as stigma, discrimination, and violence represent components of the broader context of sex work that pose formidable barriers to ensuring safe sex as well as access to prevention, testing, and treatment services (Kerrigan, Telles et al. 2008; Blankenship, Burroway et al. 2010; Reed, Gupta et al. 2010). Despite their demonstrated impact on HIV among sex workers, structural risk factors are rarely included in epidemiologic modeling scenarios used to project HIV epidemics and guide HIV prevention strategies and policy. The value of integrating the structural risk environment among at-risk populations was illustrated in a recent example with injection drug users in Ukraine, wherein elimination of police beatings was found to prevent a significant portion of HIV infections by modifying the risk environment, e.g., removing barriers to safe injection practices and enabling access to drug treatment and needle exchange programs.(Strathdee, Hallett et al. 2010)

Physical and sexual violence against sex workers, including rape by state actors as well as clients, is one example of the harmful environment that imparts HIV risk to sex workers. International concern is mounting for the alarming levels of violence experienced by sex workers perpetrated by clients, police and other actors (Sex Workers Rights Advocacy 2009; Beattie, Bhattacharjee et al. 2010; Reed, Gupta et al. 2010; Swain 2011; Decker, Wirtz et al. 2012). These abuses constitute a significant threat to the health, human rights and well-being of sex workers.

Abuse against sex workers has been linked to the risk of HIV infection (Ulibarri et al., 2009) as well as STI symptoms (Decker, McCauley et al. 2010) and infection (Cohan, Lutnick et al. 2006; Beattie, Bhattacharjee et al. 2010; Decker, Wirtz et al. 2012). Violence cannot directly cause HIV; rather it may influence risk indirectly via proximal factors such as unprotected sex (Beattie, Bhattacharjee et al. 2010; Swain 2011),(Stachowiak, Sherman et al. 2005; Rhodes, Simic et al. 2008) (Kerrigan, Telles et al. 2008; Simic and Rhodes 2009) condom failure, (Choi, Chen et al. 2008), and partners who may be at greater risk for infection, (Decker, Seage et al. 2009; Decker, McCauley et al. 2010) and injection drug use, (Ulibarri, Strathdee et al. 2011); moreover abrasions and lacerations that can result from sexual violence can facilitate HIV transmission (Draughton 2012).

Despite the demonstrated HIV impact of violence at the individual level, the role of violence against sex workers on future HIV epidemics among female sex workers remains unclear, as do the implications of violence for national HIV epidemics. New, empirical data regarding violence and HIV among sex workers enables for the first time the development of mathematical modeling approaches to inform these questions. Illustrating the urgency of understanding the impact of violence on HIV epidemics is the recent development of innovative, integrated violence-related interventions for sex workers with a demonstrated impact on reducing violence (Beattie, Bhattacharjee et al. 2010).

Despite the demonstrated associations of violence with HIV risk and infection among sex workers, and ongoing work to reduce violence against sex workers, intervention research has yet to formally document the HIV epidemic impact of reducing violence against sex workers. There exists a clear need for interventions to prevent violence against sex workers on grounds of human rights. Additionally, prioritizing a given intervention's development or implementation is often guided by estimation of its HIV epidemic impact; yet to date the potential HIV epidemic impact of violence reduction interventions among sex workers remains unclear.

To address this gap, we undertook a mathematical modeling exercise to determine the impact of reducing violence against sex workers on HIV prevalence, incidence, and new infections averted among sex workers as well as the adult populations in two low and middle income countries. The model is not based on a specific intervention, but rather it is a hypothetical exercise that depicts what could be achieved across differing HIV epidemic scenarios through a given level of reduction in violence against sex workers. Thusly, the model projects HIV incidence and prevalence trends among sex workers in response to declining prevalence of violence against female sex workers.

Methods

Using the updated Spectrum 2011 suite (v. 4.14 Beta 16), developed by Futures Institute, the research team applied the Goals projection model to Kenya and Ukraine to predict HIV incidence and prevalence among female sex workers as well as in the general adult population when the prevalence of violence against female sex workers is reduced over time. While parameters and assumptions for Goals were also available for Thailand and Brazil, the violence prevalence data from these nations used disparate referent periods (past week and past four months, respectively), and were not modeled due to concerns about comparability and assumptions of the prevalence of violence against sex workers.

Model Parameterization

Parameters and assumptions for Goals described previously (Chapter 3, Intervention Modeling Analyses) were applied to this analysis. As with the modelling of interventions, behavioural and epidemiological data for female sex workers were derived from the results of the reviews conducted for the case study chapters for countries for which we modelled the impact of violence (see country case studues for Kenya and Ukraine in Chapter 3). Similarly, other national or sex work specific data were also obtained through national reports and country experts, when necessary (see Modeling Chapter).

Unique to this analysis, the prevalence of violence was calculated using data from peer-reviewed publications for Kenya (Chersich, Luchters et al. 2007); this estimate is specific to sexual violence. For Ukraine, a weighted violence prevalence was calculated drawing on Ukraine-based data (Sex Workers Rights Advocacy 2009), as well as Russia as a proxy (Sex Workers Rights Advocacy 2009; Decker, Wirtz et al. 2012) given the small sample size for Ukraine data; this estimate reflects physical or sexual violence. The baseline prevalence reported in Table 6.1 represents the prevalence estimates of violence among sex workers in each country obtained through this review.

Table 6.1   Modeling Scenarios for Violence among Female Sex Workers in Kenya and Ukraine

Description		Kenya	Ukraine
Status quo	Baseline prevalence of violence held constant among FSW (2011–16; past year)[a]	32.4%	39.0%
	Scale-up in coverage of ART by 2016 according to country estimations (% coverage or number)[a]	85.0%	58,000
Scenario 1:	Interpolated decline in violence among FSW from 2011 levels by 14% in 2016	18.4%	25.0%
	Scale-up in coverage of ART by 2016 according to country estimations (% coverage or number)[a]	85.0%	58,000
Scenario 2:	Interpolated decline in violence among FSW from 2011 levels by 30% in 2016	2.4%	9.0%
	Scale-up in coverage of ART by 2016 according to country estimations (% coverage of number)	85.0%	58,000
Impact of FSW violence on condom non-use		69.0%	

Source: Authors.
Note: ART = antiretroviral therapy; FSW = female sex worker.
a. ART scale-up among adults based on country UNAIDS projections estimates.

Model inputs related to HIV transmission associated with violence drew on a WHO systematic review of violence and HIV risk (WHO/Shannon 2012), which identified 15 quantitative papers concerning violence and HIV risk; these papers were supplemented by a manuscript from Brazil (Kerrigan, Telles et al. 2008) that was not included in the review but included associations of violence with condom non-use. A wide range of outcomes were assessed including condom non-use, condom failure, and STI infection and symptoms. Only one study provided a direct estimate linking violence with HIV, and demonstrated the partial mediation by injection drug use (Ulibarri, Strathdee et al. 2011).   Qualitative evidence demonstrates that violence heightens HIV risk in part through pressure and overt force for unprotected sex (Stachowiak, Sherman et al. 2005; Rhodes, Simic et al. 2008; Simic and Rhodes 2009). Likely reflecting this strong conceptual underpinning, condom non-use was the outcome most consistently assessed across the manuscripts reviewed, with six of the 16 papers providing an effect estimate based on violence exposure. Thus, condom non-use during vaginal sex, including that due to client pressure, was selected as a proxy outcome for modelling purposes.

To support the requirements of the Goals model, risk or prevalence ratios are required rather than the more commonly reported odds ratio. Where not provided directly, risk ratios were calculated for the association of violence with unprotected sex. Of the six papers, two did not contain sufficient information to enable direct calculation and were excluded from further analyses (Surratt, Kurtz et al. 2005; Stulhofer, Lausevic et al. 2010). A meta-analysis, in which studies were weighted by their relative sample size, was conducted to generate a summary risk ratio for the association of violence with unprotected sex. The calculated risk ratio was 1.69 (CI: 1.27–2.25). For entry to the impact matrix, this value was then transformed to the relative decrease in condom non-use associated with violence, using the formula: $D=RR-1$. This calculation estimated a value of 69.0% increase in condom non-use associated with violence, the input needed for the Goals impact matrix.

Modeling Scenarios and Analysis Plan

In Goals, the impact of a given exposure, most often exposure to an intervention, is assessed through the change in the percent of a target population that is reached by that exposure. Given the lack of developed interventions to address violence and HIV risk among sex workers, modeling the impact of a specific violence-prevention intervention is premature. We took an alternate approach and considered violence itself as the risk exposure for the purpose of this modeling exercise. To align this purpose with the parameters of Goals, we considered the risk exposure of violence to be effectively the opposite of an intervention: we modeled the decrease in coverage, in other words, a reduction in violence exposure. Thus, violence exposure was treated as an "intervention" in the Goals model, but with an opposite process; i.e., instead of increasing coverage as would be desirable for an HIV risk reduction intervention, we modeled the decrease in coverage, in other words, a reduction in violence exposure.

Building on the associations of violence with elevated condom non-use, we were able to model violence in the "intervention" component of the Goals impact matrix, by specifying the impact of violence on condom non-use among the sex worker population in Goals. Within the Goals impact matrix, violence was the only "intervention" with a positive value in the "reduction in condom non-use" entry. This entry was made specific to the sex work population and, accordingly, on the prevalence (or "coverage" in this case) of violence was applied to the sex work population. The reductions in violence modeled herein are hypothetical and represent an illustration of the epidemic impact were violence to be reduced to a given level. Accordingly, models were designed to reflect the impact of a decrease in violence on HIV incidence and prevalence. Analysis methods were similar to those described for the primary intervention modeling (see Modeling Chapter). The impacts and coverage for all other behavioral interventions and risk populations were held constant, so that we could look specifically at the impact of violence in the absence of other types of interventions. In each modeling scenario, coverage of ART was allowed to increase according to the national estimates, acknowledging the fact that violence exists in such real world settings of expanded coverage of other HIV prevention and treatment interventions.

Table 6.1 depicts the three violence and HIV modeling scenarios applied to Kenya and Ukraine. The current prevalence (or "coverage") of violence among sex workers was used to model the status quo scenario (32.4% and 39% in Kenya and Ukraine, respectively), in which there is no change in violence between from 2011–2016. Subsequent scenarios depict the impacts of reduced prevalence ("coverage of violence") over five years; the first scenario investigates reductions in violence prevalence from baseline values to 18.4% and 25% in Kenya and Ukraine by 2016, respectively, and the second scenario investigates further reductions in violence to 2.4% and 9% in Kenya and Ukraine respectively. The levels to which violence prevalence were reduced do not imply that any level of violence is acceptable; rather, these conservative reductions in violence prevalence were selected in recognition that modifying violence is complex, and provide illustrations to reflect what gains could be achieved even with the modest reductions in violence that may be feasible in a short time frame.

Results

Kenya
Table 6.2 and Figure 6.1 depict the number of new infections observed among sex workers in Kenya when violence against sex workers is decreased from a prevalence of 32% to 18% and 2%, respectively, by 2016. There is an observed decrease in the number of new infections among sex workers for all three scenarios; this is likely attributable to the ongoing expansion of ART in the country. When violence is reduced to 18% by 2016, there is an approximate

4% reduction in new infections between 2012 and 2016 is observed, with an estimated 2,509 infections averted. Further reducing the prevalence of violence to 2% by 2016 results in almost 8% reduction in new infections among sex workers, or more than 5,300 new infections averted between 2012 and 2016 compared to the baseline scenario.

Table 6.2   New HIV Infections among Female Sex Workers in Kenya: Observations When Violence Is Reduced

Year	Baseline violence (32.4%)	Reduced violence (18.4%)		Reduced violence (2.4%)	
		New infections	Infections averted	New infections	Infections averted
2011	17,779	17,779	–	17,779	–
2012	16,139	15,949	190	15,731	408
2013	14,361	14,015	346	13,619	742
2014	13,411	12,918	493	12,356	1,055
2015	13,299	12,640	659	11,890	1,409
2016	13,063	12,242	821	11,311	1,752
Cumulative (2012–16)	70,273	67,764	2,509	64,907	5,366
Reduction	(Ref.)		3.6%		7.6%

Source: Authors.
Note: Ref. = reference.

Figure 6.1   Trends in New HIV Infections among Female Sex Workers in Kenya in the Context of Declining Prevalence of Violence

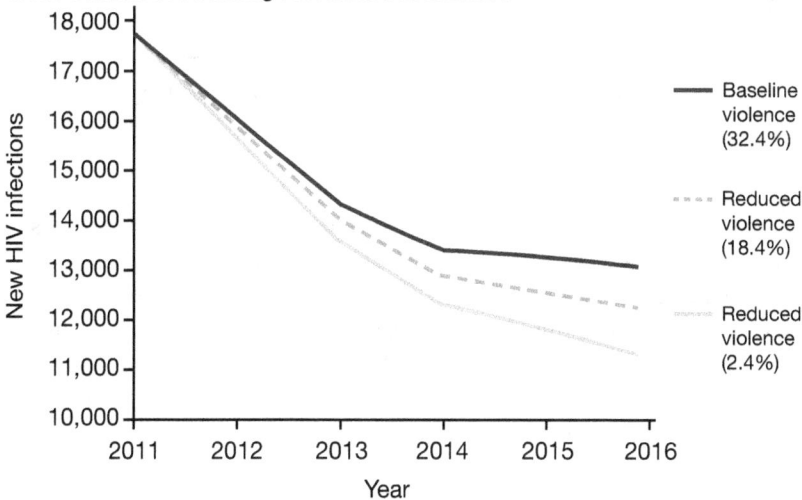

Source: Authors.

Table 6.3   HIV Prevalence among Female Sex Workers in Kenya: Observations When Violence Is Reduced

Year	Baseline violence (32.4%)	Reduced violence (18.4%)		Reduced violence (2.4%)	
		Prevalence (%)	Percent reduction	Prevalence (%)	Percent reduction
2011	33.75	33.75	–	33.75	–
2012	32.03	31.98	0.17	31.91	0.36
2013	30.11	29.97	0.47	29.81	1.01
2014	28.22	27.97	0.90	27.68	1.92
2015	26.55	26.16	1.45	25.72	3.10
2016	25.03	24.50	2.12	23.89	4.54

Source: Authors.

Figure 6.2   HIV Prevalence among Female Sex Workers in the Context of Declining Prevalence of Violence in Kenya

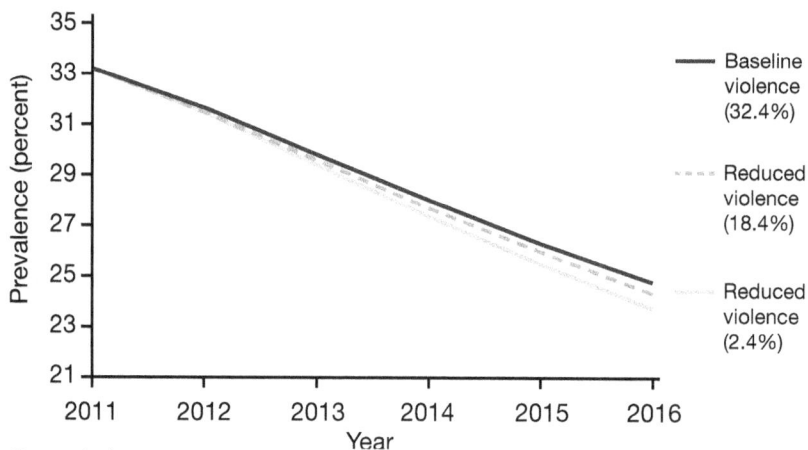

Source: Authors.

Table 6.3 and Figure 6.2 depict the HIV prevalence observed among sex workers in Kenya when violence is decreased from a baseline prevalence of 32% among female sex workers to 18.4% and 2.4%, respectively, by 2016. ART expansion among the adult population continues to play a role in the declining prevalence, assuming sex workers have equal access to treatment, as evidenced by the projected prevalence of 25% among sex workers in 2016 in the baseline scenario. However, when the prevalence of violence is reduced to 18% by 2016, the prevalence of HIV among sex workers is projected to decline further. Further reducing the prevalence of violence to 9% by 2016 results in a lower HIV prevalence among sex workers, declining to 23% compared to 25% that is observed when violence continues at its current prevalence, for a projected 4.5% reduction in HIV prevalence among sex workers. When viewing these results, it is important to recognize that HIV prevalence typically does not decline in the short terms; however, infections averted now will lead to a decline in prevalence in later years. Furthermore, ART keeps people alive and, thus the HIV prevalence elevated.

Table 6.4   New HIV Infections among the Adult Population in Kenya: Observations When Violence Is Reduced

Year	Baseline violence (32.4%)	Reduced violence (18.4%)		Reduced violence (2.4%)	
		New infections	Infections averted	New infections	Infections averted
2011	100,002	100,002	–	100,002	–
2012	90,564	90,226	338	89,840	724
2013	80,051	79,412	639	78,684	1,367
2014	74,123	73,201	922	72,153	1,970
2015	73,014	71,773	1,241	70,369	2,645
2016	71,460	69,899	1,561	68,142	3,318
Cumulative (2012–16)	389,212	384,511	4,701	379,188	10,024
Reduction	(Ref.)		1.2%		2.6%

Source: Authors.
Note: Ref. = reference.

Table 6.4 and Figure 6.3 depicts the number of new infections observed among the adult population (male and female combined) in Kenya when violence against sex workers is decreased from a prevalence of 32.4% to 18.4% and 2.4%, respectively, by 2016. There is an observed decrease in the number of new infections among the adult population for all three scenarios; this is likely attributable to the ongoing expansion of ART in the country. However, when violence is reduced to 18% by 2016, a cumulative 1% reduction in new infections between 2012 and 2016 is observed—equivalent to averting almost 4,700 new adult infections. Further reducing the prevalence of violence to 2% by 2016 results in almost 3% reduction in new infections among the adult population, when compared to the baseline scenario. In the context of a large number of people infected with HIV, this represents over 10,000 new infections averted between 2012 and 2016.

Figure 6.3   Trends in New Infections among the Adult Population in Kenya in the Context of Declining Prevalence of Violence against Female Sex Workers

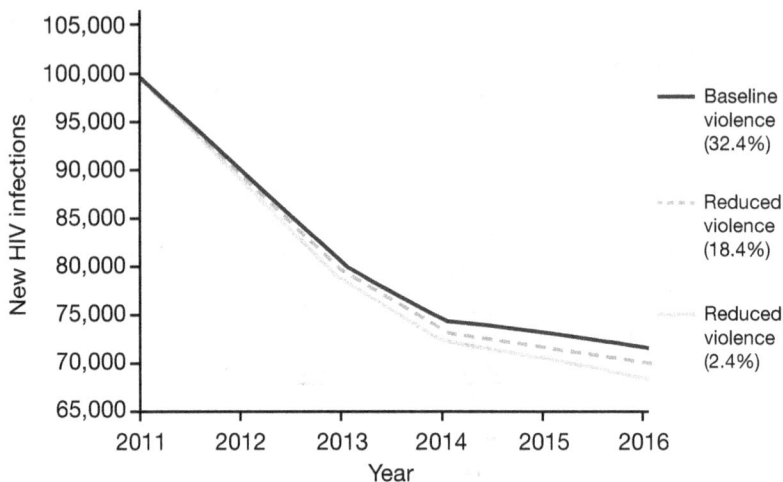

Source: Authors.

Ukraine

Table 6.5   New HIV Infections among Female Sex Workers in Ukraine: Observations When Violence Is Reduced

Year	Baseline violence (39%)	Reduced violence (25%)		Reduced violence (9%)	
		New infections	Infections averted	New infections	Infections averted
2011	3,866	3,866	–	3,866	–
2012	3,754	3,710	44	3,661	93
2013	3,650	3,564	86	3,465	185
2014	3,555	3,423	132	3,274	281
2015	3,458	3,282	176	3,082	376
2016	3,321	3,100	221	2,853	468
Cumulative (2012–16)	17,738	17,079	659	16,335	1,403
Reduction	(Ref.)		3.7%		7.9%

Source: Authors.
Note: Ref. = reference.

Table 6.5 and Figure 6.4 depict the number of new infections observed among sex workers in Ukraine when violence is decreased a prevalence of 39% among female sex workers to 25% and 9%, respectively, by 2016. There is an observed decrease in the number of new infections among sex workers for all three scenarios; this is likely attributable to the ongoing expansion of ART in the country. However, when violence is reduced to 25% by 2016, an approximate 4% reduction in new infections between 2012 and 2016 is observed. Further reducing the prevalence of violence to 9% by 2016 results in a total reduction in new infections among sex workers of almost 8%, or 1,400 new infections averted, when compared to the baseline scenario.

Figure 6.4   Trends in New HIV Infections among Female Sex Workers in the Context of Declining Prevalence of Violence in Ukraine

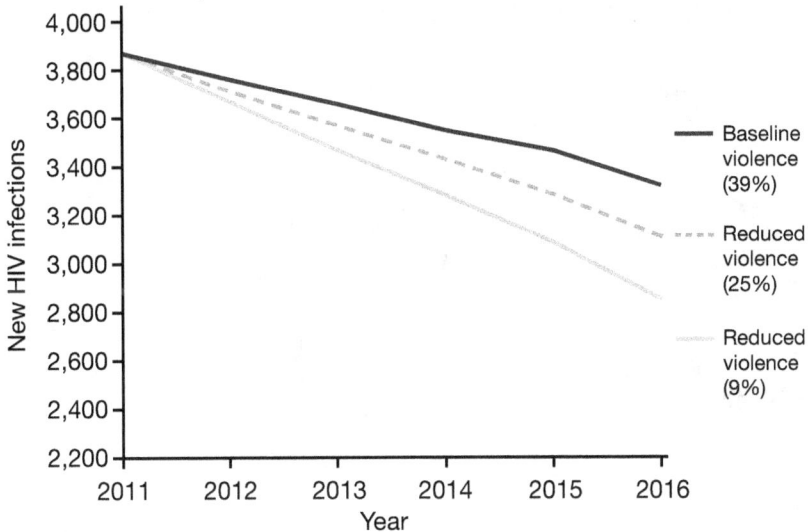

Source: Authors.

Table 6.6   HIV Prevalence among Female Sex Workers in Ukraine: Observations When Violence Is Reduced

Year	Baseline violence (39%)	Reduced violence (25%)		Reduced violence (9%)	
		Prevalence (%)	Percent reduction	Prevalence (%)	Percent reduction
2011	16.31	16.31	–	16.31	–
2012	16.21	16.17	0.25%	16.12	0.54%
2013	16.09	15.97	0.75%	15.83	1.60%
2014	15.97	15.74	1.45%	15.47	3.09%
2015	15.83	15.46	2.34%	15.05	4.98%
2016	15.66	15.13	3.38%	14.53	7.19%

Source: Authors.

Table 6.6 and Figure 6.5 depict the HIV prevalence observed among sex workers in Ukraine when violence against sex workers is decreased from a baseline prevalence of 39% to 25% and 9%, respectively, by 2016. ART expansion among the adult population continues to play a role in the declining prevalence, as evidenced by the projected prevalence of 15.7% among sex workers in 2016 in the baseline scenario. However, when violence is reduced to 25% by 2016, the prevalence of HIV among sex workers is projected to decline further. Further reducing the prevalence of violence to 9% by 2016 results in a lower HIV prevalence among sex workers, declining to 14.5% compared to 15.7% that is observed when violence continues at its current prevalence, for a projected 7.2% reduction in HIV prevalence among sex workers.

Figure 6.5   HIV Prevalence among Female Sex Workers in the Context of Declining Prevalence of Violence in Ukraine

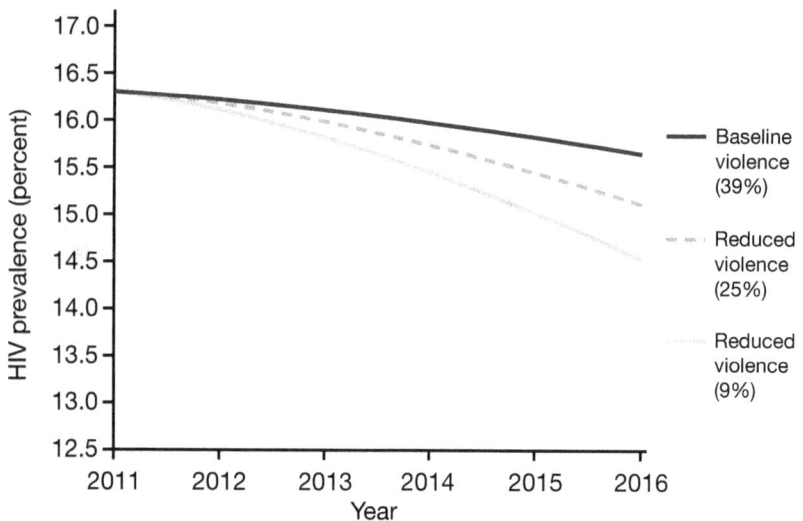

Source: Authors.

Table 6.7 and Figure 6.6 depict the number of new infections observed among the adult population (male and female combined) in Ukraine when violence is decreased from a baseline prevalence of 39% among female sex workers to 25% and 9%, respectively, by 2016. There is an observed decrease in the number of new infections among the adult population for all three scenarios; this is likely attributable to the ongoing expansion of ART in the country. However, when violence is reduced to 25% by 2016, a cumulative 2,100 infections among adults are averted; this is an approximate 1% reduction in new infections between 2012 and 2016. Further reducing the prevalence of violence to 9% by 2016 results in close to 2% reduction in new infections among the adult population, when compared to the baseline scenario. This represents approximately 4,400 new infections averted between 2012 and 2016.

Table 6.7   New HIV Infections among the Adult Population in Ukraine: Observations When Violence Is Reduced

Year	Baseline violence (39%)	Reduced violence (25%)		Reduced violence (5%)	
		New infections	Infections averted	New infections	Infections averted
2011	50,430	50,430	–	50,430	–
2012	49,609	49,484	125	49,341	268
2013	48,759	48,496	263	48,197	562
2014	47,869	47,461	408	47,001	868
2015	46,861	46,299	562	45,673	1,188
2016	45,150	44,434	716	43,643	1,507
Cumulative (2012–16)	238,248	236,174	2,074	233,855	4,393
Reduction	(Ref.)		0.9%		1.8%

Source: Authors.
Note: Ref. = reference

Figure 6.6   Trends in New Infections among Adult Population in Context of Declining Violence Against Sex Workers in Ukraine

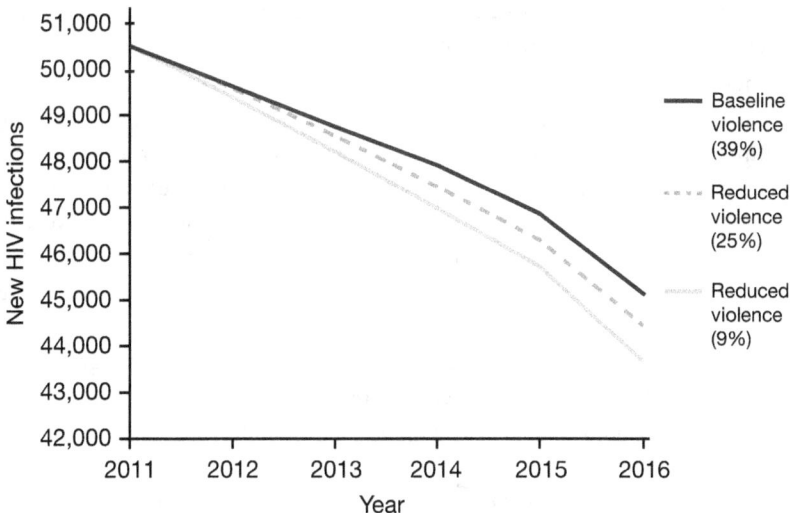

Source: Authors.

Discussion

Current findings from our modeling exercise, which depicts the gains that could be achieved were an intervention implemented and able to reduce violence to the levels evaluated, demonstrate that even in the context of expanding ART coverage, reducing violence against sex workers could achieve further declines in the HIV epidemics among both sex workers as well as adult populations. Despite differences in epidemic scenarios, and HIV prevalence among sex workers, similar patterns were observed in both Kenya and Ukraine. In Kenya, almost 5,400 (8%) HIV infections could be averted among female sex workers by reducing violence from 32.4% to 2.4% between 2012 and 2016. In Ukraine, a comparable reduction was achieved (8%), though the total number of infections averted was smaller (approximately 1,400), likely reflecting the overall lower population size and prevalence of HIV among sex workers in this setting. In both concentrated and generalized epidemics, and even where the prevalence of HIV is high among adults as in the case of Kenya, a significant number of infections are averted when violence against female sex workers is reduced.

While the cessation of violence against sex workers is a basic human right, such decreases in new infections are also of public health interest with respect to the health and well-being of a country's citizens as well as to the cost for treating new infections. This evidence highlights the impact of addressing social and structural factors in mitigating HIV, even in the context of expanding access to essential biomedical services including ART. Such interests are even more critical in low and middle income countries where programmatic resources may be limited.

These findings highlight the urgent need for interventions to prevent violence against sex workers and mitigate its impact on HIV. Existing community empowerment-based HIV prevention efforts for sex workers may serve as a useful infrastructure with which to implement anti-violence campaigns; evaluation results from a recent application of this approach in India suggest this may be a promising strategy in reducing violence (Beattie, Bhattacharjee et al. 2010). At the individual level, sex workers should be supported to discuss their experiences of violence in a safe space with counselors trained in a holistic trauma-informed approach that recognizes the multiple layers of stigma and discrimination that sex workers so often face. Evidence from other vulnerable populations demonstrates the benefits of disclosure of abuse and use of support services in buffering against self-blame and mental health consequences (Wasco, Campbell et al. 2004; Starzynski, Ullman et al. 2005; Ahrens, Stansell et al. 2010); disclosure of abuse can also enable police reporting (Ahrens, Stansell et al. 2010). Because the context of criminalization of sex work enables police and clients to perpetrate violence with impunity (Amnesty International 2006), decriminalization efforts should be explored for their potential to reduce violence. So too, police sensitization training may be a critical step in removing the demonstrated barriers faced by sex workers who have experienced violence in obtaining justice (ASWA, 2011). Finally, in addition to efforts to mitigate the immediate consequences of violence for those affected, interventions are urgently needed to modify both the abusive behavior of male perpetrators, and the climate of impunity that enables such abuse.

Our modeling results should be considered in light of several limitations. The chief limitation is that we do not model a specific intervention that is known to reduce HIV through reducing violence. The evidence clearly demonstrates associations of violence with HIV risk and infection and increasingly articulates the mechanisms underlying these patterns; consistent with the approach of the only prior investigation into the impact of reducing violence on HIV epidemics (Strathdee, Hallett et al. 2010), his modeling exercise suggests that reducing violence will reduce HIV through the mechanisms modeled. Because the causal pathways have not been confirmed, this exercise is hypothetical given the current evidence base. In addition, we do not have sufficient data to enable modeling of the historical impact of violence against sex workers on the historical HIV epidemic; thus results are limited to estimating future changes associated with reductions in violence. Therefore, these modeling exercises help to understand how violence affects the HIV epidemics in these current settings. Consistent with the Goals model, the impact of violence on HIV through condom non-use was investigated solely in reference to vaginal sex. Given the demonstrated links of violence with anal sex, (Beattie, Bhattacharjee et al. 2010; Decker, Wirtz et al. 2012) and the increased risk of HIV transmission related to anal sex (Boily, Baggaley et al. 2009; Baggaley, White et al. 2010) these findings likely represent an underestimate of the impact of violence on the HIV epidemics among female sex workers. Given the relative transmission efficiency of anal sex, estimated to be 16–18 times that observed for vaginal sex (Boily et al., 2009), inclusion of anal sex in subsequent violence-related modeling efforts is warranted to more comprehensively understand how violence impacts HIV epidemics.

These limitations in mind, our findings provide evidence that reductions in violence against sex workers confer significant benefits to this population in reducing the burden of HIV. Moreover, addressing violence as structural risk factor holds the potential to reduce HIV epidemics in broader adult populations. Current evidence bolsters recent calls to address gender-based violence (UNAIDS, 2009), and demonstrates the relevance of violence prevention as a component of international strategies to mitigate HIV. The development of violence prevention interventions is urgently needed to protect the health and human rights of sex workers and in doing so mitigate the global HIV epidemic.

References

Ahrens, C. E., J. Stansell, et al. (2010). "To tell or not to tell: the impact of disclosure on sexual assault survivors' recovery." *Violence and victims* 25 (5): 631–648.

Amnesty International (2006). *Nigeria: Rape- the Silent Weapon.* London.

Baggaley, R. F., R. G. White, et al. (2010). "HIV transmission risk through anal intercourse: systematic review, meta-analysis and implications for HIV prevention." *International Journal of Epidemiology* 39 (4): 1048–1063.

Beattie, T. S., P. Bhattacharjee, et al. (2010). "Violence against female sex workers in Karnataka state, south India: impact on health, and reductions in violence following an intervention program." *BMC Public Health* 10: 476.

Blankenship, K. M., R. Burroway, et al. (2010). "Factors associated with awareness and utilisation of a community mobilisation intervention for female sex workers in Andhra Pradesh, India." *Sexually Transmitted Infections* 86 Suppl 1: i69–75.

Boily, M. C., R. F. Baggaley, et al. (2009). "The role of heterosexual anal intercourse for HIV transmission in developing countries: are we ready to draw conclusions?" *Sexually Transmitted Infections* 85 (6): 408–410.

Chersich, M. F., S. M. Luchters, et al. (2007). "Heavy episodic drinking among Kenyan female sex workers is associated with unsafe sex, sexual violence and sexually transmitted infections." *International Journal of STD & AIDS* 18 (11): 764–769.

Choi, S. Y., K. L. Chen, et al. (2008). "Client-perpetuated violence and condom failure among female sex workers in southwestern China." *Sexually Transmitted Diseases* 35 (2): 141–146.

Cohan, D., A. Lutnick, et al. (2006). "Sex worker health: San Francisco style." *Sexually Transmitted Infections* 82 (5): 418–422.

Decker, M. R., H. L. McCauley, et al. (2010). "Violence victimisation, sexual risk and sexually transmitted infection symptoms among female sex workers in Thailand." *Sexually Transmitted Infections* 86 (3): 236–240.

Decker, M. R., G. R. Seage, 3rd, et al. (2009). "Intimate partner violence functions as both a risk marker and risk factor for women's HIV infection: findings from Indian husband-wife dyads." *Journal of Acquired Immune Deficiency Syndromes* 51 (5): 593–600.

Decker M.R., Wirtz, A. L., Baral S.D., Peryshkina A., Mogilnyi V., Weber R. A., Stachowiak J., Go, V., Beyrer C. (2012). Injection drug use, sexual risk, violence and STI/HIV among Moscow female sex workers. *Sexually Transmitted Infections.* 88 (4):278-83.

Draughton (2012). "Sexual assault injuries and increased risk for HIV transmission." *Advanced Emergency Nursing Journal* 34 (1): 82–87.

Kerrigan, D., P. Telles, et al. (2008). "Community development and HIV/STI-related vulnerability among female sex workers in Rio de Janeiro, Brazil." *Health Education Research* 23 (1): 137–145.

Reed, E., J. Gupta, et al. (2010). "The context of economic insecurity and its relation to violence and risk factors for HIV among female sex workers in Andhra Pradesh, India." *Public Health Reports* 125 Suppl 4: 81–89.

Rhodes, T., M. Simic, et al. (2008). "Police violence and sexual risk among female and transvestite sex workers in Serbia: qualitative study." *BMJ* (Clinical research ed.) 337: a811.

Sex Workers Rights Advocacy Network. (2009). *Arrest the Violence: Human rights abuses against sex workers in Central and Eastern Europe and Central Asia.*

Simic, M. and T. Rhodes (2009). "Violence, dignity and HIV vulnerability: street sex work in Serbia." *Sociology of Health & Illness* 31 (1): 1–16.

Stachowiak, J. A., S. Sherman, et al. (2005). "Health risks and power among female sex workers in Moscow." *SEICUS Report* 22 (2): 18–26.

Starzynski, L. L., S. E. Ullman, et al. (2005). "Correlates of women's sexual assault disclosure to informal and formal support sources." *Violence and Victims* 20 (4): 417–432.

Strathdee, S. A., T. B. Hallett, et al. (2010). "HIV and risk environment for injecting drug users: the past, present, and future." *The Lancet* 376 (9737): 268–284.

Stulhofer, A., D. Lausevic, et al. (2010). "HIV risks among female sex workers in Croatia and Montenegro." *Collegium Antropologicum* 34 (3): 881–886.

Surratt, H., S. Kurtz, et al. (2005). "The connections of mental health problems, violent life experiences, and the social milieu of the "stroll" with the HIV risk behaviors of female street sex workers." *Journal of Psychology and Human Sexuality* 17 (1–2): 23–44.

Swain, S., et al (2011). "Experience of violence and adverse reproductive health outcomes, HIV risks among mobile female sex workers in India." *BMC Public Health* 11 (357).

Ulibarri, M. D., S. A. Strathdee, et al. (2011). "Injection drug use as a mediator between client-perpetrated abuse and HIV status among female sex workers in two Mexico-U.S. border cities." *AIDS Behavior* 12 (1): 179–185.

Wasco, S. M., R. Campbell, et al. (2004). "A statewide evaluation of services provided to rape survivors." *Journal of Interpersonal Violence* 19 (2): 252–263.

CHAPTER 7

Sex Worker Leadership in Responding to HIV and Promoting Human Rights

Introduction

Key Themes

- Sex worker leadership has played an integral role in community empowerment-based responses to HIV prevention and human rights.
- The nature and role of sex worker participation in the response to HIV has varied across socio-political and geographic settings.
- Where sex worker rights organizations have partnered effectively with governmental actors, the response to HIV among sex workers has been particularly effective and sustainable.
- Support for sex worker rights organizations in critical to a sustained and effective response to HIV and the promotion of sex worker's rights and health.

In the earliest phases of the HIV epidemic, governments and sex workers themselves were forced to examine policies and programs that affect sex workers in sectors ranging from health to policy and criminal justice. Reviewing early responses that successfully addressed HIV among sex workers can inform the development and adaptation of future national responses. The past three decades of research on HIV among sex workers overwhelmingly confirms structural influences on HIV risk. Thus, reviewing successful early responses to HIV among sex workers is most informative in the context of considering the complex legal, policy, social, economic, and ideological backdrop to sex work, which has far-reaching implications for HIV risk. For example, stigmatizing, discriminatory climates discourage sex workers from participation in HIV prevention activities, and obtaining necessary STI and HIV testing and treatment (Whitaker, Ryan et al. 2011; Lazarus, Deering et al. 2012). Where sex workers are socially excluded and ostracized, clients and others can easily exploit their marginalized status, abuse against them is enabled, and they have minimal leverage with which to ensure successful condom negotiation. Internalized stigma and overt discrimination can impart significant limitations on sex workers ability to engage with HIV prevention services (Kerrigan, Telles et al. 2008; Blankenship, Burroway et al. 2010).

Stigma and discrimination are perpetuated by the criminalization, penalisation and other legal oppression of sex work(Ahmed, Kaplan et al. 2011) that prevails in most settings. The centrality of human rights, including non-discrimination and respect for vulnerable populations, to the HIV response targeting sex workers and other most at risk populations has been confirmed by the Joint United Nations Programme on AIDS (UNAIDS 2009). Yet thirty years into the HIV epidemic, the majority of countries' policies are largely informed on ideological terms. Even while establishing HIV prevention programs targeting sex workers, many counties retain policies that view sex work solely as a criminal offense, with 116 countries and territories criminalizing some aspect of sex work. Sex workers are arrested under national and local laws that directly prohibits sex work and related activities such as solicitation, sex exchange, and management of sex workers(Gabel 2007), as well as indirect policies including public disturbance, loitering, vagrancy, residency permits, and tax laws(Gabel 2007; OSI 2007). When condoms are used as evidence of sex work and grounds for arrest, fines, and detention, criminalization deters sex workers from carrying and using condoms, thus increasing HIV-related vulnerability.

Criminalization enables police to perpetrate abuse and humiliation, demand free sexual services, and extort fines from sex workers with impunity, and renders those who suffer violence and other human rights abuses with little legal recourse (Stachowiak, Sherman et al. 2005; Sex Workers Rights Advocacy 2009). Confirming the HIV implications of criminalization is evidence that police interference in the forms of arrest, bribes, demands for sex to avoid trouble, and taking condoms away is linked with STI symptoms (Erausquin, Reed et al. 2011). To avoid detection, sex workers may shift venues to locations in which they are more isolated and vulnerable (Shannon, Strathdee et al. 2009); evidence demonstrates that doing so can incur HIV risks such as pressure for unprotected sex(Shannon, Strathdee et al. 2009; Simic and Rhodes 2009). By driving sex work underground, criminalization is also counterproductive to community mobilization efforts to strengthen sex workers rights and promote autonomy.

Against the backdrop of the criminalization and stigmatization, sex workers suffer alarmingly high levels of physical and sexual violence at the hands of clients, police, and other actors (AIDS 2005; Chersich, Luchters et al. 2007; Choi, Chen et al. 2008; Institute 2009; Beattie, Bhattacharjee et al. 2010; Decker, McCauley et al. 2010; Go, Srikrishnan et al. 2011). These abuses constitute a significant threat to the health, human rights and well-being of sex workers. Abuse against sex workers imparts clear HIV risk (AIDS 2005), with evidence linking violence with condom non-use (Beattie, Bhattacharjee et al. 2010; Swain 2011) condom breakage (Rhodes, Simic et al. 2008; Beattie, Bhattacharjee et al. 2010), condom failure (Choi, Chen et al. 2008; Decker, McCauley et al. 2010), STI symptoms (Decker, McCauley et al. 2010) and infection (Beattie, Bhattacharjee et al. 2010; Decker, Wirtz, et al. 2012) as well as HIV infection (Ulibarri, Strathdee et al. 2011). Qualitative evidence confirms that manipulation and force are often responsible for unprotected sex; moreover recent evidence demonstrates that violence against sex workers is not limited to vaginal rape but indeed also includes anal rape (Panchanadeswaran, Johnson et al. 2008; Simic and Rhodes 2009) which confers a significantly greater risk for HIV transmission.

Taken together, these data illustrate the role of structural factors in compromising condom use and posing formidable barriers to accessing testing and treatment as well as other HIV prevention activities for sex workers. In recognition that broader social vulnerabilities can stymie HIV prevention, UNAIDS highlights and prioritizes interventions which address environmental-structural issues related to sex work and HIV prevention, in addition to ensuring universal access to comprehensive HIV prevention, treatment care and support (UNAIDS 2009).

Female sex workers continue to be burdened with HIV, with particularly large and growing epidemics in southern Africa (see Chapter 2, Epidemiology of HIV among Sex Workers. Lessons from the first twenty years of responses from the governmental and nongovernmental sectors could be useful in future interventions. To inform the development and adaptation of interventions to reduce HIV among sex workers that address structural issues influencing their risk, we review early sex worker oriented HIV prevention responses. Responses have varied greatly across countries, as have the roles of both governmental and nongovernmental actors in framing and implementing HIV prevention, treatment and care among sex workers. Responses have also varied in their ability to address underlying structural factors associated with HIV-related risk for sex workers, and ability to catalyze changes within the broader social context against which sex work and HIV risk occurs. Examples include government sponsored interventions focused on enforcing safe sex policies at brothels in the case of Thailand (Rojanapithayakorn and Hanenberg 1996) to those that empower sex workers and are led by the sex worker community such as the Sonagachi project in India (Jana, Basu et al. 2004). In numerous contexts, the role of sex worker led initiatives and civil society organizations have been essential in ensuring HIV prevention policies and programs are implemented that respect and promote the health and human rights of sex workers, largely through community empowerment-based efforts (Kerrigan, Moreno et al. 2006; Blankenship, West et al. 2008; Kerrigan, Telles et al. 2008; Reza-Paul, Beattie et al. 2008; Beattie, Bhattacharjee et al. 2010; Argento, Reza-Paul et al. 2011). Responses to HIV among sex workers can be grouped on a continuum of being almost exclusively put forth by governmental institutions using a top down approach to those that are predominantly sex worker or grass-roots initiated or rely heavily on sex worker participation. Using such a framing, Thailand and Brazil constitute examples at opposite ends of this continuum whereas Thailand's response was initiated and managed by the government with little sex worker participation, as opposed to Brazil which has been characterized by a powerful civil society response to HIV in which sex workers have historically been integrally involved in the response to HIV and treated as partners.

In this chapter, we describe a variation in responses to HIV among sex workers in three countries: Thailand, India, and Brazil. We review the nature of responses across contexts with particular attention to the level and nature of sex worker participation, types of relationships between governmental and civil society organizations, and successes and challenges in modifying the structural context surrounding HIV-related risk in the context of sex work including legal, political and social aspects of these responses, successes and challenges. Findings from these comparative country case studies indicate that sex worker leadership is critical to ensuring that social and structural factors affecting their health, human rights and well-being are understood and addressed and in generating and sustaining effective responses to HIV.

Review of National Responses

Thailand: A Government-led Response

Thailand's federal response to HIV is often touted as one of the best examples from numerous HIV prevention organizations. Its most well-known intervention strategy was the 100% condom program, which aimed to provide sufficient condoms coupled with policies to guarantee condom use among female sex workers and their clients. This campaign was launched simultaneously with widespread HIV education for the broader population.

The nuances of sex work-related legislation in Thailand may have enabled the development of the 100% condom program as an environmental intervention. The Prostitution Prevention and Suppression Act of 1996 creates offences for soliciting in public, pimping, advertising, managing sex work businesses or establishments, (Keo 2009) and associating with others for the purpose of prostitution. However the Act does not criminalize provision of premises for sex work, which may have enabled the 100% condom program to focus on venues. Given that legal protection for sex work is effectively limited to venue-based sex workers, those involved in street-based sex work, which often includes migrant sex workers, are even more heavily targeted by the police.

The "100% Condom Campaign", the Government's chief means of HIV prevention for female sex workers, unfortunately lacked meaningful input from sex workers. It was launched in the context of a looming HIV crisis after a 1989 sentinel survey suggested an extremely rapid increase in HIV among female sex workers (Ungchusak et al., 1989). The provincial government of Ratchaburi province instituted the 100% Condom Program, which mandated that sex work establishments require condom use in every sex act. The program's initial success in significantly increasing condom use and decreasing STIs attracted other provinces to implement the program. Ultimately, the national AIDS Committee, chaired by the prime minister, issued a resolution to implement the 100% Condom Campaign nationally (Unaids 2000) and by mid 1992, it was running in all provinces in Thailand, managed by local health authorities.

The program was implemented primarily through Government means, and was aimed at the commercial sex venues so as to mandate condom use. Unfortunately this approach bypassed the organizations that were already working with sex workers on issues of sexually transmitted infections and other health issues prior to the HIV epidemic. Rather, the government relied on public health officials and sex establishment owners to ensure the enforcement of the policy.

Against the backdrop of a national program that focused on condom distribution, HIV/STI testing and STI treatment, the 100% Condom Campaign entailed the distribution of approximately 60 million condoms a year free of charge, primarily to sex establishments, by the Ministry of Public Health. Mandated by the federal government, the program was implemented through municipal health structures at the provincial level. To ensure brothels enforcement of condom use, men attending STI clinics were routinely asked which brothels they visited. Brothels that were the source of repeated STIs could be fined or closed by the police (Mgbako 2008). After the program was implemented in 1992, rapid increases in condom use were observed among sex workers from 50% to 90% and upwards, with a noticeable impact on the number of new infections (Chandeying 2005).

Although Thailand successfully mitigated its HIV epidemic, there were significant unintended consequences particularly for the 100% Condom Program. Sex workers themselves were engaged neither in the conceptualization nor in the implementation of the program, which ultimately created conditions for sex workers that were considered at best coercive and in many cases abusive. The program's approach shifted power from clients, but it did not transfer that power to sex workers themselves. Rather, actors in positions of authority such as police and venue managers, who so often exploit the control they have over sex workers, found themselves with even more power to wield over sex workers. By bestowing additional authority to police and venue owners, the policy created a situation of severe human rights violations for sex workers (Loff, Overs et al. 2003). The lack of engagement of sex workers perpetuated stigma against sex workers that enabled sustained human rights violations. Further, the campaign's reliance on venue managers to implement the policy was considered evidence that sex work was not a legitimate occupation, and one fraught with disease; these attitudes reinforced stigmatization with significant harm to sex workers as a result (Center for Advocacy on and Marginalization 2008). This lack of sex worker engagement compromised the program's reach and impact as well; by not involving sex workers in the design of the program, the campaign was limited in its ability to reach those not working in designated venues who are often at even greater HIV risk.

Other issues arose as well. Despite and perhaps because of the rapid accomplishments of the program, sustainability issues surfaced as treatment was increasingly prioritized at the cost of prevention (Treerutkuarkul 2010). While the brothels that it sought to modify were the primary venues for sex work at the time, sex work over time has shifted to a broader range of venues in which the policy may not apply as directly (Hanenberg and Rojanapithayakorn 1998). Unfortunately, migrant sex workers and street-based sex workers were not targeted; as result, the gains in condom use were not as tremendous among indirect sex workers, i.e., those working outside of brothel venues (Mills, Benjarattanaporn et al. 1997). Moreover, being an environmental intervention that relied primarily on venue managers for enforcement, it did not create necessary sustainable changes in advancing the social and legal status of sex workers. To the contrary, it exacerbated impressions among potential clients and the general public that sex workers are vectors of disease. Evidence that sex workers in Thailand continue to suffer violence, discrimination and other forms of injustice (Ratinthorn, Meleis et al., 2009) and continued evidence from Thailand of client condom resistance and refusal (Decker, McCauley et al. 2010), suggests that the program did not significantly modify the underlying power dynamics for sex workers and their clients in condom negotiations. These data are illustrative of the need for further structural changes to advance the human rights of sex workers. Finally, despite the success of the program in increasing condom use, HIV was found to persist among sex workers, including those in brothels as well as those who began sex work following the implementation of the program (Kilmarx, Limpakarnjanarat et al. 1998; Kilmarx, Palanuvej et al. 1999), illustrating the challenges in ensuring consistency of the program as well as sustainability of the intervention over time.

Despite the structural change approach of the Thai Government, the program suffered significantly from its lack of meaningful engagement with the sex worker community, and created conditions that perpetuated harm. Overall, integration of, and collaboration with, sex workers could have resulted in an empowerment based approach to the 100% Condom Program. Such engagement could have achieved similar goals but through means that did not compromise the human rights of sex workers, but rather bolstered them. Collaboration with the organizations working with sex workers at the time could have also generated ways of enhancing program sustainability as well as reaching and engaging sex workers in venues other than brothels. Today, while HIV prevalence among establishments based sex workers is now less than 3 percent in Thailand (Committee. 2010), recent evidence suggests that some 18–30% of non-venue based sex workers are infected (Akarasewi 2010; Shah, Shiraishi et al. 2011).

India: Government-led Infrastructure Coupled with Sex Worker Mobilization

India's government achieved significant advances in HIV prevention and intervention infrastructure over the past two decades, with extensive prevention and surveillance efforts throughout the country. The HIV prevalence for sex workers has decreased from 10% in 2003 to 5.1% in 2007.(NACO 2007), however, significant regional variation exists with higher prevalences in Maharashtra (17.9%); Andhra Pradesh (9.7%); Nagaland (8.9%); Mizoram (7.2%); Gujarat (6.5%); West Bengal (5.9%); and Karnataka (5.3%) (2008).

While the government's response was far-reaching and multifaceted, India's HIV response to sex workers is best known for sex worker initiated efforts—the most famous of which is the Sonagachi project. Sonagachi is an occupational health-informed intervention that quickly became a catalyst for sex worker participation and collective mobilization.

The legal environment for sex workers in India is informed by a number of laws, primary of which is the Immoral Traffic and Prevention Act (IPTA). In India, sex work is not explicitly illegal, but sex workers and others who profit from sex work such as brothel owners are restricted under the IPTA, which was first enacted in 1956 as the "Suppression of Immoral Traffic Act." IPTA is the main statue addressing the criminalization of activities related to sex work and is based on the principle that sex work is exploitation and is incompatible with the dignity and self determination of those who engage in sex work (Jayasree 2004). Although IPTA focuses on trafficked women, the law is broadly applied to arrest sex workers for soliciting, rather than its charge to focus on traffickers. Technically sex workers are guaranteed human rights under the Constitution of India, though there has been limited interpretation of such rights to meaningfully improve the health and wellbeing of sex workers.

The Indian government has enacted an extensive response to HIV that targeted the general population with education, surveillance and STI/HIV testing as well as efforts specific for sex workers and other marginalized groups. The success of this response is questioned given the continued rise of HIV over the past two decades (2008). In addition to the government's efforts, a number of community-initiated responses were conducted by community-based and sex worker NGOs, the most comprehensive of which is the Sonagachi project in Kolkata. Sonagachi in effect represents a landmark example of sex work organizing and empowerment for HIV risk reduction. Sonagachi quickly gained international recognition with reports on the project emerging as early as 1993 (1993); the combination of its efficacy and international publicity enabled it to inspire similar efforts in a range of settings (Kerrigan, Moreno et al. 2006; Kerrigan, Telles et al. 2008; Reza-Paul, Beattie et al. 2008).

Government Response. The government response to HIV followed closely on the heels of the first documented cases of HIV in India in a study of female sex workers in in1986 in the city of Chennai (Simoes, Babu et al. 1987). In 1987, the government established the National AIDS Control Program (NACP) that was charged with the coordination of the national response through establishing monitoring and prevention programs including a national surveillance system, blood screening, and health education programs. During the 1990s, the Government's response was characterized by a "top down" approach with the establishment of several centralized bodies at the federal and then provincial level to build the communication, surveillance and testing and treatment infrastructure to respond to HIV.

Over time, the National AIDS Control Organization (2008), founded in 1992, expanded its surveillance system to include sex workers and other marginalized groups (Chandrasekaran 2006). The response to sex workers was heavily focused on educational campaigns and improving access to treatment, with NGOs implementing over 1,000 targeted interventions focused on high-risk populations. Although NGOs were an essential partner in implementing government funded programs, they were not involved in the development of the government's agenda.

Sex Worker Initiated Responses. Sex worker community-led interventions among female sex workers have been successful in providing this environment by addressing issues such as lack of prevention information, access to condoms, and negotiating with brokers such as brothel owners (Basu, Jana et al. 2004). For example, Sangram is an NGO based in the Sangli district, and works to further sex workers' human rights through advocacy and programming, including a sex worker initiated collective, VAMP, that has been conducting peer interventions for the past 15 years (http://www.sangram.org).

The best known HIV prevention effort in India, the Sonagachi project, was not generated by the Government, rather, it was generated by and for sex workers in 1992. Sonagachi has come to represent an innovative and powerful empowerment model for HIV risk reduction, with demonstrated success in increasing condom use and reducing STI (Basu, Jana et al. 2004; Gangopadhyay, Chanda et al. 2005). Based in Kolkata, this multi-faceted intervention began in 1992 and sought to enact sweeping changes at the community (e.g., lack of access to healthcare) and individual (e.g., skills and competencies for condom use and negotiation) levels with components including peer education for condom promotion. Notably, the Sonagachi Project is rooted in an occupation health approach, with the philosophy that HIV is an occupational health hazard and sex workers should have the right to work in nonthreatening environments. The collectivization and community organization components of the Sonagachi model evolved over time to ensure sustainability of the HIV prevention initiative, which was originally focused on more traditional HIV/STI education and clinical services (Jana, Basu et al. 2004).

The Durbar Mahila Samanwaya Committee (DMSC) was a direct outgrowth of the Sonagachi Project; in the third year of the Sonagachi Project, DMSC took over the intervention effort so as to have a fuller voice in the direction and nature of HIV prevention efforts. Today DMSC represents over 65,000 sex workers, and continues to take a labor rights approach in its advocacy to challenge factors that perpetuate stigma and social exclusion of sex workers. The intervention has demonstrated success in core HIV risk reduction outcomes at the individual level including significant increases condom use and decreased STIs; moreover it modified the broader environment in which sex work occurs with demonstrated improvements in sex workers' abilities to refuse clients and change the terms of their contracts (Swendeman, Basu et al. 2009). The structure also provided a means of identifying and addressing other social, economic and legal issues for sex workers, such as the establishment of a banking system to overcome a lengthy and complex bank account registration process that prevailed at the time and presented formidable barriers for sex workers (Evans, Jana et al. 2010).

Several features of the social and political climate of India and Kolkata in particular likely facilitated the development of this grass-roots, sex worker empowerment culture, even while the government carried out the federal HIV response. India as a whole has a rich tradition of civil activism, and Kolkata in particular is characterized by a strong spirit of collective action and mobilization to advance social goals, including ensuring labor rights for those most vulnerable to exploitation. The collective action approach of DMSC, and its goals of advancing the social and economic context for sex workers is considered to reflect the Socialist political influences and values that prevailed in the region at time and persist today (Ray 1998; Ghose, Swendeman et al. 2008).

The goals and successes of the government and grass-roots responses to HIV for sex workers in India are largely complementary, with the Sonagachi project raising awareness of labor rights for sex workers, creating changes in the working environment, and expanding condom use and HIV prevention knowledge while the government-led response included essential components including communicating HIV information, initiating surveillance systems, and scaling up testing and treatment facilities. That the DMSC quickly grew in size, capacity and impact speaks highly to the value in promoting structures for sex workers to organize with which to identify and act on their shared priorities. This collective mobilization modified the dynamics that would otherwise leave sex workers with little power relative to clients, brothel owners, managers, and others. When compared with the standard HIV risk reduction programs of NACO in recent evaluation exercises, both Sonagachi and NACO programs were found to have reduced STIs, however, the Sonagachi project additionally increased STI and HIV testing behaviors (Gangopadhyay, Chanda et al. 2005), illustrating the added value of sex worker participation and community mobilization in empowering sex workers for self protection.

Perhaps the greatest testament to the success of Sonagachi and its relevance and innovation as an empowerment-based, community-based approach is that it inspired a wide-spread response throughout India by the Bill and Melinda Gates Foundation—the Avahan India AIDS Initiative. Avahan was implemented in 2005 and partners with 134 NGOs throughout India, focusing on the six high-prevalence states, with the aim of reaching over 200,000 sex workers as well as men who have sex with men, injecting drug users, and other high-risk men through HIV prevention. The influence of Sonagachi can be felt in Avahan's grass-roots approach, focused on community ownership and extensive collaboration with community-based NGOs (Laga, Galavotti et al. 2010).

The examples of Sonagachi and the Avahan initiatives that follow illustrate that stigma and discrimination against sex workers can be overcome, and underlying power structures modified. For example in one recent structural intervention, willingness to be identified in public as a sex worker was significantly associated with greater participation in program activities (Blankenship, Biradavolu et al. 2010). This suggests that structural changes to overcome stigma and discrimination against sex workers can enable participation in HIV prevention efforts.

Simultaneously, they illustrate that the social context is not yet sufficient to enable all sex workers to comfortably come forward with their experiences. On a similar note, even in the context of community mobilization and efforts to reduce stigma, sex worker relationships with police remain tenuous. Recent evidence from Andhra Pradesh of sex workers having sex with and providing gifts or bribes to police (11% and 12% respectively) confirm that power dynamics still favor police. Even more concerning is the 7% of participants who report police taking condoms away (Erausquin, Reed et al. 2011), to the clear detriment of HIV prevention. Finally, the success of structural interventions in India appears to have inspired HIV prevention efforts that include tackling gender-based violence against sex workers. Evaluation results are promising (Beattie, Bhattacharjee et al. 2010) and suggest the capacity of structural interventions in modifying violence as a component of the broader risk environment to sex workers.

Brazil: Historical partnership between sex workers and government

The case of Brazil represents a unique example with respect to its broad, civil society based approach to the HIV epidemic and the role of sex workers therein that is closely tied to the historical period within which the epidemic emerged. In the 1980s, the country was passing through a redemocratization process after two decades of military dictatorship. The National AIDS Program was established alongside the country's universal health care system in the late 1980s, and from very early in the Program's existence, representatives of vulnerable population groups, including from the recently formed Brazilian Network of Prostitutes, were invited to participate in designing prevention actions for their peers. It exemplifies a grass-roots approach that has successfully partnered with government officials to have a profound impact on policy and thus contribute to altering the broader structure within which sex workers live and work. For example, in 2002, they successfully advocated for the inclusion of "sex work" as an official occupation in the Brazilian Occupation Classification of the Ministry of Labor, thus entitling individual sex workers to social security and other work benefits. The Network is currently advocating for the repeal of such laws that prevent many sex workers from accessing their full labor rights and has kept combating police violence and abuse at the top of their agenda (Davida 2010). Taken together, Brazil's approach of promoting the human and labor rights of sex workers is considered a key element in containing the HIV epidemic; with HIV peaking among female sex workers in the late 1990s but not rising above 20%. Today, the most recent national prevalence among female sex workers is estimated at approximately 4.8%, drawn from a study of sex workers in 10 Brazilian cities (Szwarcwald, Souza Junior et al. 2011)

The strong activism on the part of sex workers in Brazil and its impact on national policy has garnered international recognition; the most notable example of which is Brazil's denouncement of USAID funds for HIV prevention when USAID stipulated that recipient organizations have a policy explicitly opposing prostitution. The Brazilian government worked in partnership with the Brazilian Network of Prostitutes, Brazil was the only country to refuse to sign what came to be known as the 'anti-prostitution pledge' in contractual agreements, in doing so they rejected over $40 million dollars of funding for HIV prevention (Hinchberger 2005; Leite 2010). This was motivated not only to preserve their own prevention agenda, but in recognition hat an anti-prostitution approach could significantly undermine the meaningful participation of sex workers. While this action compromised prevention activities in that it limited the total amount of financial resources available for reaching sex workers, the Brazilian government funded the continuation of the planned prevention actions and established its clear autonomy in setting their own HIV prevention agenda for one of the country's most vulnerable population groups, sex workers.

Studies conducted in Brazil have confirmed the value of a community based, participatory approach to HIV prevention among sex workers. In the Ministry of Health's 2004 evaluation of eight peer education and community building intervention projects with sex workers, significant differences in consistent condom use with clients were observed between women participating in the interventions and those in the control group who were not exposed to any intervention (Health 2004). Impact data from a multi-level intervention and cohort study called, *Encontros,* that combined a social mobilization component that included community-building activities with peer education and improved clinical care found reduced odds of incident STI among sex workers actively participating in community mobilization intervention activities as opposed to those who did not (Lippman, Chinaglia et al. 2012). The cohort study followed 420 male, female, and *travesti* sex workers and also documented greater odds of reporting consistent condom use with regular clients among sex workers actively engaged in the community mobilization component of the intervention. The *Encontros* project was run out of a local STI and HIV testing and treatment center and provides an important model of a project implemented in partnership between the sex worker movement, local and international NGOs, and municipal, state, and national government STI/ HIV prevention programs.

Engagement with government offices is one of the hallmarks of the success of the civil society mobilization of sex workers; this advocacy is heavily focused on expanding labor rights and reducing stigma by seeking partnerships with institutions that are not exclusively focused on HIV, such as the Ministry of Labor and the Ministry of Culture. The powerful combination of governmental and civil society responses to sex workers catalyzed sweeping structural changes for sex workers. In more recent years, challenges, including those related to sustaining this collaboration, have begun to emerge. Contextual changes on a global and national level including the decentralization of Brazil's universal health system, the restructuring of the National AIDS Program as a Department of the Ministry of Health, decreased donor support to AIDS and sexuality related work in Brazil, and an increase in discourses with more conservative attitudes towards sex work are perceived by some in the country as negatively affecting the number and scope of projects funded with sex worker organizations that adopt a human and labor rights approach. The quality of prevention and care services continue to major concerns, as highlighted by the continued presence of stigma and discrimination as a major barrier to sex worker access to health services (Pimenta 2009). Stigma and socio-economic pressures have also been found to limit participation in community development activities (Kerrigan, Telles et al. 2008), and in an evaluation of the most recent national level project with the Brazilian Network of Prostitutes, low organizational technical capacity and a lack of sustainability of actions remained key concerns of participating NGOs at the end of project implementation (Camara 2008). Violence against sex workers persists with approximately 15% reporting abuse in the past four months (Kerrigan,

Telles et al. 2008), even in this climate of social advances and reductions in stigma. Police violence towards sex workers continues to be a major concern of the sex workers movement and commercial activities associated with prostitution (such as owning a brothel or pimping) remain illegal. Thus, as external pressures and larger structural changes have affected the organization and activism of both the NGOs and government HIV prevention actions, sex worker activists and government officials are increasingly redefining their strategies in an effort to continue to strengthen the human and labor rights approach to HIV prevention with sex workers that initially earned Brazil international recognition.

Discussion

These case studies illustrate a range of structural changes achieved and sustainability of responses based on the parties most responsible for developing and implementing HIV risk reduction efforts for sex workers. We synthesize these differences, and compare and contrast the nature of intervention targets, sustainability of responses, and level of structural change achieved based on the parties involved, and describe themes with regard to the legal, political and social backdrops to these responses. Overall, findings illustrate that sex worker leadership is critical both to creating the structural changes necessary for HIV prevention, including promotion of health, human rights and well-being, and in ensuring sustainability. Findings hold significant global relevance. As the HIV epidemic enters its third decade, and as evidence confirms the unique HIV burden of sex workers worldwide, efforts to reduce HIV risk and promote testing and treatment for sex workers remain a global priority. Achieving these goals requires continued attention to structural issues for sex workers; critical review of lessons learned in early HIV responses for sex workers serves as a powerful tool for the next generation of approaches which seek to sustain high levels of knowledge, continue to promote condom use, and ensure access to HIV testing and treatment as means to stem the continued spread of HIV.

The nature of response to HIV among sex workers appears to reflect the priorities and knowledge of the parties involved; in turn this imparts differences in the level of structural change achieved. Where sex workers are involved in shaping the HIV response, as in the cases of Brazil and Sonagachi in India, responses are comprehensive and include addressing underlying social and structural factors associated with sex workers vulnerability to HIV, and providing other health and support services to sex workers. In contrast, Thailand's approach, characterized by its predominant governmental origins, prioritized condom use as the primary focus. While it took a structural approach, it created dangerous conditions by granting further power to authority figures such as police and venue managers, with sex workers suffering exacerbated human rights violations as a result. Greater sex worker involvement in the campaign's approach could have generated a more appropriate approach that imparted the additional structural changes necessary, e.g., reducing stigma, for a comprehensive and sustained impact. In Brazil, the partnership between a new government and a prominent sex worker organization, whose mission extended far beyond that of addressing HIV among sex workers, catalyzed a response that explicitly sought social and economic rights for sex workers. Their collaboration generated policy changes at the national level, with significant reductions in stigma and enhancements to sex workers' labor rights. This broad focus is considered responsible for reductions in HIV risk associated with sex work. The case of Sonagachi represents perhaps the strongest example of role sex workers can serve once a structure is established for their participation. The intervention's initial focus was that of occupational health and safety; the broader structural changes in areas of economic and political power for sex workers, including additional intervention components such as the banking cooperative that were ultimately achieved are described as byproducts of the intervention process (Jana et al., 2004). The involvement of sex workers in this case enabled far greater structural changes than were initially envisioned. While the Brazil case illustrates the policy level change that can be achieved through sex worker and government partnership, Sonagachi illustrates the power of creating mechanisms by which sex workers can refine and expand interventions to meet the needs that individuals external to the sex work community may not readily understand.

The extent of structural change achieved through each of these responses also varies significantly based on the balance of actors involved. Thailand's early, proactive and structural response was initiated and implemented by the federal and provincial governments. While the response was a collaborative effort between several governmental sectors including public health, police, and municipal leaders that relied on national participation, it was not characterized by sex worker involvement nor was there significant sex worker initiated responses early in the Thai HIV epidemic. The intervention's environmental focus was neither designed to nor did generate sustainable structural changes beyond the context of sex work venues. Rather, it propagated the notion of sex workers as "vectors of disease" and as a result may have actually perpetuated stigma and discrimination that impede sex workers' ability to advocate for their rights (Center for Advocacy on and Marginalization 2008). In contrast, Brazil's unique case of long-standing partnership between government and sex worker networks garnered arguable the most thorough level of structural change. Brazil's case is one in which the empowerment, collectivization approach is effectively scaled up and expanded at a national level. The national policy changes it achieved were an explicit goal of this partnership, and simultaneously reduced stigma against sex workers and enhanced their labor rights. India's Sonagachi model achieved significant structural changes for Kolkata; while the model was replicated elsewhere in India (Blankenship, West et al. 2008; Argento, Reza-Paul et al. 2011), it did not generate the type of national mobilization and governmental partnership witnessed in Brazil. This contrast likely reflects the disparate goals of the initiatives; while in the case of Brazil, sex workers and policy makers joined forces for national policy change on the heels of a new government, in contrast, the economic and political power generated by the Sonagachi project are described as outgrowths of the project rather than primary objectives (Jana, Basu et al. 2004).

Significant differences are also observed in the sustainability of responses, again reflecting the level of sex worker participation. In Thailand, significant shifts in sex work away from brothels towards other types of venues were noted in the years following the implementation of the program (Hanenberg and Rojanapithayakorn 1998; Kilmarx, Limpakarnjanarat et al. 1998). Greater integration of, and collaboration with, sex workers may have generated ways of enhancing program sustainability particularly in response to the evolution of sex work in Thailand. Integration of sex workers may have also resulted in a policy approach that did not run the risk of exacerbating human rights violations for sex workers. A more collaborative approach would likely have also sought to generate a more sustainable environment within which to promote condom use via addressing the underlying social and structural factors associated with sex workers vulnerability.

In contrast, India has witnessed the gradual intertwining of a governmental approach with a sex worker empowerment model that enhances both sustainability and structural change. Sonagachi's success motivated the Gates Foundation to scale up the empowerment-based, community mobilization model via the Avahan initiative. In recognition of the need for government partnership for sustainability, Avahan's ultimate goal is to transfer the program back to "its natural owners"—India. Avahan is working closely to transition this ownership; the resulting model is intended to maximize sustainability by enabling partnership and participation for government and sex workers for continued mutual benefit. Brazil's model is one which provides a context in which HIV prevention efforts are more likely to be sustained in that a response firmly rooted in the sex worker community provides an important mechanism for ongoing communication and addressing future concerns and issues facing sex workers. However the recent challenges faced by sex workers in Brazil points to the importance of continued, long term funding that is focused as much on HIV prevention actions as strengthening the capacity of the NGOs that provide a basis for ongoing communication and addressing future concerns and issues facing sex workers.

The role of the broader social, political, and legal climate in shaping the scope and nature of sex worker participation in HIV prevention is also clear through review of the cases. The sex worker based mobilization and organization approaches notably emerged in contexts characterized by labor rights and citizens rights movements, i.e., Kolkata and Brazil. While the lack of such a political and social climate in Thailand at the time of the 100% condom program cannot be conclusively said to have impeded such a response, findings suggest the need to consider the broader social and political climate in planning efforts to promote mobilization and participation among sex workers. Settings of ongoing collectivization around labor rights or other topics may catalyze the impact of investment in sex worker participatory efforts; while climates of civic disengagement, distrust of government and protracted disempowerment may slow the process of cultivating a participatory model. These examples illustrate the need for consideration of the broader social and political climate in planning national and international responses to HIV among sex workers.

Finally, among the lessons learned from the early responses to HIV among sex workers are that the benefits are greatest to those who can participate to the fullest extent (Kerrigan, Telles et al. 2008). Even within climates characterized by overt structural changes in the forms of mobilization efforts to decrease discrimination, internalized stigma and overt discrimination pose formidable barriers to accessing HIV prevention (Kerrigan, Telles et al. 2008; Blankenship, Burroway et al. 2010). Thus the needs of the most vulnerable sex workers must be prioritized, and the limitations of both government-led and mobilization approaches recognized. The social conditions that prompt involvement in sex work are often grim, including poverty, family breakdown and abuse, low levels of education, humanitarian emergencies and post conflict situations (UNAIDS 2009). These factors may contribute to their stigma and isolation and simultaneously promote HIV risk. Because those in greatest need may be least able to participate based on documentation concerns, language barriers, and fears and instability put forth by conditions of mass migration, natural disaster and protracted civic conflict, vigilance is needed to ensure inclusion of these highest risk groups of sex workers.

Findings from the cases reviewed also illustrate gaps and provide necessary direction for the next generation of comprehensive structural responses to HIV among sex workers. Although clients constitute a primary element of the broader context of sex work, client-oriented prevention efforts remain rare. This omission can not only have consequences in affecting the trajectory of HIV epidemics among sex workers and clients' other sexual partners, but can also reinforce the deleterious stereotyping of sex workers as the sole responsible parties for HIV prevention and as "core transmitters", without any acknowledgement of clients' role in condom use negotiation and ongoing HIV transmission. Because the continued reluctance of clients to embrace condoms as an HIV prevention strategy poses significant challenges in achieving consistent condom use, reducing demand for unprotected paid sex must be a priority in the next generation of structural HIV prevention for sex workers. So too, illustrated through these early responses to HIV among sex workers is a predominant focus on identifying sex workers as such and responding to their needs through sex worker-oriented interventions. Little work has begun to identify the needs of sex workers as they exist within their underlying communities outside of sex work environments or establishments, most notably in clinical services for health issues both including and beyond HIV. The prevalence of sex work within broader samples of women is rarely studied, and little is known about how they compare with their counterparts not involved in sex work with respect to behaviors and outcomes including and beyond those related to HIV. The need to better identify and serve sex workers in a broader range of settings is evident as sex workers worldwide are increasingly relying on mobile phones, internet and other non-visible means for communication (UNAIDS 2009), and as concern emerges that many may not identify as sex workers and thus suffer limited access to sex worker-oriented HIV prevention services (UNAIDS 2009). The broader sexual and reproductive health concerns of female sex workers are increasingly recognized (Todd, Alibayeva et al. 2006; Todd, Nasir et al. 2010; Wayal, Cowan et al. 2011); sexual and reproductive health clinical settings may represent one possible community-based settings for reaching out to sex workers.

As so clearly illustrated by the cases reviewed, sex workers can benefit substantially from both national, government-led responses and community mobilization approaches, when implemented in the context of promoting human rights. Moreover, each approach stands to strengthen the other. In the absence of sex worker participation, government led responses risk unintended consequences such as those seen in Thailand, as well as threats to sustainability, particularly with the rapid evolution of sex work. Responses characterized by significant sex worker participation have achieved numerous successes in modifying the broader context, including advancing labor rights as in the case of Brazil, and creating leverage through collectivization as in the case of Sonagachi. Community-based responses in the absence of direct policy engagement can face limitations in ensuring the human and labor rights that can reduce stigma and discrimination, and providing the necessary infrastructure for STI and HIV testing. The consistent themes of stigma and discrimination, criminalization, and violence and condom-related coercion overwhelmingly illustrate the need for continued efforts to intervene on these levels to both protect the health and human rights of sex workers and to reduce the burden of HIV. The social, political and legal backdrops to sex work and HIV-related responses are relevant to understanding how, when, and why these responses occurred.

The lessons learned from these early responses to HIV among sex workers impart important lessons for the international community, including low and middle income countries with varying levels of infrastructure and emerging economies that are in the earliest phases of building an HIV response infrastructure. Current evidence that significant change can be achieved through grass-roots, civil society, sex worker community responses, and that supportive government involvement can bolster and extend these benefits through collaborative, engaged partnerships between government and community-based organizations, highlights the need to invest in developing the sex worker community infrastructure. The cases reviewed illustrate that broader socio-political factors will have an influence on the outcome of such investment, e.g., whether a community-led response can create sustainable change alone, as in the case of Sonagachi, vs. in close collaboration with the government as in the case of Brazil. The Thailand case illustrates the unintended consequences that can occur in the absence of sex worker engagement. The need to create a forum for sex workers to organize, prioritize their needs, and formally communicate with government actors is increasingly relevant for growing epidemics in which heterosexual sex and sex workers are increasingly implicated, as in the case of the Eastern Europe/Central Asia region. Sex work constitutes a dominant transmission pathway in generalized epidemics (Nagelkerke, Jha et al. 2002). So too, these lessons are relevant to generalized epidemics in which sex workers remain uniquely impacted, as in much of sub Saharan Africa. In light of the burden of HIV among sex workers in these settings, the lack of an internationally recognized response to HIV among sex workers in sub Saharan Africa is surprising and suggests the need for significant investment in this region.

National and international means of addressing structural issues for sex workers are increasingly important as HIV testing and treatment interventions are prioritized as prevention measures. Testing and treatment relies heavily on sex worker trust and access to safe clinical services, thus climates of criminalization, marginalization, harassment and abuse are inherently counterproductive to these goals. Sex worker leadership is critical to developing and sustaining the structural changes necessary for HIV prevention, including promotion of health, human rights and well-being, and should be prioritized within global efforts to mitigate HIV. As the need for relevant, effective HIV risk reduction for sex workers continues as a global priority, the international community will do well to support the development of sex worker-led organizations that can create local change and partner with governments on national interventions.

References

(1993). "NGOs and public sector collaborate in Calcutta red light district." *Global AIDSnews* : the newsletter of the World Health Organization Global Programme on AIDS (3) (3): 7.

(2008). *HIV Sentinel* Surveillance and HIV Estimation in India 2007: A Technical Brief., National AIDS Control Organization.

Ahmed, A., M. Kaplan, et al. (2011). "Criminalising consensual sexual behaviour in the context of HIV: consequences, evidence, and leadership." *Global Public Health 6* Suppl 3: S357–369.

AIDS, U. G. C. o. W. a. (2005). *Violence against sex workers and HIV prevention. Violence against women and HIV/AIDS Critical Intersections.*

Akarasewi, P. (2010). (Brief) *Overview of the HIV Epidemic and the National HIV/AIDS surveillance.*, Thailand Ministry of Public Health.

Argento, E., S. Reza-Paul, et al. (2011). "Confronting structural violence in sex work: lessons from a community-led HIV prevention project in Mysore, India." *AIDS Care* 23 (1): 69–74.

Basu, I., S. Jana, et al. (2004). "HIV prevention among sex workers in India." *Acquired Immune Deficiency Syndrome* 36 (3): 845–852.

Basu, I., S. Jana, et al. (2004). "HIV prevention among sex workers in India." *Journal of Acquired Immune Deficiency Syndrome* 36 (3): 845–852.

Beattie, T. S., P. Bhattacharjee, et al. (2010). "Violence against female sex workers in Karnataka state, south India: impact on health, and reductions in violence following an intervention program." *BMC Public Health* 10: 476.

Blankenship, K. M., M. R. Biradavolu, et al. (2010). "Challenging the stigmatization of female sex workers through a community-led structural intervention: learning from a case study of a female sex worker intervention in Andhra Pradesh, India." *AIDS Care* 22 Suppl 2 b: 1629–1636.

Blankenship, K. M., R. Burroway, et al. (2010). "Factors associated with awareness and utilisation of a community mobilisation intervention for female sex workers in Andhra Pradesh, India." *Sexually Transmitted Infections* 86 Suppl 1: i69–75.

Blankenship, K. M., B. S. West, et al. (2008). "Power, community mobilization, and condom use practices among female sex workers in Andhra Pradesh, India." *AIDS* (London, England) 22 Suppl 5 (Journal Article): S109–116.

Camara, C. (2008). *Avaliação Participativa dos Projetos Sem Vergonha.* Sao Paulo: Ministry of Health/National AIDS Program.

Center for Advocacy on, Stigma and Marginalization (2008). Rights-Based Sex Worker Empowerment Guidelines: *An Alternative HIV/AIDS Intervention Approach to the 100% Condom Use Programme.*

Chandeying, V. (2005). "Epidemiology of HIV and sexually transmitted infections in Thailand." *Sexual Health* 1: 209–216.

Chandrasekaran, P., G. Dallabetta, et al. (2006). "Containing HIV/AIDS in India: the unfinished agenda." *The Lancet Infectious Diseases* 6 (8): 508–521.

Chersich, M. F., S. M. Luchters, et al. (2007). "Heavy episodic drinking among Kenyan female sex workers is associated with unsafe sex, sexual violence and sexually transmitted infections." *International Journal of STD & AIDS* 18 (11): 764–769.

Choi, S. Y., K. L. Chen, et al. (2008). "Client-perpetuated violence and condom failure among female sex workers in southwestern China." *Sexually Transmitted Diseases* 35 (2): 141–146.

Committee., N. A. P. a. A. (2010). Country Progress Report Thailand: Reporting Period January 2008-December 2009. UNGASS (United Nations General Assembly Special Session on HIV/AIDS)

Davida (2010). *Human Rights and Female Prostitution*. Rio de Janeiro: Rede Brasileira de Prostitutas.

Decker, M. R., H. L. McCauley, et al. (2010). "Violence victimisation, sexual risk and sexually transmitted infection symptoms among female sex workers in Thailand." *Sexually Transmitted Infections* 86 (3): 236–240.

Decker, M. R., Wirtz, A. L, Baral S. D., Peryshkina A., Mogilnyi, V., Weber, R. A., Stachowiak, J., Go, V., Beyrer, C. Injection drug use, sexual risk, violence and STI/HIV among Moscow female sex workers. *Sexually Transmitted Infections.* 88(4):278-83.

Erausquin, J. T., E. Reed, et al. (2011). "Police-related experiences and HIV risk among female sex workers in Andhra Pradesh, India." *The Journal of Infectious Diseases* 204 Suppl 5: S1223–1228.

Evans, C., S. Jana, et al. (2010). "What makes a structural intervention? Reducing vulnerability to HIV in community settings, with particular reference to sex work." *Global Public Health* 5 (5): 449–461.

Gabel, L. (2007). *Legal aspects of HIV/AIDS: A guide for policy and law reform,* World Bank. Washington, DC.

Gangopadhyay, D. N., M. Chanda, et al. (2005). "Evaluation of sexually transmitted diseases/ human immunodeficiency virus intervention programs for sex workers in Calcutta, India." *Sexually Transmitted Diseases* 32(11): 680–684.

Ghose, T., D. Swendeman, et al. (2008). "Mobilizing collective identity to reduce HIV risk among sex workers in Sonagachi, India: the boundaries, consciousness, negotiation framework." *Social Science & Medicine* (1982) 67 (2): 311–320.

Go, V. F., A. K. Srikrishnan, et al. (2011). "High prevalence of forced sex among non-brothel based, wine shop centered sex workers in Chennai, India." *AIDS and Behavior* 15 (1): 163–171.

Hanenberg, R. and W. Rojanapithayakorn (1998). "Changes in prostitution and the AIDS epidemic in Thailand." *AIDS Care* 10 (1): 69–79.

Health Ministry: Brazil. (2004). Avaliação de Efetividade das Ações de Prevenção Dirigidas as Profissionais do Sexo, em Três Regiões Brasileiras Serie Estudos Pesquisas e Avaliação Brasilia, *National STD/AIDS Program.*

Hinchberger, B. (2005). "Support for sex workers leaves Brazil without US cash." *The Lancet* 366: 883–884.

Institute, Open Society. (2009). *Arrest the violence: Human rights violations against sex workers in 11 countries in Central and Eastern Europe and Central Asia.*

Jana, S., I. Basu, et al. (2004). "The Sonagachi Project: a sustainable community intervention program." *AIDS Education and Prevention: Official publication of the International Society for AIDS Education* 16 (5): 405–414.

Jayasree, A. K. (2004). "Searching for justice for body and self in a coercive environment: sex work in Kerala, India." *Reproductive Health Matters* 12 (23): 58–67.

Keo, C. (2009). Consultancy Report to Cambodian Alliance for Combating HIV/AIDS (CACHA) Hard Life For A Legal Work: *The 2008 Anti-Trafficking Law and Sex Work.*

Kerrigan, D., L. Moreno, et al. (2006). "Environmental-structural interventions to reduce HIV/STI risk among female sex workers in the Dominican Republic." *American Journal of Public Health* 96 (1): 120–125.

Kerrigan, D., P. Telles, et al. (2008). "Community development and HIV/STI-related vulnerability among female sex workers in Rio de Janeiro, Brazil." *Health Education Research* 23(1): 137–145.

Kilmarx, P. H., K. Limpakarnjanarat, et al. (1998). "HIV-1 seroconversion in a prospective study of female sex workers in northern Thailand: continued high incidence among brothel-based women." *AIDS* London, England. 12 (14): 1889–1898.

Kilmarx, P. H., T. Palanuvej, et al. (1999). "Seroprevalence of HIV among female sex workers in Bangkok: evidence of ongoing infection risk after the '100% condom program' was implemented." *Journal of Acquired Immune Deficiency Syndromes* (1999) 21 (4): 313–316.

Laga, M., C. Galavotti, et al. (2010). "The importance of sex-worker interventions: the case of Avahan in India." *Sexually Transmitted Infections* 86 Suppl 1 (Journal Article): i6–7.

Lazarus, L., K. N. Deering, et al. (2012). "Occupational stigma as a primary barrier to health care for street-based sex workers in Canada." *Culture, Health & Sexuality* 14 (2): 139–150.

Leite, G. (2010). The Impact of Collaboration: Sex Workers and Governments in Brazil. Human Trafficking, *HIV/AIDS, and the Sex Sector:* Human Rights for All. American University and Centre for Health and Gender Equality 59–68. Washington, DC.

Lippman SA, Chinaglia M, Donini AA, Diaz J, Reingold A, Kerrigan DL. Findings From Encontros: A Multilevel STI/HIV Intervention to Increase Condom Use, Reduce STI, and Change the Social Environment Among Sex Workers in Brazil. *Sexually Transmitted Diseases.* 2012 Mar; 39(3):209-16.

Loff, B., C. Overs, et al. (2003). "Can health programmes lead to mistreatment of sex workers?" *The Lancet* 361 (9373): 1982–1983.

Mgbako, C., et al. (2008). Sex Worker Empowerment Guidelines: An Alternative HIV/AIDS Intervention Approach to the 100% Condom Use Programme, *Sangram.*

Mills, S., P. Benjarattanaporn, et al. (1997). "HIV risk behavioral surveillance in Bangkok, Thailand: sexual behavior trends among eight population groups." *AIDS* (London, England) 11 Suppl 1: S43–1.

NACO. (2007). *"HIV/AIDS: Facts and Figures."* Retrieved Jan 30, 2007, from http://www.nacoonline.org.

Nagelkerke, N. J., P. Jha, et al. (2002). "Modelling HIV/AIDS epidemics in Botswana and India: impact of interventions to prevent transmission." *Bulletin of the World Health Organization* 80 (2): 89–96.

OSI (2007). "Health and Human Rights: *A Resource Guide for the Open Society Institute and Soros Foundations Network.*"

Panchanadeswaran, S., S. C. Johnson, et al. (2008). "Intimate partner violence is as important as client violence in increasing street-based female sex workers' vulnerability to HIV in India." *The International Journal on Drug Policy* 19 (2): 106–112.

Parker, R. G. (2009). "Civil society, political mobilization, and the impact of HIV scale-up on health systems in Brazil." *Acquired Immune Deficiency Syndrome* 52 Suppl 1: S49–51.

Pimenta, M. C., S. Correa, et al. (2009). Sexuality and Development: Brazilian National Response to HIV/AIDS amongst Sex Workers. *Study Report.* Rio de Janeiro, ABIA.

Ratinthorn, A., A. Meleis, et al. (2009). "Trapped in circle of threats: violence against sex workers in Thailand." *Health Care for Women International* 30 (3): 249–269.

Ray, R. (1998). "Women's movements anda political fields: a comparison of two Indian cities." *Social Problems* 45.

Reza-Paul, S., T. Beattie, et al. (2008). "Declines in risk behaviour and sexually transmitted infection prevalence following a community-led HIV preventive intervention among female sex workers in Mysore, India." *AIDS* (London, England) 22 Suppl 5: S91–100.

Rhodes, T., M. Simic, et al. (2008). "Police violence and sexual risk among female and transvestite sex workers in Serbia: Qualitative study." *BMJ* (Clinical research ed.) 337: a811.

Rojanapithayakorn, W. and R. Hanenberg (1996). "The 100% condom program in Thailand." *AIDS* 10(1): 1–7.

Sex Workers Rights Advocacy Network. (2009). *Arrest the Violence: Human rights abuses against sex workers in central and eastern Europe and central Asia.*

Shah, N. S., R. W. Shiraishi, et al. (2011). "Bridging populations-sexual risk behaviors and HIV prevalence in clients and partners of female sex workers, Bangkok, Thailand 2007." *Journal of Urban Health: Bulletin of the New York Academy of Medicine* 88(3): 533–544.

Shannon, K., S. A. Strathdee, et al. (2009). "Structural and environmental barriers to condom use negotiation with clients among female sex workers: implications for HIV-prevention strategies and policy." *American Journal of Public Health* 99 (4): 659–665.

Simic, M. and T. Rhodes (2009). "Violence, dignity and HIV vulnerability: street sex work in Serbia." *Sociology of Health & Illness* 31 (1): 1–16.

Simoes, E. A., P. G. Babu, et al. (1987). "Evidence for HTLV-III infection in prostitutes in Tamil Nadu (India)." *Indian Journal of Medical Research* 85: 335–338.

Stachowiak, J. A., S. Sherman, et al. (2005). "Health risks and power among female sex workers in Moscow." *SEICUS Report* 22 (2): 18–26.

Swain, S., et al, (2011). "Experience of violence and adverse reproductive health outcomes, HIV risks among mobile female sex workers in India." *BMC Public Health* 11 (357).

Swendeman, D., I. Basu, et al. (2009). "Empowering sex workers in India to reduce vulnerability to HIV and sexually transmitted diseases." *Social Science & Medicine* (1982) 69 (8): 1157–1166.

Szwarcwald, C., P. Souza Junior, et al. (2011). "Analysis of Data Collected by RDS Among Sex Workers in 10 Brazilian Cities, 2009: Estimation of the Prevalence of HIV, Variance, and Design Effect." *Journal of Acquired Immune Deficiency Syndromes* 57: S129–S135.

Todd, C. S., G. Alibayeva, et al. (2006). "Utilization of contraception and abortion and its relationship to HIV infection among female sex workers in Tashkent, Uzbekistan." *Contraception* 74 (4): 318–323.

Todd, C. S., A. Nasir, et al. (2010). "Contraceptive utilization and pregnancy termination among female sex workers in Afghanistan." *Journal of Women's Health* (2002) 19 (11): 2057–2062.

Treerutkuarkul, A. (2010). "Thailand's new condom crusade." *Bulletin of the World Health Organization* 88 (6): 404–405.

Ulibarri, M. D., S. A. Strathdee, et al. (2011). "Injection drug use as a mediator between client-perpetrated abuse and HIV status among female sex workers in two mexico-US border cities." *AIDS Behavior* 12 (1): 179–185.

UNAIDS (2000). *Â Evaluation of the 100% Condom Programme in Thailand,* UNAIDS Case Study.

UNAIDS (2009). *UNAIDS Guidance Note on HIV and Sex Work.* Geneva.

Wayal, S., F. Cowan, et al. (2011). "Contraceptive practices, sexual and reproductive health needs of HIV-positive and negative female sex workers in Goa, India." *Sexually Transmitted Infections* 87 (1): 58–64.

UNGASS (United Nations General Assembly Special Session on HIV/AIDS)

Whitaker, T., P. Ryan, et al. (2011). "Stigmatization among drug-using sex workers accessing support services in Dublin." *Qualitative Health Research* 21 (8): 1086–1100.

www.ingramcontent.com/pod-product-compliance
Lightning Source LLC
Chambersburg PA
CBHW070716280326
41926CB00087B/2286

Discussion

We found consistent evidence of dramatically higher levels of HIV among female sex workers compared to other women of reproductive age across geographic regions and HIV prevalence levels in lower and middle income countries. And while female sex workers have long been understood to be a population at heightened risk for HIV infection, the scope and breadth of their disproportionate risk for HIV infection had to date not been systematically documented.

The largest sample size was available from Asia with data on some 64 224 women captured. In the Asian region we found the highest magnitude of relative burden of disease (OR 29.2, 95% CI 22.2–38.4). While some countries such as Thailand showed a trend towards higher prevalence in the 1990's, surveillance data have characterized an increasingly concentrated HIV epidemic among Key populations (Ainsworth, Beyrer et al. 2003). Responses such as the 100% condom campaign have arguably been heralded as successes, though HIV prevalence remains over 10% among female sex workers and the odds of infection remain at more 10 times that of all Thai women, suggesting the need for complementary HIV prevention strategies including biomedical, such as oral or topical chemoprophylaxis or treatment as prevention, and structural .approaches (Rojanapithayakorn and Hanenberg 1996; Celentano, Nelson et al. 1998). In India, the Avahan and Sonagachi combination HIV prevention programs have had multiple targets such addressing structural issues, including community empowerment, campaigns to address stigma, and structural policy support, as well as targeting high risk sexual practices, such as increasing condom use during sex (Swendeman, Ishika et al. 2009; Laga, Galavotti et al. 2010). Both programs have been deemed to be successes and are being scaled up across the country. When reviewing the data from the last 5 years, female sex workers still carry more than a 50 fold increased odds of HIV infection in India. As HIV prevalence is a lagging indicator of prevention success, it will take time to demonstrate the benefit of these programs in terms of the absolute burden of HIV among female sex workers in India. Nonetheless, the disproportionate burden of HIV among female sex workers even in settings where progressive programs exist highlights the need to increase coverage by increasing scale and decreasing barriers to access.

HIV in Latin America and the Caribbean has remained a disease mostly concentrated among Key populations since the beginning of the epidemic (Caceres 2002). With low background prevalence and early recognition of the high risk among female sex workers in LAC, HIV prevalence is of limited magnitude among female sex workers in the region. Brazil famously declined